TREATING WORKER DISSATISFACTION DURING ECONOMIC CHANGE

TREATING WORKER DISSATISFACTION DURING ECONOMIC CHANGE

MORLEY D. GLICKEN

BENNIE C. ROBINSON

ELSEVIER

AMSTERDAM • BOSTON • HEIDELBERG • LONDON
NEW YORK • OXFORD • PARIS • SAN DIEGO
SAN FRANCISCO • SINGAPORE • SYDNEY • TOKYO
Academic Press is an imprint of Elsevier

Academic Press is an imprint of Elsevier
32 Jamestown Road, London NW1 7BY, UK
225 Wyman Street, Waltham, MA 02451, USA
525 B Street, Suite 1800, San Diego, CA 92101-4495, USA

First edition 2013

British Library Cataloguing-in-Publication Data
A catalogue record for this book is available from the British Library

Library of Congress Cataloging-in-Publication Data
A catalog record for this book is available from the Library of Congress

ISBN: 978-0-12-397006-0

For information on all Academic Press publications
visit our website at elsevierdirect.com

Typeset by MPS Limited, Chennai, India
www.adi-mps.com

Printed and bound in United States of America

12 13 14 15 16   10 9 8 7 6 5 4 3 2 1

CONTENTS

About the Authors

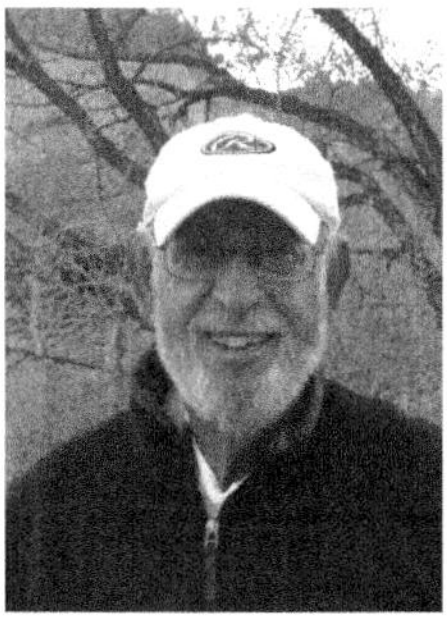

Dr. Morley Glicken is the former Dean of the Worden School of Social Service in San Antonio; the founding director of the Master of Social Work Department at California State University, San Bernardino; the past Director of the Master of Social Work Program at the University of Alabama; and the former Executive Director of Jewish Family Service of Greater Tucson. He has also held faculty positions in social work at the University of Kansas and Arizona State University.

Dr. Glicken received his BA degree in social work with a minor in psychology from the University of North Dakota and holds a Master of Social Work Degree from the University of Washington, and the Master of Public Administration and Doctor of Social Work Degrees from the University of Utah. He is a member of Phi Kappa Phi Honorary Fraternity.

Dr. Glicken has written extensively about worker stress, job dissatisfaction and worker burnout for the *Wall Street Journal* publication *National Business Employment Weekly* and currently writes for *Careercast.com* where his articles on job dissatisfaction and workaholism were part of a White Paper on worker problems in America published by Dow Jones, the parent company. He has published the following books:

Glicken, M.D. and Robinson, B. (In Press); *Treating Job Dissatisfaction During Economic Change*: Elsevier

Glicken, M.D. (Fall 2010). *Social Work in the 21st Century* (2nd edition). Sage Publications.

Glicken, M.D. (Fall 2010). *Workaholics in Retirement*. Praeger Press.

Glicken, M.D. (Fall 2009). *Evidence-Based Practice with Older Adults: A Psychosocial Perspective on Successful Aging*. Elsevier Publishers.

Glicken, M.D. (Spring 2009). *Evidence-Based Practice with Children and Adolescents: A Psychosocial Perspective*. Elsevier Publishers.

Glicken. M.D. & Haas, B. (Spring 2009). *A Simple Guide to Retirement: How to Make Retirement Work for You*. Greenwood Press.

Glicken, M.D. (Summer 2007). *A Guide to Writing for Human Service Professionals*. Rowman and Littlefield Publishers.

Glicken, M.D. (Summer 2006). *Learning from Resilient People: Lessons we can Apply to Counseling and Psychot*herapy. Sage Publications.

Glicken, M.D. (Spring 2005) *Working with Troubled Men: A Contemporary Practitioner's Guide*. Lawrence Erlbaum Publications.

Glicken, M.D. (Fall 2004). *Improving the Effectiveness of the Helping Professions: An Evidence-Based Practice Approach to Treatment* Sage Publications.

Glicken, M.D. (Fall 2004). *Using the Strengths Perspective in Social Work Practice*. Allyn and Bacon/Longman Publishers.

Glicken, M.D. (Fall 2004). *Using the Strengths Perspective in Social Work Practice: Instructor's Manual*.

Glicken, M.D. (Fall 2003). *Violent Young Children*. Allyn and Bacon/ Longman Publishers.

Glicken, M.D. and Sechrest, D. (Fall 2003). *The Role of the Helping Professions in Treating the Victims and Perpetrators of Violence*. Allyn and Bacon/Longman Publishers.

Glicken. M.D. (Fall 2003). *Social Research: A Simple Guide*. Allyn and Bacon/Longman Publishers.

Dr Glicken has published over 50 articles in professional journals and has written extensively on clinical and management subjects. He has held clinical social work licenses in Alabama and Kansas and is a member of the Academy of Certified Social Workers. He is currently Professor Emeritus in Social Work at California State University, San Bernardino and Executive Director of the Institute for Personal Growth: A Research, Treatment, and Training Institute in Tucson, Arizona offering consulting services in counseling, research, and management.

More information about Dr. Glicken may be obtained on his website: www.morleyglicken.com. A listing of all of his books may be found on Amazon.com at: https://authorcentral.amazon.com/v/1973805540 and he can be contacted by email at: mglicken@msn.com.

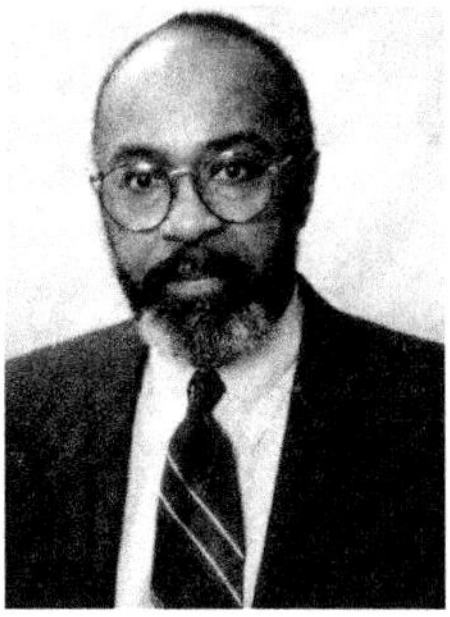

Dr. Bennie C. Robinson (PhD, University of Denver; MSW, Indiana University and BA, Roosevelt University) is the former Director of Community Programming for FIBCO Family Services Inc. in Phoenix Arizona. He is currently a Community Affiliate with the Southwest Interdisciplinary Research Center, at Arizona State University in Phoenix. He teaches in the Arizona State University, College of Public Programs, School of Social Work and is an Honors Disciplinary Faculty member in the Barrett Honors College at Arizona State. He previously served as Professor and Chairperson of the Division of Social Work and Criminal Justice at Kentucky State University. Prior to this period he was a faculty member at the University of Kentucky and conducted a number of community based research studies and published 12 longitudinal Ethnographic Studies for the *Comprehensive Child Development Program* (*CCDP,* US Department of Health and Human Services, 1991-1994. Earlier, Dr. Robinson served as Assistant City Manager and Director of Community Assistance for the City of Cincinnati and received many awards and recognitions. He was a Regional Representative for the US Department of Health, Education and Welfare; District Administrator for the Illinois Department of Children and Family Services and Consultant/Clinical Social Worker for the Chicago Department of Health.

PREFACE

In the current economy, companies, non-profits, and public organizations are expected to respond quickly to changing market needs and ever-decreasing funding to stay vibrant. What that means is that organizations constantly reorganize—not just every year but sometimes as frequently as every six months. Workers live in a constant state of change that includes new processes, new procedures, new bosses, and new organizational structures where they are often measured on goals that were typically set before the changing economy and then never modified. As a result, there is very little loyalty to workers who may have been valued in the past. The new emphasis in the workplace is on "what have you done for me lately?" This changing dynamic in the workplace has undoubtedly increased worker dissatisfaction, lowered morale, and often led to burnout in workers who were previously satisfied with their jobs and were productive.

To understand how the new dynamic in the workplace has affected workers and productivity, the book focuses on the most current research evaluating worker difficulties as a result of the changing pressures in the workplace and what can be done by workers, managers, HR professionals, and therapists to reduce the stressors that often result when workers feel demeaned, misused, overworked, and under constant pressure to perform.

Part One of the book sets the stage with a discussion of the current economic climate and how it impacts the public and private sectors, how organizations react to it, and how the new work climate affects employees. Part Two lays out the most current research on what organizations and workers can do to improve the workplace, reduce stress, and improve worker coping skills and performance. Case studies and guidelines are used extensively throughout the book. Part Three contains material related to best management practices to reduce workplace problems and includes chapters on competency-based management, behavioral evaluations, and the important issues of hiring and termination. Part Four is an overview of best practices to treat a variety of workplace problems and includes material on quality of life therapy and research on life and job satisfaction. Part Four concludes with a chapter on prevention and our view of what the ideal workplace will look like in the future.

The authors are social work educators who have managed large organizations and have years of experience as therapists and managers dealing with workplace problems. We write this book because of our concern for the American workforce, which is often underpaid, overworked, underappreciated and, when it comes to unionized workers, ridiculed. We also write the book for managers who often work under tremendous pressure that affects their personal lives and are as subject to the same stress, unhappiness at work, and burnout as the workers they manage. Downsizing, letting people go, firing workers you've known for years—by any name it's hurtful and all too common in this time of world-wide economic upheaval.

Not everyone who works suffers from many of the problems we discuss in the book, which makes it all the more important that we remember the large number of unemployed workers in America, the many workers who toil in dangerous workplaces, the older workers who get downsized and have no hope of ever finding a new job, the workers whose unemployment compensation has run out, and the new graduates who face unfulfilling futures doing work which neither excites nor inspires them. Their anguish should motivate all of us to open our hearts and minds to new ideas, to new treatment approaches, and, in Bertrand Russell's words, to have "unbearable sympathy for the suffering of others."

PART *One*

Understanding and Identifying Work-Related Problems

CHAPTER 1

The Serious Problems in the American Workplace

INTRODUCTION

This is a book about what goes wrong on the job and what can be done to right it. It is written for workers, human resource managers, middle managers, and therapists specializing in work-related problems. Both authors are social work educators who have extensive managerial experience. We write this book because of our concern that work is becoming a joyless, stressful, and oppressive experience for too many workers and managers. This chapter provides data about job unhappiness and burnout that should be a wakeup call to organizations that think workers are in an endless supply and are unconcerned with the costs associated with finding, training, and keeping new workers.

As both managers and employees, we are sensitive to both populations and strive to make the book as applicable and useful as we can. We are also therapists and will provide information we trust you will find helpful in dealing with work-related problems that increasingly affect many workplaces in the midst of a down economy that places extra pressure on everyone to work harder and longer and to receive less in return.

To make this task easier for you, the reader, we will include the latest research, give real experiences of others dealing with problems in the workplace, and offer suggestions and solutions we hope you will find of value. And we will cover a number of work-related problems in the book, including worker burnout, job dissatisfaction and low morale, unemployment and under-employment, harassment and bias toward women and minorities, workplace violence, workers who are work-addicted, and many others.

THE LANDSCAPE OF WORK IN THE CURRENT ECONOMY

The economic climate in the United States is in its worst condition since the Great Depression. Although the official unemployment rate at the end of December, 2011 was 8.5%, a Gallup poll (Jan. 5, 2012)

Treating Worker Dissatisfaction During Economic Change
DOI: http://dx.doi.org/10.1016/B978-0-12-397006-0.00001-4

wrote that "Underemployment, a measure that combines the percentage of workers who are unemployed with the percentage working part-time but wanting full-time work, was 18.2% in December, 2011" (p. 1). While this is down somewhat from December, 2010, Gallup believes that there is little reason for optimism and that many workers who are no longer receiving unemployment compensation, and who have stopped looking for jobs, are not reported in the official unemployment calculations and that the actual rate of unemployment in the country is far higher.

Lawrence Summers, President Clinton's Treasury Secretary and one of President Obama's economic advisors, notes that recent surveys have found that 40% of Americans believe that capitalism and the free market economy are incapable of sustaining the relatively high employment rates of the past and writes, "Few would confidently bet that the US or Europe will see a return to full employment as previously defined within the next 5 years. The economies of both are likely to be constrained by demand for a long time. One in six American men between 25 and 54 are likely to be out of work even after the US economy recovers" (Summers, January 9, 2012, p. 1). *The Economist* (2010, p. 1) also believes that unemployment will be a long-term problem and states:

> *... policymakers need urgently to think beyond stimulus measures, and also to adopt more targeted policies to help the millions stuck in the wrong place with the wrong skills. Otherwise, even a return to brisk economic growth (something that scarcely looks likely right now) will not be enough to rescue them from the breadline.*

Unemployment has severe social, emotional, and financial consequences. A study of 1,200 unemployed workers reported by Deprez (September 3, 2009) for *Bloomberg Business News* found that overwhelming majorities of the survey's respondents said they feel or have experienced anxiety, helplessness, depression, and stress after being without a job. Many said they have experienced sleeping problems and strained relationships and have avoided social situations as a result of their job loss. Still others described diminished hopes of finding employment at older ages, and feelings that advanced degrees are useless or have caused potential employers to think they're overqualified. Some said they have questioned their self-identity after they had allowed their professional careers to define them, and some reported difficulty finding credit to begin new businesses (p. 1).

Davidson (April 16, 2012) reports that lawsuits filed by workers against employers rose 32% against the same data in 2008. The main complaints in the lawsuits were that workers put in more time than their 40 hours without overtime pay and were forced to work off the clock. Other complaints included having jobs misclassified as exempt from overtime requirements and that, because of smartphones and other devices, work bled into personal time. The major complaint, however, is that productivity per worker hour more than doubled in 2009 and 2010 because companies ignored labor laws that prohibit practices that violate a worker's rights. Many of the lawsuits are class action suits where numerous employees are represented, forcing the Department of Labor to hire 300 more investigators to protect workers, particularly those "in high risk industries that employ low-wage and vulnerable workers such as those in hotels and restaurant work" (p. 2A).

EXAMPLES OF BAD WORKPLACE EXPERIENCES

The following are examples of how badly done the termination experience can be.

- Matt Cooper, an executive at Accolo, a recruitment outsourcing company, wrote in the *New York Times* (January 31, 2009) that when the company began having financial problems and downsizing became necessary, upper level executives called employees into a conference room, one at a time, told them they were fired, and had them walk to their offices, pack up their personal items, and immediately leave. One of his co-workers was so frightened of being called in that he hid in his cubicle until a vice president of the company found him and told him the bad news.
- Jean Colette, a supervising OR nurse at a New Jersey Hospital told me that every June, 50 people are fired across staff lines. The hospital decides if their salaries and benefits are consistent with the quality of their work. Because the fiscal year runs July 1st to June 30th, the director of each department calls people into their office on June 29th and gives them the bad news and a severance packet. Because older and more experienced workers make better salaries and are usually more effective at their jobs, it's often the very best people who get fired. Anxiety is so bad in June, Colette told me, that almost nothing gets done.
- Amber Elefson, a public health professional working for a non-profit in San Diego (her identity has been changed to protect her ability to network), and pregnant with her first child, asked her employer if her job was secure and was told that it was. Two weeks later, amid glowing reviews of her work and praise for special projects she had done, she was terminated because of severe budget constraints.

Fortunately, she had heeded the advice to continue networking and was able to move on to a new job, almost seamlessly, but she remains skeptical about the ability of supervisors to foresee the future. "When they need to fire you," she told me, "management often makes quick decisions. Program or front-line staff is cut first. Because mid-level managers haven't been privy to higher level budget discussions, it often comes as a shock." Ms. Elefson told me her supervisor "drove two hours and cried when she told me I was being terminated. She said that it was the most difficult thing she had done in 30 years as a professional."

To add to the emotional impact of unemployment, the study reported by Deprez (September 3, 2009, p. 1) found that many of the laid off workers had no advanced information about their job security and consequently had little time to prepare emotionally or financially. The report notes that:

- 60% of the respondents received no advance warning of their layoff;
- 84% received no severance package or other compensation;
- 43% of those unemployed reported having received unemployment benefits in the past year;
- 61% described themselves as "very concerned" their benefits would expire before they found a job.

To further complicate matters, the average wage of US workers has not been keeping pace. In 1997, the average wage in the United States was 11th-highest among all nations. The difference between the highest wage country, Switzerland, and the United States was $7.00 an hour. In December, 2011 the United States had slipped to 14th among all nations but the differential between the country with the highest hourly wage, Norway ($57.53/hour), and the United States ($34.74/hour) was fully $22.79 an hour (Bureau of Labor Statistics, December, 2011). Part of the cost per hour differential is related to benefits. In European countries the average benefit is 40% of compensation whereas in the United States it is 33%, leaving a much greater amount of direct costs to US workers in health insurance, lower vacation and sick days allowed, and benefits we have never seen in the United States, including 35-hour work-weeks and up to 9 months in leave to care for newly born children.

Writing for *Yahoo Finance*, Snyder (July 15, 2010) believes that the middle class is not only being systematically wiped out of existence in America, but that more American workers are actually moving into poverty because of low wages, and provides the following data as evidence:

- Eighty-three percent of all US stocks are in the hands of 1% of the people.
- Sixty-one percent of Americans "always or usually" live paycheck to paycheck, which was up from 49% in 2008 and 43% in 2007.
- Sixty-six percent of the income growth between 2001 and 2007 went to the top 1% of all Americans.
- Thirty-six percent of Americans say that they don't contribute anything to retirement savings.
- A staggering 43% of Americans have less than $10,000 saved up for retirement.
- Twenty-four percent of American workers say that they have postponed their planned retirement age in the past year.
- Over 1.4 million Americans filed for personal bankruptcy in 2009, which represented a 32% increase over 2008.
- Only the top 5% of US households have earned enough additional income to match the rise in housing costs since 1975.
- For the first time in US history, banks own a greater share of residential housing net worth in the United States than all individual Americans put together.
- In 1950, the ratio of the average executive's paycheck to the average worker's paycheck was about 30 to 1. Since the year 2000, that ratio has exploded to between 300 and 500 to one.
- As of 2007, the bottom 80% of American households held about 7% of the liquid financial assets.
- The bottom 50% of income earners in the United States now collectively own less than 1% of the nation's wealth.
- Average Wall Street bonuses for 2009 were up 17% when compared with 2008.
- In the United States, the average federal worker now earns 60% MORE than the average worker in the private sector.
- The top 1% of US households own nearly twice as much of America's corporate wealth as they did just 15 years ago.
- In America today, the average time needed to find a job has risen to a record 35.2 weeks.
- More than 40% of Americans who actually are employed are now working in service jobs, which are often very low paying.
- For the first time in US history, more than 40 million Americans are on food stamps, and the US Department of Agriculture projected that number would go up to 43 million Americans in 2011.

- This is what American workers now must compete against: in China a garment worker makes approximately 86 cents an hour and in Cambodia a garment worker makes approximately 22 cents an hour.
- Approximately 21% of all children in the United States are living below the poverty line in 2010—the highest rate in 20 years.
- Despite the financial crisis, the number of millionaires in the United States rose a whopping 16% to 7.8 million in 2009.
- The top 10% of Americans now earn around 50% of our national income.

But more telling than the data is the feedback we get from workers. Here's what one worker told us: "I work for a large corporation and, believe me, there is no compassion, loyalty or any values that used to encourage people to work for them. They don't seem to understand how much more money they could make if employees and customers were treated well." Joan Wright, an IT supervisor from Boulder, Colorado told us,

> *Fifteen year-ago I lost my job at a large defense company and was outsourced to a contractor. In the process I lost a good chunk of my pension. In the new setting I never meet management. We have computer conferences and even though I manage 15 people I've never once spoken directly to my immediate supervisor whose office is several thousand miles away. It would be nice to have someone tell me "nice job" or to congratulate me in person on the tough and demanding assignments I have and carry out on time and under budget but it hasn't happened to me in fifteen years. In this outsourced company, the bottom line is all that matters and older workers are expendable. We have no job protection and no clear cut incentives to perform well other than the constant thought that we'll be fired on some unknown and unseen manager's whim. The idea of anyone caring about us is laughable and we joke that what we experience in this faceless corporation is like the science fiction films we watch where everything is controlled by robots and computers. I'm 60 and all I hope is that I make it another six years to get my maximum social security check. My 401 K is in the toilet, my house is under water, and my pension is worth half of what it was worth a few years ago. Ask me about whether I'm satisfied? I'm just plain scared and holding on and hoping someone doesn't decide I'm expendable.*

A CRISIS IN LEADERSHIP

At a time when public and private managers should be at their very best, a number of researchers report the often dismal competencies of American managers. Stensaker, Meyer, Falkenberg, and Haueng (2001) argue that managers who institute "excessive change" often have disgruntled workers.

The authors describe excessive change as "Change [that] creates initiative overload and organizational chaos, both of which provoke strong resistance from the people most affected" (p. G6). Situations that lead to excessive change include change when change isn't needed, change for the sake of change, and change where one element of the organization is changed, but others are not. The result is middle management stress, worker unhappiness, and a general decline in the quality of services. Many workers we interviewed complained that regulations and policies change so frequently that they cannot keep up and blame management for creating a workplace in which workers never have sufficient knowledge to do the job because the policies that govern their work are always in flux. Workers also complain that they are frequently left out of the decision-making process and feel neglected and ignored by supervisors.

Ghoshal (2005) argues that too many management theories used in American organizations view organizations and workers in a way suggesting an ideology that is "essentially grounded in a set of pessimistic assumptions about both individuals and institutions—a 'gloomy vision' that views the primary purpose of social theory as one of solving the 'negative problem' of restricting the social costs arising from human imperfections" (p. 76). According to Ghoshal, the result of this pessimistic view of workers and organizations is that management has virtually no impact on whether an organization functions well or badly. Citing a review of 31 studies of organizational leadership by Dalton, Daily, Ellstrand, and Johnson (1998), the researchers found no difference in organizational performance based on who occupied leadership roles. According to the authors, the reason for this is that most labor is performed at much lower levels and that organizational health is in the hands of workers and not managers. When workers are treated well and feel a part of the organization, performance is predictably better. Although it may seem counterintuitive that good managers lack better results than bad managers, Ghoshal points to the number of corporate scandals since 1998 and reminds us that most of the managers involved were thought to be not only good managers, but great ones.

One of the reasons for poor managerial impact on performance of organizations is the way managers are chosen. Cook and Emler (1999) studied the issue of technical skills versus integrity (moral qualities suggesting ethical behavior and sensitivity to the feelings of others) and found that top to bottom hiring (hiring done at the highest level with minimal input from subordinates) focused on technical competence with only low to moderate concern for the integrity of the manager. Bottom to top decision-making (subordinates choosing managers) was made with a high-level concern for managerial integrity and only moderate concern for technical competence. Subordinates worried that a manager lacking in integrity would mistreat them, while upper management worried that high levels of integrity might interfere with getting the job done. The authors write, "If the effectiveness of managers is a function of how they treat their subordinates and whether they will be treated fairly, that promises to them will be kept, that their welfare will be considered, that they will be told the truth—then conventional top-down methods of selection will systematically under-select the best potential performers" (Cook and Emler, 1999, p. 439).

ETHICAL ISSUES IN MANAGERIAL PRACTICE

Menzel (1999) suggests that an important criticism of American management is that from CEOs, to supervisors, to low-level bureaucrats, many workers in the public and private non-profit sectors have developed a "morally mute" position where they fail to act in ways that help organizations and, instead, stay silent when it comes to issues that trouble organizations, particularly those involving the unethical behavior of higher-ups. In describing this atmosphere of moral muteness, Mitchell (1999, p. 16) writes,

> *Not much impartial scientific method is to be discerned in our administrative practices. The poisonous atmosphere of city government, the crooked secrets of state administration, the confusion, sinecurism, and corruption ever and again discovered in the bureau at Washington forbid us to believe that any clear conceptions [of public management] are as yet very widely current in the United States.*

While Menzel believes that precious little has been done to make managers more aware of ethical behavior, he acknowledges that legislation to enforce morally positive behavior has produced dubious results. There is, according to Menzel, even the suggestion that by stating in law or policies punishable offenses, that this has allowed managers to define ethics as behaviors and practices that do not break the law.

Pfeffer (2005) worries that what is taught in schools with management specializations tends to create a reduced level of ethical behavior in students. Williams, Barrett, and Brabston (2000) report that "The link between an organization's size and illegal activity becomes stronger as the percentage of top management team members possessing an MBA degree ... rises" (p. 706).

McCabe and Trevino (1995) found that business school students placed "the least importance on knowledge and understanding, economic and racial justice, and the significance of developing a meaningful philosophy of life" (p. 211) and that "business majors report almost 50% more [cheating] violations than any of their peer groups and almost twice as many violations as the average student in our study" (p. 210).

In its position paper on supervision in social work, The American Board of Examiners in Clinical Social Work, the ABE (2004, p. 5) is very critical of supervision in many public social service and mental health settings. Among those criticisms are the following.

1. Changes in many work settings have forced some clinicians to seek outside supervision at their own expense and at the risk of circumventing the responsibilities inherent in the relationship of a clinician and a formal organization-based supervisor. These arrangements raise issues of accountability, confidentiality and liability, which need to be addressed by regulatory agencies, service agencies, and professional associations.
2. There are inadequate and inconsistent standards for regulation and training of clinical social work supervisors.
3. It is difficult to achieve the necessary training to become an advanced practitioner in clinical social work with the current lack of financial support for supervision in social work agencies, the limited coursework in supervision in graduate schools of social work, and insufficient post-masters' training opportunities.

A WORKER REFLECTION ON AN ETHICAL LAPSE IN AN ORGANIZATION: DIRE CONSEQUENCES FOR THE WORKER

When organizations are functioning well, decisions are usually made with consideration of their ethical and moral results, but when organizations are in crisis, as many currently are today, unethical decision-making often takes place. Christensen and Kohls (2003) point out that when organizations are in crisis, they experience continuous turmoil causing crisis after crisis that creates "constant stresses for management and employees" that ultimately increase unethical decisions, worker dissatisfaction, and burnout. The following example shows how even academics are faced with ethical decisions that may affect their careers.

Dr Margo Kingston, a PhD level historian taught at a private church-sponsored college in the mid-west. Several students in one of her classes alerted her to the fact that two students were bragging that they had cheated on her essay test. She found a way to document the students' cheating on the mid-term and final exams and decided to fail them. She reported their cheating to the Dean of the College but, instead of supporting her, he wanted her to give the students a "D" for the semester. Other students in her class were indignant because they had worked very hard for their grades. She told the Dean that she would not change the grade. The Dean then confided in her that the father of one of the students was currently serving on the state Supreme Court and was a major donor to her university. The message was clear: change the grade or the father would stop contributing to the college.

She told the senior author, "I was changed by the experience. I saw myself as a person of integrity and honor. As a result of the conflict I experienced between my standards and the standards of administration I was denied tenure and never again found a position in an American university. I underwent years of therapy for depression. Several marriages failed. I learned that my experiences were far from unique, which led to much greater understanding of power politics at all levels of society. I have not given up my ideals, but I am now more cautious and strategic in my thinking. I am no longer naïve but the experience has made me feel more empathy for the ethical conflicts I see other people increasingly experiencing in our society."

In their review of the literature on crisis and unethical behavior, Christensen and Kohls (2003) found that organizational crises limit cognitive abilities, reduce consultation with others in a good position to give advice, and limit sources of information because of time constraints. All of this, the researchers found, increases levels of stress and the potential for unethical decision-making which may have very negative future consequences for everyone involved in the decision.

Bodtker, Jameson, and Katz (2001) argue that managers often demonstrate limited ability to handle the type of conflict in the workplace that often leads to more serious problems including ethical issues. Rather than using it to create new ways of providing services and developing practice theory, managers tend to stifle conflict or use short-term remedies to keep emerging conflict from developing. The authors write (p. 259):

We contend [there is] a western bias that views emotions as counterproductive and a normative belief that conflict is dysfunctional. While academic research has debunked this myth by demonstrating the utility of conflict for achieving productive outcomes such as more vigilant problem solving, the fact remains that many people prefer to avoid or hide conflict. In this paper we offer the argument that to be in conflict is to be emotionally charged. This is especially true in the workplace, where organizational norms explicitly or implicitly tell us what we are supposed to feel (and the emotional expression that is appropriate). To manage conflict more effectively, managers must attend to the role of emotions in conflict and conflict management. By doing so, opportunities for using generative conflict management strategies which serve to stimulate conflict for long-term gain rather than suppressing conflict or leaving it to simmer will develop.

HOW THE CHANGING WORKPLACE AFFECTS WORKERS

It may seem logical to think that, in a bad economy, workers would be appreciative of having any job, however bad the working conditions, and that just having a source of income would lead to high rates of productivity and job satisfaction. Instead, current information suggests just the opposite.

The Conference Board Research Group (Weaver, 2012) found that in more than 22 years of studying the issue, "even Americans who are lucky enough to have work in this economy are becoming more unhappy with their jobs and that only 45 percent of Americans are satisfied with their work" (p. 1), a 20% decrease since a similar study was made 4 years earlier (p. 1). According to the Conference Board Group, workers have grown increasingly unhappy because, fewer workers consider their jobs to be interesting, incomes haven't kept up with the cost of living, and health care costs have substantially reduced a worker's take home pay, when they are lucky enough to even have decent health care coverage.

The Board concludes that "if the job satisfaction trend is not reversed, it could stifle innovation and hurt America's competitiveness and productivity. And it could make unhappy older workers less inclined to take the time to share their knowledge and skills with younger workers" (p. 1).

A Presidential report, "Work in America" (Presidential Commission on Work, 1973) found that unhappy workers suffer from physical and emotional problems related to their jobs in far greater numbers than do satisfied workers. Reported problems include depression, anxiety, headaches, backaches, ulcers, substance abuse, marital discord, violence, and other physical and emotional problems related to increased levels of stress.

The following data come from CareerBuilder.com surveys of American workers (Lorenz, 2009).

- American workers have the least amount of vacation time of any modern, developed society.
- In 2007, 20% of workers said they would be checking in with office while on vacation.
- More than half of workers say they work under a great deal of stress, and 77% say they feel burned out on the job.

- Forty-four percent of working moms admit to being preoccupied about work while at home and one-fourth say they bring home projects at least 1 day a week.
- Nineteen percent of working moms reported they often or always work weekends.
- Thirty-seven percent of all working dads said they would consider the option of taking a new job with less pay if it offered a better work/life balance.
- Thirty-six percent of working dads reported they bring work home at least 1 day a week, and 30% say they often or always work weekends.

Noting declining rates of job satisfaction in an environment where people work more hours and have less time off to renew themselves or to have a personal life, the American Management Association (2007) reports the following.

- Compared with workers in developed nations such as France and Norway, which have high rates of productivity, US workers log many more work hours.
- There is a strong feeling among US workers that they must work more hours to get ahead in their careers because managers often judge performance largely in terms of hours spent working and are often unwilling to ask for a decrease in hours for fear they'll be branded as indolent or uncommitted to their job, a dynamic that can lead to overwork, burnout, and a range of problems that stem from burnout.
- Burnout was cited as the primary reason for employee turnover by three-quarters of US workers surveyed in 2006.
- US workers feel so consumed by work that they often skip vacations entirely, often out of fear that when they return, they won't have a job. In 2006, US workers stockpiled an estimated total of 574 million unused vacation days in 2006.

Another measure of job dissatisfaction is worker turnover, Wolfe (June 10, 2010) reports that yearly turnover in North American jobs consistently ranges between 25% and 30% on average. With estimates for the true cost of turnover ranging from 25% for entry level jobs to 250% or more of annual salary for senior management, Wolfe believes that these high rates of turnover take valuable managerial time away from projects, resources, and profits to reinvest for growth and innovation. As an example of what high turnover rates cost organizations, the Canadian Grocery Human Resource Council (CGHRC) reported an overall employee turnover rate of 38.7% in the grocery industry at a cost of finding, interviewing, training, and equipping a new hire of a minimum of $1,500 per frontline employee. Factoring in that nearly four out of every 10 new employees leave each year, a grocery store with a net margin of 1.5–3% would have to sell $60,000 worth of groceries to recover the cost of losing a single employee.

THE CHANGING WORK ETHIC

Mirhaydari (2012) reports that the number of men in the labor force has been steadily declining from 87.5% in 1945 to 70% in 2011 and writes "many qualified workers seem to be turning up their noses at jobs they see as demeaning, or that don't pay what they need, and they are deciding instead to leave the workforce, trying to strike out on their own or retire" (p. 1). Looking closely at the jobs data, Miraydari sees an across-the-board erosion of America's "can-do" spirit, a change that will affect corporate profits, Federal Reserve policy, and the overall shape of the nation's economy for years to come.

In a provocative article in the *Wall Street Journal*, Murray (2012) argues that in March 2008, months before the economic crisis in fall 2008, and at a time when employment was still fairly robust, a large number of white working-class men with high-school diplomas or less were unavailable for work and were considered to be the long-term unemployed who no longer were actively looking for work. Murray states that the rate of those who had taken themselves out of the labor pool went from 3% in 1968 to 12% in 2008 and writes "Twelve percent may not sound like much until you think that we're talking about men in the prime of life, in their 30's and 40's, when according to hallowed American traditions, every American man is working or looking for work" (p. C2). Murray notes that among college-educated white males the rate of long-term unemployed in March 2008 was 3%. He concludes that large numbers of white working-class males have opted out of traditional American beliefs about work, supporting families, marriage, and community values, and points to a marriage rate that has been steadily falling from 94% of white working-class males and females studied in the 1960s to 48% in March 2008, and sees no compelling evidence that marriage rates or the desire to work will improve.

Murray goes on to point out that more than half of the births to American women under 30 occur outside marriage and that the fastest growth of children born to single women in the last two decades has occurred among white women in their 20s, further evidence of major changes in the way Americans view family life and added economic stressors on single women.

Murray (2012) believes that the extensive welfare programs created in the 1960s reduced incentives for less-educated white and minority citizens to maintain traditional work and community values, and that those in the affluent middle and upper classes have a responsibility to speak out about the loss of virtuous behavior. It's not too late to change the trend, according to Murray, but as a result of a substantial change in the culture regarding work and civic values, he believes that in 2012, "America is falling apart" (p. C1).

We don't agree with Murray and believe that tax laws benefiting the rich, the loss of adequate paying jobs, and the lack of quality education and training have caused many working-class Americans to give up. Whichever reason you believe is responsible for high rates of long-term unemployment, many Americans across race, ethnicity, and social class lack a strong work ethic.

Both authors of this book are educators. We have seen a rapid decline in university standards and a significant increase in grade inflation, where As are so common that anything less than a grade of A often brings with it a student grade grievance. The mean undergraduate grade point average at a university at which one of the authors taught was 3.6 on a 4.0 scale, an increase from 2.3 just 15 years earlier. A colleague of ours was fired from a teaching position because he was told his tests were too difficult and that student morale was affected. Over three million jobs went unfilled in America in 2011 during our current economic crisis with high unemployment, because employers could not find qualified American workers—often because technology is considered too difficult by many US students and young adults. In a *Wall Street Journal* report, Madigan (2011) wrote that 40% of small businesses studied said it was "not easy at all" to find good help. Only 14% said hiring good workers was "very" or "extremely" easy. The report notes that in addition to finding workers with good technical skills, it was very difficult to hire workers who were punctual and reliable. Almost one-third of the respondents said they had seen very few qualified applicants for their firms' open positions, even though business owners were increasing compensation.

We will address the problems of the declining work ethic in more detail in the final chapter but we agree with Murray that a new work ethic is in order and that those of us who hold a bully pulpit because of our achievements and positions have a responsibility to use it to begin the revitalization of the workplace and urge more comprehensive changes in education and, perhaps, even in parenting.

Before we end the chapter, we present a more positive view of the workplace from a high-level manufacturing executive.

An Industrial Sector Executive Discusses the Impact of Culture on Worker Satisfaction and Productivity

Jacob Fox is a high-level executive with over 30 years of experience managing many thousands of industrial workers in the United States and Canada, Germany, Japan, and Mexico. He is in a unique position to answer questions about the workforce and whether the work ethic is stronger in some countries than it is in others.

Fox believes that workers are primarily influenced by the culture they grow up in. When products are not well made it's less the fault of workers than basic flaws in the design of a product often caused by budgetary restrictions. In describing workers in each of the five countries, he believes that American and Canadian workers are highly individualistic and are most productive when their needs and aspirations coincide with those of the organization. North American workers want to build quality products but are often unable to because funding is insufficient in many industrial sectors to adequately do the job.

Japanese workers have been socialized to practice harmony and cooperation and to be dedicated and disciplined workers able to work together as loyal team members. They have fewer unproductive and openly dissatisfied workers than America because the culture they live in values cooperation and using one's energies to advance the goals of the company. German workers believe in precision and unity of purpose and have a high degree of satisfaction when the products they build are very high in quality. They also have a long tradition of trade unions which provide a stable, well paid, and respected work force.

Mexican workers are generally without unions or legal rights, have no job protection, have low wages, and can be terminated at any time for any reasons. Because of the difficulties of life in Mexico and the lack of suitable employment, they work very hard and are highly productive even though they are poorly paid, have no job protection, and have few legal rights. When asked if nonexistent legal rights led to strikes and other indications of worker discontent in Mexico, he said that in his experience, labor unrest seldom happened in modern day Mexico.

When asked about removing manufacturing jobs from the United States and Canada and moving production to other countries with lower costs, Fox believes that most company executives are loyal to North American workers and want to keep manufacturing employment in the

United States and Canada if at all possible. Although unions are often blamed for the loss of manufacturing jobs, Fox believes that unions help in the creation of employee rights but have also demanded raises and benefits that have become unsustainable because of global competition. It takes two sides to negotiate a contract and both union and management share an equal responsibility for having created unsustainable manufacturing costs. However, in countries where workers have more rights and where the issue of how they are treated can have legal ramifications, unions serve an important function by agreeing to steps the company must take before a worker can be terminated. But given the poor economy, unions have become much more cooperative with management to make certain that companies continue to be profitable and that jobs are retained.

Fox believes that many outsourced manufacturing jobs will ultimately return to the United States because costs are going up in low-wage countries and the cost of shipping often makes a product more expensive than if it were built in the United States. He also believes that it's not in America's best interest to rely so heavily on foreign-made goods, since our national survival depends on a robust industrial sector where vital products are built at home and are not susceptible to economic, political, climate, and military problems elsewhere.

We wondered about his view of Employee Assistance Programs (EAPs) and whether they present a company with good value. He stated emphatically that EAPs are vital to aiding union/management relationships and often help troubled workers retain their jobs and resolve work-related or personal problems that might otherwise lead to reduced effectiveness and job loss. Once a worker loses a job and becomes overly dependent on social programs, Fox believes that it reduces the motivation to seek new employment or to upgrade skills.

As a country, Fox believes we face a challenge to reinvigorate the long-term unemployed. Reducing dependence of welfare and unemployment compensation is one solution that will likely take place because of spiraling and unsustainable costs; but, to make certain that jobs are available, Fox believes that we should strongly support goods made in North America. Those industries, when revitalized, will ultimately lead us to more jobs and better economic times.

SUMMARY

This introductory chapter spells out the many and varied problems in the current workplace and confirms that worker dissatisfaction is at an all-time high. Reasons for worker unhappiness are related to the poor economy and the increase in stress as fewer workers take on much more of the workload. Beyond the demand for workers to work harder and to take on more assignments is the increasing awareness that some employers are taking advantage of workers and not compensating them fairly. This is borne out in data showing that workers are often asked to work extra hours off the clock and that there has been a substantial increase in the number of law suits alleging that workers have not been paid for work exceeding 40 hours. The chapter also points out that American workers are paid as much as $20 or more per hour less in salaries and benefits than is the norm for European companies. Many organizations blame unions for the loss of industrial jobs and unfair demands made in labor negotiations, but as one high-level executive told us, unions and management are now working cooperatively to improve production and save jobs. Keeping jobs in the US that are vital to our national survival is something that will keep American jobs at home and bolster an economy in the doldrums.

REFERENCES

American Board of Examiners in Clinical Social Work (2004). Clinical supervision: A practice specialty of clinical social work. *A position statement of the American Board of Examiners in Clinical Social Work*. Retrieved on the Internet, May 12, 2006 at <www.abecsw.org>.

American Management Association (2007). *Addressing worker burnout (2007)*. Retrieved January 4, 2011 at: Addressingworker-burnout.aspx

Bodtker, A. M., & Jameson, J. K. (2001). Emotion in conflict formation and its transformation: Application to organizational conflict management. *International Journal of Conflict Management, 12*(Issue 3), 259–276.

Bureau of Labor Statistics (Dec. 2011). *International comparisons of hourly compensation costs in manufacturing*, 2010. Retrieved January 11, 2012 at: <http://www.bls.gov/news.release/ichcc.nr0.htmn>.

Christensen, R. L. & Kohls, J. (2003). *Ethical decision making in times of organizational crisis a framework for analysis*. Retrieved from the Internet January 13, 2012 at: <http://citeseerx.ist.psu.edu/viewdoc/summary?doi = 10.1.1.94.1956>.

Cook, T., & Emler, N. (1999). Bottom-up versus top-down evaluations of candidates' managerial potential: An experimental study. *Journal of Occupational & Organizational Psychology, 72*(Issue 4), 423–440.

Cooper, M. (Jan 31, 2009). *Handing out the pink slips can hurt, too*. Retrieved from the Internet April 27, 2012 at: <http://www.nytimes.com/2009/02/01/business/01pre.html?_r = 1>.

Dalton, D. R., Daily, C. M., Ellstrand, A. E., & Johnson, J. L. (1998). Meta-analytic reviews of board composition, leadership structure, and financial performance. *Strategic Management Journal, 19*, 269–290.

Davidson, P. (2012). *Overworked and underpaid? USA Today, 30*(no. 150), 1–2A.

Deprez, E. E. (Sept 3, 2009). Bloomberg business week. *Study Shows Psychological Impact of Unemployment*. Retrieved from the Internet January 6, 2012 at <http://www.businessweek.com/bwdaily/dnflash/content/sep2009/db2009092_648686.htm>.

Gallup (January 5, 2012). *Gallup finds U.S. unemployment holding at 8.5% in December.* Retrieved from the Internet January 12, 2012 at: <http://www.gallup.com/poll/151898/Gallup-Finds-Unemployment-Holding-December.aspx>.

Ghoshal, S. (2005). Bad management theories are destroying good management practices. *Academy of Management Learning & Education, 4*(Issue 1), 75–92.

Lorenz, M. (Dec 17, 2009). *5 Signs of job burnout and what to do about it.* Retrieved from the Internet August 14, 2012 at: <http://msn.careerbuilder.com/Article/CB-655-The-Workplace-5-Signs-of-Job-Burnout-and-What-to-Do-About-It/>.

Madigan, K. (November 8, 2011). *A good worker is hard to find.* Retrieved February 16, 2012 at: <http://blogs.wsj.com/economics/2011/11/08/small-business-a-good-worker-is-hard-to-find/>.

McCabe, D. L., & Trevino, L. K. (1995). Cheating among business students: A challenge for business leaders and educators. *Journal of Management Education, 19*, 205–218.

Menzel, D. C. (1999). The morally mute manager: Fact or fiction? *Public Personnel Management, 28*(Issue 4), 515–528.

Mirhaydari, A. *Are American workers getting lazy*? Retrieved March 21, 2012 at: <http://money.msn.com/investing/are-american-workers-getting-lazy-mirhaydari.aspx>.

Mitchell, C. E. (1999). Violating the public trust: The ethical and moral obligations of government officials. *Public Personnel Management, 28*, 27–38.

Murray, C. (March 16, 2012). *Why economics can't explain our cultural divide.* Retrieved April 4, 2012 at: <http://online.wsj.com/article/SB10001424052702304692804577281582403394206.html?KEYWORDS = charles + murray>.

Pfeffer, J. (2005). Why do bad management theories persist? A comment on Ghoshal. *Academy of Management Learning & Education, 4*(Issue 1), 78–95.

Presidential Commission on Work (1973). *Work in America.* Cambridge, MA: MIT Press.

Snyder, M. (July 15, 2010). *The middle class in America is radically shrinking.* Retrieved from the Internet January 13, 2012 at: <http://finance.yahoo.com/tech-ticker/the-u.s.-middle-class-is-being-wiped-out-here's-the-stats-to-prove-it-520657.html?tickers = %5EDJI,%5EGSPC,SPY,MCD,WMT,XRT,DIA>.

Stensaker, I., Meyer, C., Falkenberg, J., Haueng, A.-C. (2001). Excessive change: Unintended consequences of strategic change. *Academy of Management Proceedings*, p. G 1-7.

Summers, L. (January 9, 2012). *Why isn't capitalism working?* Retrieved from the Internet January 12, 2012 at: <http://blogs.reuters.com/lawrencesummers/2012/01/09/why-isnt-capitalism-working/01>.

The Economist (August 26, 2010). *Joblessness in America.* Retrieved from the Internet January 6, 2012 at: <http://www.economist.com/node/16888999>.

Weaver, J. (2012). *Job stress, burnout on the rise: Layoffs, long hours taking their toll on workers.* Retrieved January 24, 2012 at: <http://www.msnbc.msn.com/id/3072410/ns/business-us_business/t/job-stress-burnout-rise/>.

Williams, R. J., Barrett, J. D., & Brabston, M. (2000). Managers' business school education and military service: Possible links to corporate criminal activity. *Human Relations, 53*, 6.

FURTHER READING

Bureau of Labor Statistics. (December 21, 2011). International comparisons of hourly compensation costs in manufacturing, 2010. *United States Department of Labor.* Retrieved January 11, 2012 from <http://www.bls.gov/news.release/ichcc.nr0.htm>.

Jacobe, D. (January 5, 2012). *Gallup finds U.S. unemployment holding at 8.5% in December.* Retrieved January 12, 2012 from <http://www.gallup.com/poll/151898/Gallup-Finds-Unemployment-Holding-December.aspx>.

Snyder, M. (July 15, 2010). *The middle class in America is radically shrinking.* Retrieved January 13, 2012 from <http://finance.yahoo.com/tech-ticker/the-u.s.-middle-class-is-being-wiped-out-here's-the-stats-to-prove-it-520657.html?tickers = %5EDJI, %5EGSPC,SPY,MCD,WMT,XRT,DIA>.

Summers, L. (January 9, 2012). *Why isn't capitalism working?* Retrieved January 12, 2012 from <http://blogs.reuters.com/lawrencesummers/2012/01/09/why-isnt-capitalism-working/>.

Weaver, J. (2012). *Job stress, burnout on the rise: Layoffs, long hours taking their toll on workers.* Retrieved January 24, 2012 from <http://www.msnbc.msn.com/id/3072410/ns/business-us_business/t/job-stress-burnout-rise/>.

CHAPTER 2

Understanding Job Stress, Job Dissatisfaction, and Worker Burnout

INTRODUCTION

This chapter discusses three main issues related to work-related problems: job stress and the reasons behind it, worker dissatisfaction and the many personal and work-related reasons people become unhappy at work, and worker burnout and the many signs that workers are beginning to develop symptoms of depression on the job. Additionally, the chapter provides several personal reflections by workers with job stress and burnout. Finally, the chapter includes major instruments to measure all three issues and, by way of understanding what the instruments measure, the chapter includes a discussion of intrinsic and extrinsic factors in job satisfaction and considers three main theories of management leadership and their potential impact on stress, job satisfaction, and burnout: Theories X, Y, and Z.

JOB STRESS

The National Institute for Occupational Safety and Health (NIOSH) defines job stress as "the harmful physical and emotional responses that occur when the requirements of the job do not match the capabilities, resources, or needs of the worker" (NIOSH, 1999, p. 1). Job stress is sometimes confused with job challenge, but challenge energizes us emotionally and physically and motivates us. When we master a challenge, we are often satisfied with our work. Job stress, on the other hand, has harmful physical and emotional consequences when not handled well or when it is difficult to change because workers have no control over it. The NIOSH report (p. 5) offers the following job conditions as ones that may lead to stress:

- **The design of tasks**: Heavy workload, infrequent rest breaks, long work hours and shiftwork; hectic and routine tasks that have little inherent meaning, do not utilize workers' skills, and provide little sense of control.

Treating Worker Dissatisfaction During Economic Change
DOI: http://dx.doi.org/10.1016/B978-0-12-397006-0.00002-6

- **Management style:** Lack of participation by workers in decision-making, poor communication in the organization, lack of family-friendly policies. (Chapters 8 and 9 of this book propose approaches to management intended to reduce worker stress.)
- **Interpersonal relationships:** Poor social environment and lack of support or help from co-workers and supervisors.
- **Work roles:** Conflicting or uncertain job expectations, too much responsibility, too many "hats to wear."
- **Career concerns:** Job insecurity and lack of opportunity for growth, advancement, or promotion; rapid changes for which workers are unprepared.
- **Environmental conditions:** Unpleasant or dangerous physical conditions such as crowding, noise, air pollution, or ergonomic problems.

Storey and Billingham (2001) have a similar but slightly different idea of what produces workplace stress and suggest the following potential conditions in the workplace that may lead to stress:

- **The physical climate of a workplace:** Poor working conditions can cause stress. This may include overcrowding, unbearable levels of noise, immoderate temperatures in a building, long commutes to get to work, unsafe conditions on the job, poorly built or uncomfortable office space, and smells that can be offensive.
- **The worker's role in the organization:** Four factors influence role issues: role conflict or incompatibility between one's values and beliefs and those of the organization; uncertainty about duties and responsibilities; too much to accomplish and too little time to do it; an expectation that work must be done which is beyond a worker's level of ability.
- **Work relationships:** Because human service work often takes place in a team context, teams provide both relief from stress and an increase in stress because teams are not always supportive of individual colleagues.
- **Organizational structure and climate:** The extent to which a worker can be involved in and influence decision-making processes can have a significant positive or negative effect. All too often organizations make changes without consulting workers and face morale problems as a result. Asking workers to take on more decision-making for the organization than they can handle also has potential for increasing stress.
- **The impact of one's personal life on work and the interface between work and home:** Workers are affected by their jobs when stress becomes high. Similarly, their work is affected when personal problems seep over into the workplace. Marital and relationship

problems, financial difficulties, substance abuse and health problems can all negatively affect work and increase stress.

Karasek (1979) found that two work-related elements contribute to job stress: the demands of the job and how much freedom workers have to meet those demands. If job demands are high and freedom to resolve those demands in ways that fit an individual's coping style is low, workers experience high job strain. Beehr (1995) found that ambiguous work assignments and conflict with others are additional reasons for job stress. Sutherland and Cooper (1988) report that job stress substantially increases with the existence of job insecurity, under-promotions, over-promotions, and hindered ambition.

Personal problems that are not connected to work can also add to work stress. These include marital and relationship issues untreated depression and anxiety, other more serious mental health conditions, substance abuse, undiagnosed medical problems, anger issues (which are discussed in greater detail in the chapter on workplace violence), deep insecurities that affect performance and relationship with others on the job, and a number of other issues that can impact job performance. In the chapter on treatment, we will include treatment suggestions for all three conditions: stress, job unhappiness, and burnout.

The University of Massachusetts, Lowell (U. Mass. Lowell Center for the Promotion of Health in the New England Workplace, 2012, p. 1) reports that studies indicate a strong relationship between workplace stress and the development of cardiovascular problems such as hypertension and myocardial infarction. The report notes that "... up to 23 percent of heart disease related deaths per year could be prevented if the levels of job strain in the most stressful occupations were reduced to average levels seen in other occupations" (p. 1). The report explains that work stressors can trigger cardiovascular disease (CVD) and other chronic health problems and points to three main areas of the body:

- Changes in physiological processes that increase the risk for CVD—high cholesterol, high blood pressure, high blood sugar, weakened immune response, high cortisol, and changes in appetite and digestive patterns;
- Changes in behavior that increase the risk for CVD—low physical activity levels, excessive coffee consumption, smoking, poor dietary habits.
- Development of mental health conditions—anxiety and depression—that independently increase the risk for a range of chronic health conditions, including CVD, obesity, stroke, atherosclerosis, arrhythmias, and myocardial infarction.

The American Institute of Stress (2012, p. 1) reports the following data on workplace stress.

- Sixty-five percent of workers said that workplace stress had caused difficulties, and more than 10% described these as having major effects.
- Ten percent said they work in an atmosphere where physical violence has occurred because of job stress; and, in this group, 42% report that yelling and other verbal abuse is common.
- Twenty-nine percent had yelled at co-workers because of workplace stress, 14% said they work where machinery or equipment has been damaged because of workplace rage, and 2% admitted that they had actually personally struck someone.
- Nineteen percent, or almost one in five, respondents had quit a previous position because of job stress, and nearly one in four have been driven to tears because of workplace stress.
- Sixty-two percent routinely find that they end the day with work-related neck pain, 44% reported stressed-out eyes, 38% complained of hurting hands, and 34% reported difficulty in sleeping because they were too stressed-out.
- Twelve percent had called in sick because of job stress.
- Over half said they often spend 12-hour days on work-related duties, and an equal number frequently skip lunch because of the stress of job demands.

Sometimes stress occurs when you fail to understand underlying issues on a job and how petty jealousies about you and the work you do can lead to very stressful experiences even when your work is at a high level, as this story from a business consultant demonstrates:

A Personal Reflection on Job Stress: A Business Consultant Tries to Help a Family-Owned Business

I am a long time business consultant. Recently, I worked with a mother-daughter team who had successfully created a unique fabric store sewing school. The mother started the business and the daughter stepped in later to try to save it when it began to fail. I was brought in much later to introduce a new product line.

Although I have a friendly relationship with the mother, I primarily report to the daughter, who has turned the business into a profitable and thriving one. Together, the daughter and I developed and launched a new product line. After a very successful sales launch, I was feeling very good about the work I'd done until I got verbally lambasted by the mother concerning one of the new sewing tools we were launching. She blamed me for creating something that wasn't good for the end-user or the business, and said that I had to live with myself hurting a business she had put so much time and effort into creating. She, in essence, threw a temper tantrum. It turns out she is extremely jealous of her daughter and her accomplishments. Because she could see how successful the new products would be, all that jealousy surfaced and I was in the firing line.

Often the success of a business leads to jealousies and pettiness that I'm never aware of until it surfaces. We somehow have the illusion that families who work together support each other but, quite often, that's not the case. I find that people often torpedo my best efforts even when it leads to successful business ventures because I haven't understood that, all along, they often have deep resentment toward me because their failure becomes my success. That's one of the biggest stressors in my work. I still replay in my mind the mother accusing me of ruining the business and now I have second thoughts about new situations and wonder whether there is something going on that I'm not aware of that will end up in a stressful and hurtful confrontation or, an attempt to undermine everything I've done to help the business.

JOB DISSATISFACTION

When job stress becomes increasingly difficult to control, it often leads to job dissatisfaction. The most commonly used definition of job satisfaction is given by Locke (1975) who defined it as "... a pleasurable or positive emotional state resulting from the appraisal of one's job or job experiences" (p. 1304). This definition implies that not only do we evaluate satisfaction as an emotional state but that we think about those aspects of the job that make us satisfied and dissatisfied.

Morale refers to how a worker appraises the work experience in the future. It's possible for a worker to have good job satisfaction with a current position but to have their morale affected because of future perceptions of the job. A worker may feel that they've learned as much as they can about a job and that to continue doing it will result in boredom or to feel that future salary increases or promotional opportunities are limited.

Early studies of job satisfaction and productivity resulted in very limited evidence to support a relationship between the two. Iaffaldano & Muchinsky (1985) concluded that the relationship was at best trivial, illusory, and nothing more than a management fad. However, more recent research has found these conclusions to be incorrect.

Harrison, Newman, and Roth (2006) reported that low job satisfaction is a very strong predictor of absenteeism, lateness, reduced productivity, high staff turnover, and low morale. These behaviors often have a profound impact on other employees and can be cumulative throughout an organization. Believing that getting rid of an unhappy employee will reduce job dissatisfaction in an organization fails to consider that the open unhappiness of one worker may not take into account other workers who keep their unhappiness to themselves but have all the symptoms and behaviors of job dissatisfaction.

Organ (1988) found that job unhappiness negatively affects organizational citizenship, a behavior that may undermine the morale of others and create organization-wide withdrawal from the extra effort that may be needed to keep the organization functioning during difficult times. Judge, Thoresen, Bono, & Patton (2001) note that job satisfaction is particularly important for professional workers performing complex jobs. Judge and Watanabe (1994) found that job dissatisfaction had a spillover effect and negatively impacted personal life, often resulting in increased levels of depression, minor illness, alcohol and drug use and, in some cases, disrupted domestic relationships and family violence. Although some might argue that spillover has more to do with personal traits of the worker, Wheaton (1990) found that the evidence clearly shows that what workers experience on the job has a clear spillover effect and, when the experience is bad, work may negatively affect mental health.

This is not to say that the job itself is always the reason workers experience job distress and unhappiness. Selecting workers ill-suited for a job, or a mismatch between the worker's personal goals and ways of working with those of the organization, may increase job unhappiness. Key personality traits can also influence job satisfaction. Judge, Bono, and Locke (2000) report that a worker's positive or negative self-evaluation influences job satisfaction, as does extraversion and conscientiousness. Workers with very positive evaluations of themselves and who are also outgoing and conscientious often have high levels of job satisfaction.

Hofstede (1980, 1985) found that the country of origin and culture of a worker often influences their fit within an organization. The researcher said that there were four cross-cultural behaviors that influenced comfort with an organization and work output: (1) whether they view themselves as individuals with distinct needs and aspirations or part of a large whole; (2) their willingness to take risks or just to do what they were told to do; (3) their comfort with a top-down organizational structure or a desire to have a more equal power distribution, and (4) their passivity or assertiveness in achieving success. For example, Saari and Judge (2004) found that workers in the United States were high on individualism, wanted equality in the workplace, and were high on risk-taking, whereas workers in Mexico were low on individualism, high on the notion of power coming from top management, and low on risk-taking. Keep in mind, however, that as workers assimilate in the United States their work-related behavior becomes more like that of native-born Americans. Nonetheless, it's useful to think that culture and country of origin may affect the way workers view their place in an organization and, consequently, their job satisfaction.

One of the primary reasons for worker unhappiness is explained by the concept of workplace inequity. Taris, Kalimo, and Schaufeli (2002) found that an imbalance in equity, or a feeling that a worker was being treated unfairly, resulted in "emotional exhaustion, cynicism, lack of professional efficacy, sickness, absence, and health complaints" (p. 297). Adams (1963, 1965) believed that people pursue a balance between their work inputs—such as time, attention, skills, and effort—and the rewards of their work, including status, appreciation, gratitude, and pay. According to Adams, any disturbance in that balance will have negative outcomes because workers receive less than what they believe they are entitled to.

WORKER BURNOUT

Tracy's study of workers aboard cruise ships describes burnout as "a general wearing out or alienation from the pressures of work" (Tracy, 2000, p. 6). Burnout is generally thought to be the end result of job dissatisfaction and low morale. To be burned out is not the same as being burned up. Workers who are burned out can have renewing experiences and time-outs that bring back their motivation to work and satisfaction with their jobs. Burned up workers are so depressed and unmotivated with their jobs that it may be difficult or impossible to improve motivation and performance. Burn up happens when burnout goes untreated for too long a period of time. Think of burn up as the final stages of a long-term clinical depression.

Maslach (1993) described three dimensions of worker burnout: (a) emotional exhaustion; (b) depersonalization, defined as a negative attitude towards customers and clients, a personal detachment, or loss of ideals; and (c) reduced personal accomplishment and commitment to the profession. Farber (1990) suggests three types of burned out workers: frenetic, under-challenged, and worn out. The characteristics of each type are as follows.

- **Frenetic type**: The frenetic type of worker is highly dedicated and committed to their work. Feelings of dissatisfaction cause them to work even harder. Frenetic workers are often tenacious, energetic, and invested in their work and might be considered highly idealistic by most colleagues. Additionally, they are often unable to acknowledge failure, and they set unrealistically high goals for themselves. When those goals are not met, they often feel great negativity about themselves, neglect their own personal needs, and respond to themselves and others with anxiety, irritability, and depression. Glicken (2010) called these workers "idealistic workaholics."
- **Under-challenged type**: The under-challenged worker has lost interest in his or her occupation and does their work in a superficial way. They have little motivation, see no new challenges, and lack a desire to be more involved on the job. Behaviors associated with the under-challenged worker are indifference, an unwillingness to develop as a person, obsession with finding new jobs and new careers without actually following through, and often complaining about how monotonous the work is and how bored they are.
- **Worn-out type**: The worn-out worker has lost all optimism about his or her job, including even considering other work or new assignments. They have essentially given up, neglected their work-related responsibilities, feel no control over the situation, often feel depressed, and have difficulties performing assigned work tasks. Farber believes that worn-out workers are often the byproducts of inflexible, rigid, bureaucratic organizations where everything is done following arcane rules and procedures no one really knows or understands and that hide the fact that there is unfairness in almost all the decisions made regarding salaries, promotions, and work assignments. Workers at greatest risk of this type of burnout often work in large organizations providing little recognition, support, or appreciation for their work.

Freudenberger and North (1985) believe that burnout often shows itself in the following phases:

1. The need to prove oneself on the job.
2. Taking on increasing amounts of work to the point of work's becoming a compulsion.
3. Neglecting personal needs.

4. Knowing they are working too hard, beginning to have physical symptoms of overwork, but being unable to do anything about it.
5. Being consumed by work, which leaves them isolated from others.
6. An increase in social isolation, sarcasm with others, and a tendency to blame the work for their increasing sense of isolation.
7. Withdrawal, beginning to use substances to cope, and a tendency to do the job by the book.
8. Obvious behavioral changes noted by others.
9. Behavior at work becoming mechanical and robotic.
10. Inner emptiness and exaggerated activities involving food, substances, and sex.
11. Depression.
12. Physical and emotional collapse.

Lorenz (2009, p. 1) provides the following signs of burnout:

- Crankiness, irritability, and an inability to get along with co-workers you used to get along with just fine;
- Coming to work late, wanting to leave early, dreading coming to work at all, watching the clock, and counting the minutes until you leave;
- A sense of apathy and a lack of motivation; no longer wanting to be challenged;
- No longer interested in interacting socially with co-workers;
- Feeling exhausted much of the time, having headaches, feeling tension in all of your muscles, and having trouble sleeping.

A Personal Reflection on Worker Burnout: A Judge Confronts the Limitations of Her Job

Linda Morgan is a superior court judge in a state in the northeast. She told us that as caseloads have increased and judicial discretion has been taken away from judges because of strict sentencing guidelines handed down by legislatures, many judges are experiencing burnout and retiring early. In her own experience an example she cited was a young man charged with possession of illegal drugs. Should she impose prison time or probation on the son who is taking care of his elderly mother (who sits weepy eyed in the back of the courtroom)? He claims he is going to school to become a nurse. She doubts that he will make it since he was caught with enough marijuana to show that, although he is not a dealer, he is very likely a heavy user. Heavy drug use, she suspects with considerable past experience with drug users, will not bode well for academic work.

The guidelines for the amount of marijuana found in his possession calls for a prison sentence, but who will take care of the elderly mother? If she sentences him to probation, she faces judicial scrutiny and possible sanctions in her appointed job because her decision would be contrary to the guidelines imposed by a strongly anti-drug-use legislature.

She told me that "His face reflected what so many others tell me in their eyes: A pleading to be released, a desire to do better for themselves, if only in this moment. I, of course, have heard it all before. I know of all the jobs that are starting "tomorrow," of all the children that need them to be "out" so they can provide for their families, and even the ones who just look at me as only a shell of the person they once were. But for today, at this hour, at this time, I believe him and yet I must sentence him to jail time. It eats away at me. I go home and look at the calendar and wonder if I can make it for three more years until I can retire. I'm not sure that I can."

WAYS OF DETERMINING JOB DISSATISFACTION AND WORKER BURNOUT: THEORIES X, Y, AND Z

There are a number of well-accepted ways to determine job dissatisfaction and worker burnout. The following are a few, and more instruments may be found on the book's website.

Job Satisfaction

The Job Descriptive Index (JDI; Smith, Kendall, & Hulin, 1969) is the most frequently used measure. The JDI measure five major factors associated with job satisfaction: the nature of the work itself, compensations and benefits, attitudes towards supervisors, relations with co-workers, and opportunities for promotion. To understand how the JDI and similar instruments can give us an understanding of the level of job satisfaction across all occupations, Table 2.1 shows data reported by Bryner (2007) on a 2006 national study of 27,000 workers conducted at the University of Chicago, which provides, for a range of occupations, the percentage of workers in each occupation who are satisfied with their work.

Intrinsic and Extrinsic Motivators

On average, 47% of all workers surveyed by Bryner (2007) said they were satisfied with their jobs and 33% reported being very happy. Table 2.1 shows that many of the most highly satisfied workers are also only moderately paid (clergy, teachers, authors). The reason for this may have to do

Table 2.1 Percentage of Workers, by Occupation, who are Satisfied with their Work

Occupation	Percent satisfied
The Top 10	
Clergy	87
Firefighters	80
Physical therapists	78
Authors	74
Special education teachers	70
Teachers	69
Education administrators	68
Painters and sculptors	67
Psychologists	67
Security and financial services salespersons	65
Operating engineers	64
Office supervisors	61
The Bottom 10	
Laborers, except construction	21
Apparel clothing salespersons	24
Handpackers and packagers	24
Food preparers	24
Roofers	25
Cashiers	25
Furniture and home-furnishing salespersons	25
Bartenders	26
Freight, stock, and material handlers	26
Waiters and servers	27

Source: Bryner (2007).

with the satisfaction they experience from the work itself rather than the salary and benefits they receive. Herzberg (1973) argued that *intrinsic aspects* of the work (whether the work itself gives you pleasure) leads to being satisfied, while *extrinsic aspects* of the job such as salary and benefits prevent workers from being dissatisfied. In order for salary and benefits to keep workers from being dissatisfied they must regularly increase. Failure to do so leads to job dissatisfaction.

Herzberg's contribution to our understanding of job satisfaction is that the motivation to work hard, and ultimately job satisfaction, comes from within. The organization's task is to utilize workers in ways that facilitate their internal motivation, or the satisfaction derived from the work itself and the contribution they make to the organization. This crucial finding offers management a better way to use people by hiring workers who are motivated by the work itself rather than assuming workers are only interested in money. The belief that extrinsic factors motivate workers requires management to continually up the ante with increasingly better pay and benefits to get results. During times of economic trouble when added salary and benefits aren't available, in organizations that use money as a motivator, lack of salary increases can precipitate reduced job satisfaction.

Theories X, Y, and Z

Theory X and Y

McGregor (1960) suggested that the use of incentives to motivate workers could best be understood by the leadership style of an organization's managers and suggested two distinct types of leadership styles: Theory X and Theory Y. The Theory X leadership style is very authoritarian and assumes that workers are largely lazy, lacking in motivation, require a high level of supervision to make certain the work gets done, and require substantial salary and benefit incentives to work hard. On the other hand, the Theory Y leadership style assumes that employees are driven, ambitious, and want to accept larger roles within the organization. This leadership style encourages creativity in the workforce based on the belief that productivity increases when employees have the opportunity to face new work-related challenges. This leadership style is often found in workplaces that prize employees who think and use their creative abilities over those who can simply repeat a task. Under Theory X, the leadership style is likely to be autocratic, which may create resistance on the part of workers. Communication flow is downward from manager to the subordinates. Theory Y leadership styles value worker participation and empowerment which, it is hoped, will result in workers seeking more responsibility and commitment to organizational goals.

Theory X has been criticized for being out of touch with workers who have been socialized by a society that values participation and resents punitive practices like the carrot and stick approach used in Theory X (the carrot if you do what you're told to do and the stick if you don't). Theory Y has been criticized because, in the hands of a less than competent manager, it can become chaotic with lines of authority so unclear that nothing gets done. An additional criticism of Theory Y is that it is nothing more than a subtle form of manipulation with management giving workers the illusion of having freedom when actually they don't. Without shared economic benefits for their productivity then, goes the criticism, workers have simply been manipulated into working harder for limited economic benefits.

Theory Z

One additional leadership style that affects motivation to work and job satisfaction is Theory Z (Ouchi, 1981). This theory, also known as the Japanese approach to management, focuses on increasing employee loyalty to the organization by providing a job for life with a strong focus on the well-being of the employee, both on and off the job. According to Ouchi, Theory Z management tends to promote stable employment, high productivity, and high employee morale and satisfaction. Whether this approach can be sustained in difficult economic times is questionable since even Japanese companies have laid workers off and changed their policy of lifetime job security as a result of the poor worldwide economy.

Determining Burnout

The Maslach Burnout Inventory (MBI; Maslach & Jackson, 1986) is the most well accepted and frequently used way of determining burnout. The MBI consists of 22 questions and three subscales which measure interrelated aspects of burnout, including emotional exhaustion (EE), depersonalization, and personal accomplishment. The MBI takes 10–15 minutes to complete; in some busy settings this may lead to either socially desirable answers (answers the test taker thinks are the most positive or negative but do not actually represent his or her true feelings) or answers that are not well thought through. Instead, Hansen (2010) found that asking workers just one question—"Are you emotionally exhausted?"—was as effective in determining burnout as giving the entire instrument. Measures of depression such as the Center for Epidemiologic Studies Depression Scale (CES-D), which is free and can be found on the book website, may be just as good a measure of burnout as the MBI, which can be expensive to give since there is a fee for each copy used.

A concept that is increasingly used in the helping, medical, and teaching professions is compassion fatigue. Compassion fatigue refers to a decline in the ability to experience joy or to feel and care for others, and occurs in professionals who expend a great deal of energy and compassion on others, yet get little positive feedback or inner peace for their labors. Compassion fatigue may also be seen as an extreme form of stress in which the professional begins to experience secondary traumatic stress because of the physical and emotional trauma of taking care of people in dire need.

However, all the surveys and instruments to measure burnout seem less likely to spot it than carefully listening to workers talk about their depressed feelings toward their jobs and observing their behavior, their productivity, and the many signs of burnout mentioned earlier in the chapter. Careful observation and honest discussions could lead to changes in work assignments, strategic timeouts from work, or retraining for new assignments. All of these as well as personal counseling would help to reduce the number of cases in which burnout enters a final stage in which the worker is completely burned up.

Personal Observation: A Worker Confronts the Realization That Her Burnout Stems From an Incorrect Career Choice

Lynn Packer, a former Marriage and Family Counselor from Thousand Oaks, California told us, "I knew I wasn't suited for a career as a therapist. I'd sit listening to people complain about their problems at work and at home and I'd get up in the morning grumbling that I didn't want to go to work, arrive late, and leave early. I was one step away from an exit interview".

"I finally had to admit that I was the problem, not the clients who were pouring their hearts out to me. I was a proponent of 'just do it' therapy long before Nike entered the picture. I couldn't understand why anyone who was so unhappy in their lives just didn't change it. Finally, I took my own advice and left. I planned my exit. It took over a year before I left and I made sure not to burn any bridges. I applied to law school, got accepted, and I was off to the races. Now, no more waking up to 'I don't want to go to work.' Now it's 'did I malpractice yesterday?' but I'm far happier and more successful at work. I think my early life ideas about a career were influenced by my own personal problems and a belief that helping others would be a way of helping myself. I didn't realize that once I dealt with those problems, that counseling would bore me".

"I'm glad I didn't wait around and become cynical and pessimistic like a lot of people I know who stick with a career way longer than they should. And I have to admit that my training and experience as a counselor have taught me a great deal about human behavior that comes in very handy as a lawyer, so I don't feel that I wasted my time getting my degree. I do think that you shouldn't always blame organizations for burnout but you should recognize that people come to jobs with their own issues and that before the next job or the job after that also ends in burnout, you have to be honest with yourself, get the necessary help and change whatever past ways of thinking about work continue to end in burnout."

SUMMARY

This chapter defines three types of work-related problems that impact a worker's performance: job stress, job dissatisfaction, and worker burnout. It is suggested that the three move in tandem with one another, with job stress leading to job dissatisfaction, and dissatisfaction, unless corrected, leading to burnout. Many researchers believe that burnout is a type of depression that saps motivation to work. All three conditions impact work effectiveness and often intrude into the personal lives of workers. Instruments to measure stress, dissatisfaction, and burnout are provided, but in the case of burnout a simple question asking workers if they are depressed can have the same impact as the use of a burnout instrument. Supervisors observing worker attitudes and performance can often identify all three conditions on the basis of simple behaviors such as tardiness, missing work with vague reasons, decline in the quality and quantity of work, and a thorough lack of enthusiasm. Early research suggesting that unhappy workers had the same level of productivity as happy ones has been thoroughly debunked in later research showing that job unhappiness not only affects productivity but may have a negative impact on health, mental health, and personal and family lives. Several workers gave their personal descriptions of how it feels to have each of the three work-related conditions discussed in the chapter.

REFERENCES

Adams, J. S. (1963). Toward an understanding of inequity. *Journal of Abnormal and Social Psychology, 67*, 422–436.

Adams, J. S. (1965). Inequity in social exchange. In L. Berkowitz (Ed.), *Advances in Experimental Social Psychology* (2, pp. 267–299). New York: Academic Press.

American Institute of Stress. (2012). *What is workplace stress*? Retrieved August 14, 2012 from <http://www.stress.org/>.

Beehr, T. A. (1995). *Psychological stress in the workplace*. London: Routledge.

Bryner, J. (17 April 2007). *Survey reveals most satisfying jobs*. Retrieved from the Internet January 24, 2012 at: <http://www.livescience.com/1431-survey-reveals-satisfying-jobs.html>.

Farber, B. A. (1990). Burnout in psychotherapist: Incidence, types, and trends. *Psychotherapy in Private Practice, 8*, 35–44.

Freudenberger, H. J., & North, G. (1985). *Women's Burnout: How to Spot It, How to Reverse It, and How to Prevent It*. New York: Doubleday.

Glicken, M. D. (2010). *Workaholics in Retirement*. Santa Barbara, CA: Praeger Press.

Hansen, V. (2010). Can a single question effectively screen for burnout in Australian cancer care workers? *BMC Health Services Research, 10*, 341.

Harrison, D., Newman, D., & Roth, P. (2006). How important are job attitudes? *Academy of Management Journal, 49*(2), 305–325.

Herzberg, F. (1973). *Work and the Nature of Man*. New York: Signet.

Hofstede, G. (1980). *Culture's consequences: International differences in work-related values.* Newbury Park, CA: Sage.

Hofstede, G. (1985). The interaction between national and organizational value systems. *Journal of Management Studies, 22*, 347–357.

Iaffaldano, M. R., & Muchinsky, P. M. (1985). Job satisfaction and job performance: A meta-analysis. *Psychological Bulletin, 97*, 251–273.

Judge, T. A., & Watanabe, S. (1994). Individual differences in the nature of the relationship between job and life satisfaction. *Journal of Occupational and Organizational Psychology, 67*, 101–107.

Judge, T. A., Bono, J. E., & Locke, E. A. (2000). Personality and job satisfaction: The mediating role of job characteristics. *Journal of Applied Psychology, 85*, 237–249.

Judge, T. A., Thoresen, C. J., Bono, J. E., & Patton, G. K. (2001). The job satisfaction–job performance relationship: A qualitative and quantitative review. *Psychological Bulletin, 127*, 376–407.

Karasek, R. A., Jr. (1979). Job demands, job decision latitude and mental strain: Implications for job redesign. *Administrative Science Quarterly, 24*, 285–308.

Locke, E. A. (1975). The nature and causes of job satisfaction. In M. D. Dinette (Ed.), *The Handbook of Industrial and Organizational Psychology.* Chicago: Rand-McNally.

Lorenz, K. (2009). *Five signs of job burnout and what to do about it.* Retrieved from the Internet January 3, 2012 at <http://msn.careerbuilder.com/Article/CB-655-The-Workplace-5-Signs-of-Job-Burnout-and-What-to-Do-About-It/>.

Maslach, C. (1993). Burnout: A multidimensional perspective. In W. B. Schaufeli, C. Maslach, & T. Marek (Eds.), *Professional burnout: Recent developments in theory and research.* Washington, DC: Taylor & Francis.

Maslach, C, & Jackson, SE (1986). *Maslach Burnout Inventory Manual* (2nd edition). Palo Alto, CA: Consulting Psychologists Press.

Mass U. Lowell Center for the Promotion of Health in the New England Workplace. (2012). *Stress at work*. Retrieved January 19, 2012 at: <http://www.uml.edu/centers/cph-new/job-stress/research.html>.

McGregor, D. (1960). *The Human Side of the Enterprise.* New York: McGraw-Hill, Inc.

NIOSH (1999). *Stress at work*, Publication 99-101. Retrieved from the Internet January 19, 2012 at: <http://www.cdc.gov/niosh/docs/99-101/>.

Organ, D. W. (1988). A restatement of the satisfaction-performance hypothesis. *Journal of Management, 14*, 547–557.

Ouchi, W. G. (1981). *Theory Z.* New York: Avon Books.

Saari, L. M, & Judge, T. A. (2004). Employee attitudes and job satisfaction. *Human Resource Management, Winter 2004, 43*(No. 4), 395–407.

Smith, P. C., Kendall, L. M., & Hulin, C. L. (1969). *The Measurement of Satisfaction in Work and Retirement.* Chicago: Rand McNally.

Storey, J., & Billingham, J. (2001). Occupational stress and social work. *Social Work Education, 20*(6), 659–670.

Sutherland, V. J., & Cooper, C. L. (1988). Sources of work stress. In J. J. Hurrell, Jr, L. R. Murphy, S. L. Sauter, & C. L. Cooper (Eds.), *Occupational stress: Issues and Developments in Research* (pp. 3–40). London: Taylor & Francis.

Taris, T. W., Kalimo, R., & Schaufeli, W. B. (2002). Inequity at work: Its measurement and association with worker health. *Work & Stress, 16*(4), 287–301.

Tracy, S. (2000). Becoming a character for commerce emotion. *Management Communication Quarterly,* 14. *113*, 1–12.

Wheaton, B. (1990). Life transitions, role histories, and mental health. *American Sociological Review, 55*, 209–223.

FURTHER READING

CES-D depression scale to measure the degree of worker burnout. Retrieved April 20, 2012 from <http://www.chcr.brown.edu/pcoc/cesdscale.pdf>.

Job Stress Inventory: Retrieved March 11, 2012 from <http://www.arborfamilycounseling.com/archives/Library/workplacescreenings/screenings/jobstressinventory.pdf >.

The Job Descriptive Index (JDI). Retrieved April 20, 2012 from <http://www.bgsu.edu/departments/psych/io/jdi/page54706.html>.

The Maslich Burnout Inventory (MBI). Retrieved April 25, 2012 from <http://www.mindgarden.com/products/mbi.htm>.

The Professional Quality of Life Scale: Compassion satisfaction, burnout and compassion, fatigue/secondary trauma scales. Retrieved January 12, 2012 from <http://www.compassionfatigue.org/pages/ProQOLManualOct05.pdf >.

PART Two

Major Work-Related Problems that Lead to Job Dissatisfaction and Burnout

CHAPTER 3

Teamwork and Cooperative Work Assignments Sometimes Lead to Job Dissatisfaction

INTRODUCTION

Cooperative work and working in teams are currently much in vogue as ways of getting the job done. The impact of Japanese management techniques, so successful in assuring quality and high productivity, has strongly influenced the way we think about work. However, as many of us know from long and unproductive meetings, committee work, team teaching, and other cooperative ventures, workers often do rather badly when it comes to teamwork. This chapter will discuss why many workers, both professional and non-professional, have problems with cooperative work and what we can do to improve the functioning of teams.

DEFINITIONS AND DISCUSSION

Mason (1998) describes a team as a "group of people coming together to share their expertise to accomplish a specific outcome" (p. 30). Although not everything is best done in teams and some functions are better given to individuals, many workers share similar assignments and can learn from one another through support, direct feedback, and help in problem-solving. Even though teamwork is often a better way for organizational goals and objectives to be met, many problems exist that often interfere with cooperative work. Mason suggests that those impediments include confused work objectives, unclear roles for members of the team, poor decision-making on the part of supervisors and workers, and personality differences. A good deal of what makes or breaks a team is appropriate feedback from supervisors to workers and back. Although some people lack the ability to work cooperatively and are better when working alone, "People skills can be taught, then practiced, with feedback. Team members can give each other daily feedback on what a person's doing right and wrong" (Mason, 1998, p. 31).

Treating Worker Dissatisfaction During Economic Change
DOI: http://dx.doi.org/10.1016/B978-0-12-397006-0.00003-8

Who is the best person to lead a team? Mason believes it is the one who is most versatile and can communicate with everyone. "Versatility means you're providing information the way a different person hears it. It's called interpersonal reciprocity. If someone gives me information the way I want to receive it I feel bound to want to follow them" (Mason, 1998, p. 32). According to Mason, versatility also means that you share information with others in a way that provides open and honest interaction and that you don't hoard important information. Versatility implies that supervisors provide feedback including follow-up, rewards, and recognition for well-done work both individually and in the team.

Adam Smith (1937, pp. 7—10) believed that teamwork was a superior way of dividing labor because it improve quality, as groups make work more efficient, save time, and increase skill for all workers since competence can be passed on from one worker to another. Alchian and Demsetz (1972) argue that teams influence each other's levels of performance and maintain high levels of productivity. Holmstrom and Milgrom (1991) studied the meaning of the term "teamwork" and believe the term embodies the notion of a "help effort" to other workers. It is this help effort that increases the effectiveness of work done in teams. Itoh (1991) believes that the driving force behind teams is that they tend to take lower-performing workers and increase their productivity by increasing their willingness to compete with higher-performing workers. Lin (1997) found the claim that teams divide and conquer workers not to be true and writes, "The findings in this paper weaken a long-held claim that division of labor is little more than a capitalist device to 'divide and conquer' workers.... this paper shows that the practice of division of labor may have a distinct incentive effect that makes its adoption attractive in certain circumstances" (p. 422).

WHAT MAKES TEAMS WORK

Wisner (2001, p. 58) believes that the important factors involved in making teams work include the following: (1) A senior leader who shares information and is supportive in good and bad times; (2) An ongoing assessment of communications, feedback, morale and performance; (3) A road map that describes where the team is going, how best to get there, and how to resolve problems and impediments when they arise; (4) A long-term view that gives the team a chance to solidify; (5) Comprehensive training that adds to the team's ability to work well together and to develop all the skills necessary to succeed; (6) When members of the team aren't working cooperatively, well-functioning teams have the skill to determine who should go, who should stay, and who should be added to the team to make it work.

Teams need to understand boundaries or the process becomes chaotic. This has been a real problem in organizations that give workers maximum autonomy, as in university settings where getting faculty to keep posted office hours can become contentious. Boundaries and rules apply to everyone, and the team works only when everyone accepts them and behaves accordingly. The team needs positive feedback and recognition to function well. Singling out individuals rather than focusing on group achievement can, in some cases, cause a loss of morale and increased team conflict. Care needs to be taken in the way feedback and rewards are given by praising the work of the group before mentioning specific workers.

It is important to identify reasons the team is or is not working well and to create indicators that tell us where the team does well and where it doesn't. The indicators should be developed in part by the team so it can own up to problems but still reap the benefits of positive results. The indicators, however, should be bottom line indicators that really matter. In an article written on merit pay Glicken (1986) points out how well workers can develop indicators of performance that are irrelevant and that end up making poorly performing workers look positively marvelous.

LaFasto and Larson (2002) interviewed 6,000 team members and team leaders to find out what made teams work well. Their conclusion is that team leadership is the key ingredient in successful teams and that the following six dimensions of team leadership influence successful team functioning:

- The ability of leadership to focus on the goal, otherwise the issue of performance gets confused.
- A willingness to develop a collaborative climate, because it makes communication safe.
- The capacity to build confidence, because confident workers are creative and productive and add to the team's overall performance.
- The ability to demonstrate sufficient technical know-how so that team members can come to the leader for solutions to problems that might be outside the team's knowledge base.
- The ability to set priorities, otherwise important issues related to the function of the team might get lost.
- The capacity to manage issues of performance, otherwise the team begins to lose its level of achievement.

A Personal Reflection on Teams and the Importance of Good Leadership

The following story is provided by Michelle Collette, RN, a highly experienced OR supervisor in a large teaching hospital in the North East of the United States.

"I was part of a team that was pulled together to implement education for a change in care delivery in our department. We were informed that a person who had no experience in our area would be our team leader. Our group assignment was to come up with a spreadsheet identifying all of the education that the department would need to implement the new policy and procedures. We were given two 4-hour meetings as a group to complete the assignment but completed it in one 4-hour session and were pretty pleased with ourselves. We were told by our administrator that our part was done and that our leader would contact some people who were identified as content experts to add their input to the plan. All of us left the meeting saying 'great, that's done and it wasn't as painful as we expected it to be.'

About a month later our leader called us into another 4-hour meeting. We were all confused about the reason for the meeting but, of course, we went as we were told. Our leader informed us that we were delinquent. We asked what that meant. He said that no one had contacted the other content experts for their input and we are all in trouble. We responded by saying that he was assigned to do that. A lively discussion followed and our leader decided he would do it but he was very unhappy about it. Once again we left the meeting thinking the work was completed.

Fast forward another month and we all got summoned to an emergency meeting about the original assignment and we were once again informed that we were delinquent because we hadn't turned over our standards and procedures to the 'educational designers.' We asked what educational designers were, where did they come from, what they needed, and why we hadn't been told? In response, our leader informed us that this is the way it was done in the military and why didn't we know what educational designers were? I have been an educator for 26 years and I'm still not sure what an educational designer is. Another lively discussion followed and we turned in what was asked of us (we had the items needed anyway).

I think what happened was that our leader (fresh out of the military) thought that the world functions like the military and failed to fully explain the expectations of the group or his role and just assumed that we knew what he wanted. I don't think he really knew, either. The interesting thing is that all the team members interpreted things the same way because we all had a similar mindset as nurses about what needed to be done. The leader was transferred to a different department but like so many meetings I've attended over the years, there's often a disconnect in the process, and what might have been easily done by a motivated and experienced group of people in a short period of time often gets extended into a long drawn out process where a couple of people could have done the assignment quickly. In terms of lost patient care and misuse of time, it's inexcusable."

TEAMWORK AND GENERATION X WORKERS

Karp, Sirias, and Arnold (1999) discuss teamwork and Generation X, or what has become known as the "slacker generation" of workers born between 1963 and 1982. Generation X workers have sometimes been characterized as lazy, arrogant, unreliable, cynical, and particularly oriented to self rather than to teams. According to the authors, the lack of a team orientation turns out to be untrue. GEN XERS work well in teams "if it's a high-performing team composed of strong, diverse individuals, focused on delivering results, who create flexible linkages to work as an entire team, in isolation or in different configurations, depending on the task. They are looking for authentic team synergy rather than conformance to group norms" (p. 30). The authors also note that while GEN XERS have the ability to work in teams, they may not necessarily accept some of the limiting expectations of organizational life. To bring them together as a team capable of working with a mix of older and younger workers, the authors propose the following strategies and tactics:

1. Identify a worker's strengths and interests and emphasize the attributes they bring to the team, which may include a fresh perspective, high technological ability, adaptability to change, resilience, and enthusiasm.
2. Encourage individual identity since XERS may be fiercely independent.
3. Integrate perspectives. XERS use the team to support their individual efforts and relationships, while boomers see supporting the team as their primary, individual role. Both perspectives must be discussed and valued as the team moves forward.
4. Provide personal support and offer feedback, frequently, quickly, and when it's needed.
5. Create a dialogue among team members that allows the team to delegate responsibilities and to frequently review and revise how the team is working.

6. Share information, recognizing that XERS have grown up with PCs and are used to getting immediate feedback. If you don't provide it, you will be seen as hoarding needed data and you will inhibit productivity.
7. Focus on results since XERS are often quite pragmatic.
8. Motivate with the work. XERS are not motivated by pep talks about the greater good of the organization. Their motivation comes from within and has to do with the intrinsic nature of the team's work.
9. Reward team and individual contributions. XERS are tuned in to "what's in it for me" (WIIFM); but let the team decide the best way to provide for individual contributions and consider non-financial incentives such as trips, training opportunities, flexible work schedules, and work from home, as options.

FAULT LINES IN TEAMWORK THAT LEAD TO CONFLICT AND LOWERED PRODUCTIVITY

Li and Hambrick (2005) studied what they call fault lines or variables that negatively influence group performance and found that the larger a factional fault line (the amount of significant demographic difference in a team), the greater the emotional conflict in a group. Large fault lines also give rise to task conflict, or intellectual opposition among members concerning the content of the tasks being performed. When team members are of widely differing backgrounds, they bring divergent experiences and frames of reference to problem-solving, which each member takes to be valid. As a result of differing experiences, members may disagree on supervisory policies, risk-taking, control systems, urgency, and other factors. Factions that differ widely in their backgrounds diverge in completing tasks and in their knowledge of alternatives and their estimates of consequences attached to alternatives. These differences will emerge as task conflict.

The authors found that the larger a factional fault line, the greater the task conflict in a group, leading to behavioral disintegration. Conflict can be thought of as emotional or cognitive, and it negatively impacts communication, collaboration, and social interaction. Hambrick (1994) developed the concept of behavioral integration to explain why some groups function well while others don't. Behavioral integration has three indicators: how well information is exchanged, collaborative behavior, and joint decision-making. Disintegration is an expected by-product of conflict in a group. If emotional conflict is great, and members dislike each other, they try to avoid each other and compartmentalize their tasks.

In further findings, Li and Hambrick (2005) report that the greater the emotional conflict in a group, the greater the team conflict. While conflict can be healthy, especially when there are explicit norms that support debate and contention, a very high level of task conflict can cause member dissatisfaction and withdrawal from group efforts. Jehn (1995) found that task conflict was negatively related to member satisfaction, intention to remain in a group, and group production. In a meta-analysis of worker conflict studies, DeDreu & Weingart (2003) found a negative association between task conflict and both member satisfaction and group performance. According to the authors, a high level of task conflict—accompanied by intense disagreement and possibly even outright arguments—drives members apart. The ensuing tension will become highly stressful, and group members may insulate their activities from each other. In this vein, Hambrick, Li, and Tsui (2001) reported an instance of a factional joint venture management group in which conflict led to behavioral disintegration so severe that "They sharply reduced their interactions; decision-making became rigid and mechanical and several scheduled management meetings were cancelled" (pp. 1046–1047).

Another finding by Li and Hambrick (2005) is that the greater the task conflict in a group, the greater the behavioral disintegration. Social psychologists have long noted the positive effects on group performance of the main elements of behavioral integration: communication, collaboration, and joint decision-making. Shaw wrote that, "if a group is to function effectively, its members must be able to communicate easily and efficiently" (1981, p. 150). Similarly, Hambrick (1995) concluded from field interviews that behavioral disintegration generally led to group problems including failure to exchange key information, poor coordination of activities, and difficulty in formulating and implementing responses to environmental shifts. Behavioral disintegration within a group will be negatively associated with subsequent group performance.

The greater the emotional conflict in a group, the lower the subsequent group performance. The greater the task conflict in a group, the lower the subsequent group performance. Emotional conflict and task conflict bring about behavioral disintegration. As Li and Hambrick (2005) note, "Although diversity within a group can yield benefits (e.g., Jehn, Northcraft, & Neale, 1999) prior research indicates that heterogeneity often impairs group functioning (Williams & O'Reilly, 1998)" (p. 798). The authors go on to say that "even though factional groups are often formed out of a belief that the two sets of members possess valuable complementarities, we can anticipate that large demographic fault lines between factions will engender group dysfunction" (p. 798).

While the authors caution that much more research is needed to predict which fault lines, specific to a population of workers, will lead to conflict, they did find that the following variables lead to team deterioration and low performance: "Age differences were positively related to task conflict; tenure differences were positively associated with emotional and task conflict; gender differences were positively related to emotional conflict and behavioral disintegration; and ethnic differences were positively related to all three process variables" (Li and Hambrick, 2005, p. 809).

Raver and Gelfand (2005) indicate that one of the primary reasons for gender conflict is sexual harassment. Noting the harmful impact of sexual harassment on the functioning of teams, the authors write (p. 395):

> *Our results demonstrated that at the team level, ambient sexual harassment was positively related to relationship and task conflict. We also found that ambient sexual hostility was negatively related to team cohesion and team financial performance. Team relationship conflict and cohesion mediated the relationship between ambient sexual hostility and team financial performance, suggesting that harassment may have far-reaching implications for teams' performance through its influence on everyday team processes. Overall, these results extend the extant literature by demonstrating that sexual harassment is significantly associated with indicators of teams' functioning and performance.*

Where does that leave us regarding group diversity? And given the realities that most human service agencies value diversity, aren't we going to have a certain amount of discord in teams and shouldn't we do something to keep it at a minimum for the sake of our clients? Self, Holt, and Schaninger Jr. (2005) suggest that organizational loyalty and concern for clients can often overcome conflict in groups with diverse compositions. They believe that when workers are given sufficient input about the purpose of teams and their potential for improving the services they offer, even highly diverse groups can function well. Rehling (2004, pp. 480–482) says that conversational styles that create conflict can be modified with help from supervisors to reduce conflict. She indicates in her research that group conflict may be reduced when group members are asked to:

1. Recognize the sources of a worker's own conversational style habits.
2. Help workers monitor themselves to avoid the downsides of the conversational style that they habitually use with a project team that may create conflict within the team.
3. Apply everyday ethics to conversational behaviors.

4. Help workers flex their own style to adapt more to others'.
5. Recognize how others express their backgrounds and their opinions through their conversational styles.
6. Recognize others' preferred conversational styles without judging.
7. Identify how others define the group or occasion to choose between conversational styles.
8. Practice actively listening to others.

DOES TEAMWORK LEAD TO HIGHER PRODUCTIVITY AND BETTER WORKER PERFORMANCE?

Wisner (2001) reports that Bell Atlantic Corporation conducted an extensive research study on the benefits of placing workers in teams. In particular, they were interested in three key success factors: productivity, service quality, and employee satisfaction. Bell found that all three factors were increased by teamwork. They achieved this success by developing an organizational structure that included the following:

1. An office committee made up of supervisors and managers to identify, coordinate, and communicate team needs.
2. Physically grouping team members together and changing furniture to remove high walls.
3. Training workers and supervisors in team processes, cooperative communication, and problem-solving skills.
4. Holding weekly team meetings to discuss results, solve problems, or to cross-train team members.
5. A performance feedback system that provided individual results, team results, and summary data about other teams' performance. This created an environment of acknowledgment and learning that many workers applauded. The feedback system also helped to identify "best practice" workers, who were then asked to share their skills with other team members.

While productivity went up rather dramatically in this study, so did worker satisfaction. When comparing the non-grouped workers with teamed workers, Bell discovered that: the number of employee suggestions increased; employees participated more in meetings; employees took more initiative in identifying and solving problems; and some employees volunteered to take on additional assignments in the office.

Bell decided to find out why teaming improved work to such a degree. Their conclusions were that: teams provided common goals through joint decision-making; employees could work together to solve problems; the decision-making process was much more in real time rather than being delayed by long discussion held by managers who then, when decisions were made, told workers what to do; the team structure promoted cross-training; the physical proximity between team members increased learning since team members could observe how their colleagues handled problems; team members could turn to others on their team for help and advice.

WHY TEAMS SOMETIMES DON'T WORK

Teams that include different professions doing the same job have built-in conflict because each profession has a different way of functioning that might not be acceptable to everyone on the team. Teams composed of different professions (doctors, social workers, psychologists) often have someone who needs convincing or is unwilling to go the extra mile for a client. Cynicism about group members can create conflict and a sense that someone is going to have to do more of the work if the client is to be helped.

Although supervisors should know about group dynamics, they often include members who are so disparate in their personalities, competencies, and attitudes that the group fails to function well. Once a group begins, supervisors sometimes believe that their responsibility for seeing that it works well is limited.

Rewards that benefit the group may not fully benefit the best team members, who may believe that the group has actually held them back from doing their best work and from being differentially and fairly rewarded. Many workers believe that teams can be terribly time-consuming and often unproductive. Group members may be passive-aggressive about group attendance. When they aren't present, the group doesn't function well, because it thinks the missing workers are manipulating the group.

High turnover rates in many agencies make teams impractical since individual team members may be employed for such a brief amount of time that they are never fully integrated into the group and the group ultimately loses cohesion. Many human service workers have little actual training in working in groups or with cooperative styles of learning although this can easily be rectified by graduate schools that teach students about group treatment, offer a good deal more about group dynamics, and encourage field experiences that teach students to lead and function within both clinical and non-practice task groups.

Mason (1998) provides a description of a contentious team meeting that sounds painfully familiar. She describes a highly competent supervisor trying to supervise a group of very able professionals whom she is trying to keep on budget and mission, with no success. Every time she asks the team questions about client satisfaction in human service work, productivity, or paperwork, she's told, in many different ways, that she's interfering with the work they do with clients and that the clients are all doing better than ever, although there is absolutely no evidence provided or any reason to believe this. Secretly, Mason suggests, the workers hate the way the supervisor dresses and tell jokes about her she has heard from others. And further, she's agreed that decisions on this team are all made by consensus—"no dictating please, we're professionals!" But what she's really thinking is that a good dictator is just what is needed to get these workers rolling. She's also thinking, "Do it! And do it right!" (Er, please.) In short, she's thinking that teams don't work. "How can they work with so many different personalities jostling against one another like 3-year-olds set loose on a tray of baked goods?" (Mason, 1998, p. 33). But, as Mason points out, people have a long history of working together. She notes that "we got here as a species by collaborating with one another. Teams are almost in the genes, but admittedly a number of barriers get in the way such as confused objectives, unclear roles, poor decision making, and personality differences" (p. 33). Knock down these barriers, she advises, to give your team a clear chance to be successful.

Glover (2002) believes that one of the reasons teams don't always work well is the tendency to focus on group composition and whether people are compatible with one another rather than focusing on whether they'll get the job done. She writes, "Team-building can be detrimental to longer-term development because it can make a team appear too close-knit and make new members feel excluded" (p. 38). Glover reports that in studies of teams, emotional intelligence is a significant factor in their success. She recommends that teams include members who are practical, grounded, have a good sense of how things work, and know what should be done to complete the job. She reports that in research on whether teams work well, work groups of six to eight members represent optimal size and seem to work best. Teams are present-oriented but also work in the context of what may need to be done in the future. Too many groups, she notes, do well with current projects but are ill-equipped to deal with new challenges or longer-term issues that are likely to define predictable future problems. While leadership should be clear and the direction taken compelling, team members resent and often actively resist leaders who, while being pacesetters, also need to micro-manage the team's functioning.

A Personal Reflection About Groups: A Student Learns about Leading a Group

My (Dr Glicken) second-year graduate social work field placement was in the rehabilitation unit of a large teaching hospital. My supervisor correctly wanted me to have a group experience. Two internationally known professionals, a psychiatrist and a psychologist, led a group of recently disabled people who were in the hospital for medical treatment, but also to help them learn to cope emotionally with their serious disabilities. My supervisor allowed me to join the group as an observer. My job was to watch, discuss group dynamics with my supervisor, and to keep my mouth shut, a wise rule since my mouth was very large and uninformed at that moment in time. I was 21 years old.

I was also to meet with the two clinicians and my supervisor after each session to discuss group dynamics, treatment strategies, and to learn to work with different professions. To our dismay, the psychiatrist and psychologist developed a bitter antagonism toward one another. The psychologist was a behaviorist and the psychiatrist was a Freudian. One wanted to change behavior, the other thought behavior only changed if you understood it. Suddenly, the two stopped coming to group sessions and I was left on my own to treat some very antisocial and profoundly disabled patients. One of the patients had tried to steal a car parked on a steep hill, released the emergency brake, and as the car began racing downhill with him on the hood, the patient was slammed into a tree where his leg was crushed and later amputated. When he joined the group, he was wheeling himself down the hall of the hospital at night stealing money and sexually abusing the female patients. I was to get him to stop.

My supervisor asked that the four of us meet to get the two professionals to return to the group. Clearly, an untrained Master of Social Work (MSW) student couldn't handle such a troubled and difficult group of patients. Neither showed up for the meeting but each let it be known that they'd speak to us without the other present. When we met, each berated the other while my supervisor tried to get the discussion back on track. Impossible. The animosity was just too great. They both said, finally, that I should run the group but to keep my mouth shut and let the group do the work, which is exactly what I did.

I told the group that the two professionals had time conflicts (many people sniggered. It was no great secret that they disliked each other), and that given the fact that I was just a student, could we figure out if the group was important enough to continue and, if it was, how could we make it work?

After much discussion it was agreed that the group was very important, that the members only needed me to book the room and make sure there was coffee and cookies and, for darn sure, to keep my mouth shut. I did and the group, much to my amazement, began to work superbly. There was a great deal of talk among the mental health professionals at the hospital about what a wise young man I was and how much potential I had.

Word got back to the two professionals that the group was going very well without them and that a lowly student ... me ... was working magic. They both came back to the group, the group stopped functioning well because they inhibited its development, and I learned a valuable set of lessons about groups. They are:

- Too many leaders may create conflict.
- Leadership requires cooperation and acceptance of group goals.
- Sometimes group members can develop their own style without you doing anything.
- Give a group an assignment and they may surprise you by doing it well with very little interference on your part, but let them know you can help if they need it.
- Asking a group what they want your role to be is often a very good strategy.
- Keeping silent, or at least talking as little as possible, may be a very effective way to run groups since it forces groups to develop their own unique style.
- You can never know enough about groups, and time should be spent in learning about group dynamics and group strategies.

You be the Manager

You have overall supervisory responsibility for a staff of 50 professionals in a community drug and alcohol treatment center. You have been receiving complaints from the professional staff that whenever a support staff member misses a day or takes sick leave or vacation time, no one provides services in place of the missing support staff member. In the past, the agency has had floaters who take over when a support staff member is gone, but agency budget constraints have made that policy impossible to continue. Support staff had been good about covering for one another in the absence of a staff member. However, low morale and the lack of decent salary increases had begun to eat away at cooperative efforts, and, as complaints from the professional staff have increased, you've decided to institute a more specific plan which assigns coverage whenever a staff member is gone.

In effect, the system you've designed breaks the support staff into three teams of four people each. Whenever a team member is gone, the team meets at the beginning of the workday and decides on the staff member who will cover for the absent person. The system isn't working and there is a great deal of passive-aggressive behavior and blaming others for the failure of the system.

You decide to have a pep talk with the staff members complete with team names, symbols, and coffee mugs with inscribed names of the team and the person. You even include a morale-boosting speech from the agency director who explains that he knows how hard everyone is working, but that covering for one another is the only way the agency can make it through these perilous times. You overhear one of the support staff members, who makes $25,000 a year and has to pay $200 a month for medical insurance, say to a friend that while the support staff is working its tail off without salary increases, the director gets 15% a year salary increases and, according to the agency's bookkeeper, makes $125,000 a year. The speech falls flat and the problem intensifies. When a staff member is gone, the professional staff suffers and productivity falls. What used to be a sick leave system that wasn't misused has now become a mental health day system where staff members take sick leave to miss going to work and believe that if the agency isn't going to treat them well, that taking unneeded sick leave is a way of rewarding themselves while getting back at the agency.

Questions

1. Do you believe that salary increases would improve morale and lead to better cooperative efforts on the part of staff?
2. Is there a way to stop the use of sick leave when staff aren't sick but feel they deserve a mental health day?
3. The approach used by the supervisor failed to get at underlying issues. What might a better approach have been to help staff deal with the reasons staff coverage has become such a problem?
4. How would you deal with the type of passive-aggressive behavior described in the case?
5. The lack of a cooperative spirit suggests a problem of agency identity and loyalty. Should we expect support staff to feel the same loyalty and identity to the agency as the professional staff?

SUMMARY

This chapter discusses teamwork and other cooperative efforts and whether teams provide the benefits we often think they do. Ways of organizing teams are discussed and impediments to effective teamwork are identified. Fault lines are the problems that sometimes occur among a diverse workforce where culture, gender, race and ethnicity may actually inhibit the team from coming together and working effectively. The material presented isn't meant to discourage diversity but to make the reader aware of some of the underlying problems that exist in a culturally and ethnically diverse workforce and to resolve issues as they arise to prevent the team from failing. A case is provided showing what happens when professionals fail to work together as a team. By way of a case study, you were asked to consider the problem of non-professional staff members failing to provide coverage when a staff member was absent, its impact on provision of services, and the possible cause.

REFERENCES

Alchian, A., & Demsetz, H. (1972). Production, information, costs and economic organization. *American Economic Review, 62*, 777–795.

DeDreu, C., & Weingart, L. (2003). Task versus relationship conflict, team performance, and team member satisfaction: a meta-analysis. *Journal of Applied Psychology, 88*, 741–749.

Glicken, M. D. (1986). *Improving productivity through merit* (pp. 361–366). *Public Personnel Administration: Policies and Practices for Personnel Service.* Paramus, NJ: Prentice Hall.

Glover, C. (2002). Variations on a team. *People Management, 8*(3), 36–39.

Hambrick, D. C. (1994). Top management groups: A conceptual integration and reconsideration of the "team" label. In B. M. Straw, & L. L. Cummings (Eds.), *Research in Organizational Behavior* (16, pp. 171–213). Greenwich, CT: JAI Press.

Hambrick, D. C. (1995). Fragmentation and the other problems CEOs have with their top management teams. *California Management Review, 37*(Spring), 110–127.

Holmstrom, B., & Milgrom, P. (1991). Multitask principal-agent analyses: incentive contracts, asset ownership, and job design. *The Journal of Law, Economics, & Organization*, 7, 24–52.

Itoh, H. (1991). Incentive to help in multi-agent situations. *Econometrica, 59*(3), 611–636.

Jehn, K (1995). A multimethod examination of the benefits and detriments of intragroup conflict. *Administrative Science Quarterly, 40*, 256–282.

Jehn, K. A., Northcraft, G. B., & Neale, M. A. (1999). What differences make a difference: a field study of diversity, conflict, and performance in workgroups. *Administrative Science Quarterly, 44*, 741–763.

Karp, H., Sirias, D., & Arnold, K. (1999). Teams: why generation X marks the spot. *Journal for Quality and Participation, 22*, 30–32.

LaFasto, F., & Larson, C. (2002). *When teams work best: 6,000 team members and leaders tell what it takes to succeed* Thousand Oaks, CA: Sage.

Li, J., & Hambrick, D. C. (2005). Factional groups: a new vantage on demographic, faultlines, conflict, and disintegration of groups. *Academy of Management Journal, 48*(5), 794–813.

Lin, Y. (1997). Division of labor in teams. *Journal of Economics & Management Strategy, 6*(2), 403–423.

Mason, L. (1998). *Do teams work? Outlook, 66*(3), 30–34.

Raver, J. L., & Gelfand, M. J. (2005). Beyond the individual victim: linking sexual harassment, team processes, and team performance. *Academy of Management Journal, 48*(3), 387–401.

Rehling, L. (2004). Improving teamwork through awareness of conversational styles. *San Francisco State University Business Communication Quarterly, 67*(4), 475–482.

Smith, A. (1937). *The wealth of nations.* New York: Modern Library.

Williams, K. Y., & O'Reilly, C. A. (1998). Demography and diversity in organizations: A review of 40 years of research. In B. Shaw, & R. Sutton (Eds.), *Research in Organizational Behavior* (20, pp. 77–140). Greenwich, CT: JAI Press.

Wisner P. (2001, Feb). Does teaming pay off? *Strategic Finance 82*(8), 58–64.

FURTHER READING

Anon (n.d.). *Teamwork in the classroom: Collaborative learning.* NDT Resource Center. Retrieved April 20, 2012 from <http://www.ndt-ed.org/TeachingResources/ClassroomTips/Teamwork.htm>.

Bradford, J.A. (n.d.). *Why competitive individualism needs to be replaced by teamwork.* Retrieved April 16, 2012 at: <http://www.cct.umb.edu/effteamwork.html>.

Clements, D., Dault, M., & Priest, A. (2007). *Healthcarepapers,* 7(Spring), 26–34 Retrieved April 25, 2012 from <http://www.longwoods.com/content/18669>.

Murphy, D. (March 1, 2008). *Teamwork can boost manufacturing productivity.* Retrieved April 15, 2012 from <http://www.gsb.stanford.edu/news/research/shawteams.shtml>.

Various authors (n.d.). Teamwork: A number of articles exploring various aspects of teamwork. *Buzzle.* Retrieved April 18, 2012 from <http://www.buzzle.com/articles/teamwork/>.

CHAPTER 4

Sexual Harassment in the Workplace

BACKGROUND OF SEXUAL HARASSMENT

Sexual harassment is relevant to the issues of concern that relate to the recent economic downturn in several ways. During the downturn, sexual harassment in the workplace is an important issue that needs to be addressed forthrightly. It was included here because it is a subjective workplace-related measure that can also be objectively observed. Despite various other intervening factors, sexual harassment can be measured by the number of claims filed before and after the economic downturn.

One observation of this subject was set forth by Dziech and Weiner (1990) and Boland (2002) who described how the term sexual harassment came about. In a report by Rowe (1996), it was found that various terms describing inappropriate sexual behavior had been discussed by women's groups in the early 1970s. During that period a number of organizations began to more critically define the issue and developed policies and procedures that addressed various aspects of the problem. Brownmiller (1999) described how several groups, including the Working Women's Institute in 1976, eventually suggested that the term sexual harassment suitably embraced a broad range of both subtle and very offensive behavior. As a result of considerable effort, the term "sexual harassment" became gradually accepted. Bowers and Hook (2002) pointed out that the term was largely unused until the early 1990s. Sexual harassment during that period became an intense and broader public issue when, in 1991, Anita Hill witnessed and testified against Supreme Court Justice Nominee Clarence Thomas.

As a result of the unclear definition of sexual harassment, there is no precise method to determine how people who have been victimized can clearly classify the feelings and discomfort that they have experienced as sexual harassment. A further difficulty raised by several authors is how the behavior of a sexual harasser could be directly related to the negative psychological and physical outcomes often experienced by victims. There

Treating Worker Dissatisfaction During Economic Change
DOI: http://dx.doi.org/10.1016/B978-0-12-397006-0.00004-X

are further problems of distinguishing how sexual harassment is perceived and differentiated among people of different classes, races, sexual orientations, or cultural groups.

DEFINITION OF SEXUAL HARASSMENT IN THE WORKPLACE

The evolution of sexual harassment has eventually led to a specific use of the term as it relates to the workplace (see, e.g., Wikipedia). In the workplace, sexual harassment is described as an exercise of power and control. It could occur in the form of casual comments, threats of negative personnel actions, or direct physical abuse of a sexual nature. Other writers agree that sexual harassment is difficult to define because it does not have to be of an explicit sexual nature and can be expressed by generally offensive remarks and comments that are often subjective.

Koss (1990) reported that, prior to 1990, US National data on sexual harassment in the workplace were not routinely collected. It is therefore difficult to obtain accurate numbers on its prevalence or impact during that period. Koss did find that in 1993 it was estimated that 50% of all women workers would experience some form of sexual harassment during their working lives. The extent of workplace sexual harassment was also difficult to clearly determine because victims could not recognize or label it accurately, or would willingly report it.

Victims often feared that they would be blamed for initiating the unwanted behavior and that nothing would be done if they complained. A main fear of many victims was that by reporting sexual harassment, some form of retaliation would follow. Many victims would therefore simply continue to live with the harassment situation. Women often have to decide if it is worth leaving their jobs and risking serious financial hardship, acquiring a poor work history or obtaining negative job references (Koss, 1990).

Victims who speak out against sexual harassment in the workplace are sometimes labeled as troublemakers or simply looking for attention (Fitzgerald, 2003). It has been found that sexually harassed workers who complain may risk hostility and isolation from colleagues, supervisors, and even friends. Retaliation sometimes occurs when a sexual harassment victim receives a disciplinary action as a result of the harassment claim.

Contemporary legal writers have explained how sexual harassment progressed as an illegal activity. The government ruling by the US Equal Opportunity Commission (2012a) defines sexual harassment as follows.

- It is unlawful to harass a person (an applicant or employee) because of that person's sex. Harassment can include "sexual harassment" or unwelcomed sexual advances, requests for sexual favors, and other verbal or physical harassment of a sexual nature.
- Harassment does not have to be of a sexual nature, however, and can include offensive remarks about a person's sex. For example, it is illegal to harass a woman by making offensive comments about women in general. Both victim and the harasser can be either a woman or a man, and the victim and harasser can be the same sex.

The US Equal Opportunity Commission (2012a) recently explained that the law does not prohibit non-serious teasing, offhand comments, or isolated incidents. Harassment becomes illegal when it is frequent or severe and creates a hostile work environment or results in an adverse employment decision. The harasser can be a supervisor, supervisor in another area, a co-worker, or someone who is not an employee of the employer.

Preventing sexual harassment and defending employees from sexual harassment charges have become key reasons for legal decision-making in many organizations. Ebeid, Kaul, Neumann, and Shane (2003) wrote how management has been primarily concerned with workplace discrimination and due process. Sexual harassment issues related to emotional abuse that is inflicted on employees by supervisors or managers are seldom addressed. The organizational climate can become more sexually abusive when it permits or tolerates this type of abusive treatment by supervisors, managers, and employees.

From an international perspective, the Commission of the European Union in 2002 agreed that sexual harassment in the workplace can have a negative effect upon workers' health, morale and performance (Zippel, 2006). Anxiety and stress created by sexual harassment in the workplace can also result in worker absenteeism or seeking other employment. Besides the adverse consequences of sexual harassment on workers themselves it can also have a damaging impact on co-workers, significant others, and the organization itself.

Although there are numerous types of sexual harassers, Langelan (1993) identified several distinct classes who can be found in the workplace. One of these classes was described as public harassers who are sometimes seen in the workplace as people who exhibit extremely aggressive sexual behavior. They can be identified by their nasty sexual innuendos and strongly suggestive sexual attitudes toward people in the workplace. Another class is recognized as a private harasser, who presents a respectable and professional demeanor, but harasses victims when a discreet opportunity presents itself. For example, when they are alone with their target, such as in a private office, their demeanor often becomes aggressive or disrespectful. Another common class of harasser was described as a dominance harasser, such as an employee who engages in harassing behavior as a means of boosting their ego. The final category was identified as strategic or territorial harassers who are primarily interested in maintaining workplace privileges or advantages.

SEXUAL HARASSMENT DURING THE ECONOMIC DOWNTURN

The recent economic downturn brought with it some dramatic changes in the number and variety of sexual harassment incidents. Quite a few writers, including Vanderbilt University economist Joni Hersch (2011), have investigated the impact of sexual harassment in the workplace during the recent economic downturn. Hersch reported that most of the economic data indicate that the economic downturn and its effect on high unemployment will likely persist for an indefinite period. Hersch noted from earlier studies that during a time of very high and persistent unemployment, people are more fearful of leaving jobs and/or filing complaints of sexual harassment.

Hersch reviewed many recent claims filed with the Equal Employment Opportunities Commission and compared the claims and filings of sexual harassment by sex, age group, and industry. Consistent with other findings, Hersch was able to confirm that sexual harassment during the economic downturn increased for both men and women, but the actual incidences of claims and fillings were not available. Hersch's analyses of EEOC data during the same period indicated that, although many claims were not filed, claims for women showed they were six times more likely to be harassed than their male counterparts. It was also reported that they were most likely to be sexually harassed in workplaces that employed small numbers of women.

Sexual harassment as it relates to the economic downturn has been found to have important consequences for problems beyond just financial insecurity. As economically devastating as sexual harassment has been for employees in the workplace, other serious social and psychologically related factors have become exacerbated as well. Lessons learned before the current economic downturn found prevention to be valuable in combating sexual harassment in a male-dominated workplace. Bernstein (1994) suggested that some of the following guidelines may be useful for preventing sexual harassment:

- Clear anti-harassment policies that are effectively communicated;
- Special training and education for managers and supervisors;
- Designated ombudspersons to deal with reported complaints;
- Formal grievance procedures and alternatives to them;
- Disciplinary treatment of those who violate the policies.

Sexual harassment needs to be openly addressed and treated as a serious and legitimate workplace issue (Kauppinen-Toropainen & Gruber, 1993; Cole et al., 1997). During the recent economic downturn the impact of sexual harassment may be even more difficult to determine. Because workers may fear reporting sexual harassment, there may be a greater possibility that they will become the next person blamed, humiliated, or fired.

During normal economic cycles or when major economic downturns occur, sexual harassment is always unacceptable and should never be tolerated. There are a number of effective ways for offended and victimized people to mediate the negative effects of workplace sexual harassment, whether it is psychological, physical, or social. Other writers have found that victims can remain affected or return to more normal socialization, reestablish positive personal relationships, regain social approval, and recover the ability to be productive in educational and work environments.

Many writers have recommended that immediate psychological and legal counseling should be provided in the event that sexual harassment has been determined. Self-treatment may not adequately release stress or remove trauma. Simply reporting to authorities may not resolve a problem. If treatment is ignored or delayed, further injury may lead to more harmful psychological, social, or other negative circumstances.

The following list includes some of the common psychological, academic, professional, financial, and social effects of sexual harassment:

- Psychological stress and health impairment;
- Decreased work or school performance as a result of stress conditions; increased absenteeism in fear of harassment repetition;
- Firing and refusal for a job opportunity, which can lead to loss of job or career, loss of income;
- Having to drop courses, change academic plans, or leave school (loss of tuition) in fear of harassment repetition and/or as a result of stress;
- Being objectified and humiliated by scrutiny and gossip;

- Having one's personal life offered up for public scrutiny—the victim becomes the "accused," and his or her dress, lifestyle, and private life will often come under attack;
- Becoming publicly sexualized (i.e., groups of people "evaluate" the victim to establish if he or she is "worth" the sexual attention or the risk to the harasser's career);
- Defamation of character and reputation;
- Loss of trust in environments similar to that where the harassment occurred;
- Loss of trust in the types of people that occupy similar positions as the harasser or his or her colleagues, especially where they are not supportive or in case of difficulties or stress on peer relationships or relationships with colleagues;
- Effects on sexual life and relationships—can put extreme stress upon relationships, sometimes resulting in divorce;
- Weakening of support network, or being ostracized from professional or academic circles (friends, colleagues, or family may distance themselves from the victim, or shun him or her altogether);
- Having to relocate to another city, another job, or another school;
- Loss of references/recommendations.

TYPES OF SEXUAL HARASSMENT IN THE WORKPLACE

Sexual harassments can occur in a variety of circumstances and situations. But most often the harasser is in a position of power or authority over the victim. This can be due to differences in age, or social, political, educational, or employment relationships. Some harassers may expect to gain power or authority in the form of a promotion.

Many types of harassment have been described by various writers. A number of relationships and circumstances were described by Heyman (1994), which include the following.

- The harasser can be anyone, such as a client, a co-worker, a parent or legal guardian, relative, a teacher or professor, a student, a friend, or a stranger.
- The victim does not have to be the person directly harassed but can be a witness of such behavior who finds the behavior offensive and is affected by it.
- The place of harassment occurrence may be school, university, workplace, or other locations.

- The harasser may be completely unaware that his or her behavior is offensive or constitutes sexual harassment or may be completely unaware that his or her actions could be unlawful.
- The harassment may be a one-time occurrence but more often it has a type of repetitiveness.
- Adverse effects on the target are common in the form of stress and social withdrawal, sleep and eating difficulties, overall health impairment, etc.
- The victim and harasser can be of any gender.

SEXUAL HARASSMENT OF WOMEN IN THE WORKPLACE

Case Example

A letter was written by a prominent feminist lawyer who represented a former corporate consultant. In 1998 the company agreed to pay $34 million to female workers at a plant where the work environment was anything but normal. The company was charged with allowing a hostile work environment for women since at least 1990. In addition to the $34 million, the company paid out several more million in individual suits.

"The women were routinely fondled, verbally abused, and subjected to obscene jokes, behavior, and graffiti. One male worker even fired an air gun between a female's legs. The abusive work environment caused many women to quit. Others were simply denied promotions when they refused to grant sexual favors.

"The silver lining in this cloud is that the company has impressively cleaned up its tarnished reputation. The company immediately hired a former Secretary of Labor. The former Secretary of Labor overhauled the anti-sexual harassment and complaint system, which now boasts a zero tolerance policy." (Legalzoom, 2012)

Based upon an overall social or economic perspective, sexual harassment deprives women of fair and active participation in the workplace. Equally important, hundreds of millions of dollars are lost as a result of sexual harassment that prevents educational and professional opportunities for female workers (Boland, 2002). Over time, numerous governmental and legal attempts have been made to reduce the incidence of sexual harassment of women in the workplace. The US Equal Employment Opportunity Commission (EEOC) (2012b) reported that in 2011 a total of 11,364 sexual harassment claims were filed with the EEOC, state agencies, and local Fair Employment Practices agencies. It was also reported that women filed 83.7% of these claims. Damages that were awarded based on claims other than litigation, totaled approximately $52.3 million.

Previous findings show that there are significant incentives for employers to prevent sexual harassment of women in the workplace. A history of legal decisions has also established sexual harassment of women as a special form of discrimination under Title VII. When employers are found guilty of sexual harassment or allowing it to happen, they can be forced to pay substantial damages. Besides leading to the imposition of legal and monetary penalties, sexual harassment of women can also lead to lower productivity, absenteeism, employee turnover, lower morale, and negative publicity for the company.

Piotrkowski (1998) and others reported that sexual harassment began to be recognized as a serious problem as more women began to work outside of the home. In a work setting the victim often has little control and there is always the possibility of retaliation and fear of losing one's livelihood. Workplace sexual harassment may also have special health consequences for women that can be serious and qualify as a workplace health and safety issue (Bernstein, 1994).

MacKinnon (1979) noted that the nature of sexual harassment toward women has been established for a long period of time as being directly related to power and control. Sexual harassment in the workplace is often the use of power directed towards a specific woman and can involve unwanted sexual comments, seductive behavior, propositions, and pressure for dates. Having power in the workplace can also take a more harmful form through touching, sexual coercion, bribery, physical assault, and sometimes even rape. In the case of a "hostile environment" sexual harassment can involve jokes, taunts, and other sexually charged comments. This is quite often viewed as acceptable demeaning behavior toward women. Pornographic or sexually explicit posters and literature and crude sexual gestures are also part of this environment. Gender sexual harassment can involve sexual harassment in the form of remarks or behavior that offends the dignity of women or men.

Case Example

On some occasions a claimant in sexual harassment cases will receive large compensation for damages. A Labor Law Center blog reported that top executives at a trucking company in Illinois "practiced sexual harassment of female employees that included inappropriate touching and sexual jokes. The women were also required to entertain the company's customers and potential clients at a number of strip clubs in Chicago. After the case was examined, the women were granted more than $1 million in damages."

Cole et al. (1997) explained that, like other workplace stressors, sexual harassment can have negative effects on a woman's health that are sometimes very serious. It is obvious that when sexual harassment is severe, such as with rape or attempted rape, women can be seriously traumatized. But even where sexual harassment is less severe, women can have numerous psychological and other health-related problems. Women may become fearful, depressed, and lack the ability to cope. Other symptoms can be physical, such as stomach aches, headaches, nausea, and trauma. Women may exhibit behavioral problems such as sleeplessness, sexual problems, and difficulties in their relations with other people.

A report by the Ms. Foundation for Women (2012a) describes how women are bearing the brunt of the recent economic crisis. The Community Voices for the Economy and Lake Research Partners Survey reported that two-thirds of Americans stated that the economic downturn continues to have a definite impact on their lives. The impact of sexual harassment on women in the workplace will most likely be related to this crisis. This is especially relevant for low-income women and women of color. It is difficult to determine the effect that sexual harassment in the workplace has on women based upon these findings. A key indicator of recent economic security is the percentage of Americans who report living paycheck to paycheck all or most of the time. This indicator was found to be up by five points over 2010 to 49%. The increase among low-income women was especially devastating with 77% reporting living paycheck to paycheck. This represented a 17-point jump from the previous year.

Highlights from the survey include the following.

- Seventy-one percent of women and 65% of men reported that the economic downturn had some or a great deal of impact on their families.
- Nearly half of all Americans (46%) remain concerned that they or someone in their household could be out of a job in the next 12 months.
- Low-income women continue to feel the greatest impact from the downturn, with 80% saying it has had some or a great deal of impact, compared with 73% of low-income men.

- Other groups experiencing a particularly strong impact are: Latinas (74%), single mothers (73%), and women without a college degree (74%).

Anika Rahman (Ms. Foundation for Women, 2012b) used the term "womancession" to indicate that, since the economic downturn, women were losing jobs faster than men, mainly because of drastic cuts in areas like education and health care. These were the areas where women make up the majority of the workforce. In the state and local public sector, women are affected by the attacks on public-sector unions. Women suffer most from cuts to social services because they're more likely to be poor and care for children and the elderly.

SEXUAL HARASSMENT OF MEN IN THE WORKPLACE

Calvasina, Calvasina, and Calvasina (2011) and others who studied the current economic downturn discovered a growing trend of sexual harassment complaints from men. It was reported that a total of 16.4% of all sexual harassment claims, or 2,094 claims, were filed by men in fiscal 2009. This finding was shown to be up from 15.4%, or 1,869 claims, in fiscal 2006, as reported by the US Equal Employment Opportunity Commission. From January 2009 to December 2011, 3.44 million men lost jobs they had held for at least 3 years, compared with 2.68 million women, according to the Bureau of Labor Statistics (2012).

Attorney David McManus (Mattioli, 2010) and others cited a spike in employment litigation claims that occurred during previous economic downturns. The increase in sexual harassment claims filed by men during the current economic downturn could be related to the type of work that primarily involves men. Jobs such as manufacturing and construction have been hit exceptionally hard by the economic downturn.

Typically, male victims experience less serious behavior such as groping and unwanted sexual advances. Attorney Ron Chapman (Mattioli, 2010) reported that employment lawyers found that vulgar "locker room" type behavior and horseplay with sexual connotations has increasingly been the subject of claims. Several employment lawyers found that, in the past when jobs were harder to obtain, many forms of litigation, especially relating to discrimination, increased. Greg Grant (Mattioli, 2010), an attorney in Washington, DC, stated that "in the past, men who were victims of harassment might have sought other job opportunities rather than filing harassment claims."

Other experts on sexual harassment matters say that the numbers of claims are still under-reported. This is felt to be mainly due to the stigma associated with men who are sexually harassed. Mattioli (2010) found that, although companies have educated employees about sexual harassment for a long time, some are beginning to make their messages more male-focused during the economic downturn. They are increasingly recognizing a need to develop safeguards to prevent potential litigation.

Case Example

The New York Times in 2007 reported the case of a major hedge-fund company founded in the early 1990 s, as a "$14 billion group company." A scandal erupted when a former employee filed suit against his supervisor who was said to have forced him into taking female hormones and wearing female clothing. This was in order "to eliminate the trader's aggressive male attitude so he could become a more obedient and detail-oriented player" at work. The company vehemently denied the charges but no settlement was reached in the case.

SEXUAL HARASSMENT PERPETRATORS

Kim and Fiske (1999) supported the view that, whatever form it takes, sexual harassment is predominantly about male dominance and superiority. A number of earlier writers generally support that belief. MacKinnon (1979) indicated that the unequal status of women in the workplace can sometimes lead to sexual harassment. It was explained by Benson (1984) and Grauerholz (1989) that even men in inferior social and economic roles sense that they can harass women, which indicates an example of male feelings of dominance.

Tangri, Burt, and Johnson (1982) described sexual harassment as a means of carrying out unequal male–female interactions based upon established sex status norms. This is intended to maintain male dominance in the workplace and can often lead to economic discrimination and emotional distress. This behavior may also cause women to become intimidated, discouraged, or lead to termination from work. Burgess and Borgida (1997) reported that women view unwanted sexual attention as more harassing, threatening, inappropriate, and uncomfortable than do men.

Matchen and DeSouza (2000) studied a unique perception of sexual harassment in the university setting. It is normally assumed that professors would likely be the sexual harassment perpetrators. These scholars found that professors may also be victims of sexual harassment from students. They discovered that male professors receive casual unwanted sexual attention, but appear to experience actual sexual harassment from students at about the same rate as females. The authors suggest that future areas of study should look at men who are being harassed by women and other men and why they do not report it (Waldo, Berdahl, & Fitzgerald, 1998). The authors also suggested that there might be a need to develop explicit policies that discourage sexual activity by either faculty or students. Faculty members also need to know that they can take action if a student is sexually harassing them, regardless of the sex or gender of the perpetrator.

SEXUAL HARASSMENT AND ORGANIZATIONS

Much of the literature dealing with workplace management theory and practice deals with employment discrimination and due process. Workplace issues of sexual harassment and related emotional abuse of employees by supervisors or managers are seldom addressed. An organization becomes a sexually abusive environment when it permits or tolerates this behavior by employees, supervisors, or managers. The media regularly report incidences of maltreatment and violence facing society, such as child, domestic, or elderly abuse. Although it is extremely important, workplace sexual harassment and emotional abuse are rarely mentioned.

As a greater number of employees become emotionally and physically harmed as a result of sexual harassment, employers are beginning to reexamine their workplace management practices. The level of workplace stress has also been intensified by the economic downturn, mergers, and restructuring. Many organizations have felt a need to eliminate more jobs, resulting in a greater increase in workplace stress and sexual harassment. Workplace sexual harassment is becoming a greater organizational problem, and employers are beginning to realize its consequences for management, employees, and families.

Methods of dealing with sexual harassment as a management problem and a source of increased litigation have been studied by various investigators. Several found that there can be very significant costs to the employer (Fitzgerald & Ormerod, 1993; Gutek, 1985; Kauppinen-Toropainen & Gruber, 1993). Companies have attempted to address the problem through various prevention strategies. Employers established sexual harassment policies, grievance procedures, and a number of sexual harassment awareness-training programs. Some approaches have been utilized to address the company's culture, with respect to gender bias and the identification of potential harassment. Some researchers explained this as an effort to make the workplace more conscious of sexual harassment issues. Companies have been aware of these approaches for a long period, but have not taken necessary actions once sexual harassment has been identified (Roberts & Mann, 2012). Recent news reports indicate that sexual harassment has involved the highest levels of management, but they appear unsure of how to adequately address it.

Schickman (1996) and other writers have seen sexual harassment result in a loss of employee morale, diminished productivity, and the decline of a company's public image. Given the current economic downturn, companies need to recognize and seriously address the new legal grounds available to victims. The cost of sexual harassment to victims is high and is becoming more costly to businesses. Despite the high stakes involved in sexual harassment, many employers continue to be unwilling or unable to protect their own interests and those of their employees.

Boland (2002) and others found that when organizations, including hospitals, colleges, and various other institutions, neglect to take positive measures that provide psychological counseling and support, sexual harassment-related problems can lead to:

- Decreased productivity and increased team conflict;
- Decreased study/job satisfaction;
- Loss of students/staff—loss of students who leave school, and staff resignations to avoid harassment; resignations/firings of alleged harassers;
- Decreased productivity and/or increased absenteeism by staff or students experiencing harassment;
- Reduced success in meeting academic and financial goals;
- Increased health care costs and sick pay costs because of the health consequences of harassment and/or retaliation;
- Undermining of ethical standards and discipline in the organization in general if harassment is permitted;
- Damage to a company's or school's image if the problem is ignored or not treated properly;
- High jury awards for the employee, and attorney fees and litigation costs, if the problem is ignored or not treated properly (in case of firing the victim) when the complainants are advised to and do take the issue to court.

Reichers and Schneider (1990) indicated that an organizational climate should reflect absolute non-tolerance for sexual harassment. Policies and procedures in the workplace environment are necessary to eliminate the conditions in which sexual harassment is likely to occur. Challenges remain for a more informed understanding of what policies, procedures, and strategies are needed to address this issue.

As another way of addressing sexual harassment, organizations may actively promote ethics standards within their organizations. Joseph (2000) listed some of the potential benefits of an effective ethics program:

- Fostering a more satisfying and productive working environment;
- Building and sustaining your organization's reputation within the communities in which you operate;
- Maintaining the trust of members to ensure continued self-regulation;
- Legitimizing open discussion of ethical issues;
- Providing ethical guidance and resources for employees prior to making difficult decisions;
- Aligning the work efforts of staff with the organization's broader mission and vision.

Gretchen Winter, vice president of business practices at Baxter International, stated that ethics standards programs are designed to affect how people think about and address ethical issues that arise on the job (Joseph, 2000). She felt that offering employees ethics training, and resources, can create a positive work environment in which employees can acknowledge that they have an ethical dilemma. This is designed to guide employees in working through such dilemmas before making unethical decisions.

Winter felt that ethical guidelines in the form of policies and practices offer employees the basic tools they need to take informed risks on behalf of their organizations. She stated that everyone benefits by steering employees away from ethical risk-taking and into more productive and appropriate kinds of behavior. Joseph (2000) noted that there is no substitute for clear procedures and sanctions, but he recommended a set of ethics standards that promote the following:

- Less observed misconduct at work;
- Greater willingness to report misconduct;
- Greater satisfaction with the organization's response to reported misconduct;
- Greater overall satisfaction with the organization;
- Greater likelihood of "feeling valued" by the organization.

GUIDELINES FOR A SEXUAL HARASSMENT POLICY IN THE WORKPLACE

Some employers have provided general policies that can also address sexual harassment issues during the current economic downturn and include the following principles.

- Demonstrate a renewed commitment to eradicate and prevent sexual harassment.
- Provide a clear definition of sexual harassment including both the giving of a favor or with the expectation of a returned favor, or *quid pro quo*, and a hostile work environment.
- Include enforceable penalties that the employer will impose for substantiated sexual harassment conduct.
- Provide a detailed outline of the grievance procedure employees should use.
- Develop and make qualified resource or contact persons available for consultation.
- Make an expressed commitment to keep all sexual harassment complaints and personnel actions confidential.

The US Equal Employment Opportunity Commission (1990) set forth principles that address sexual harassment:

- An expressed commitment to eradicate and prevent sexual harassment;
- A definition of sexual harassment including both *quid pro quo* and hostile work environment;
- An explanation of penalties that the employer will impose for substantiated sexual harassment conduct;
- A detailed outline of the grievance procedure employees should use;
- Additional resource or contact persons available for consultation;
- A clear commitment to keep all sexual harassment complaints and personnel actions confidential.

During the current economic downturn it is important that a company's basic policies incorporate these guidelines.

Case Example

The American Academy of Pediatrics (AAP) described the broad and varied setting in which its constituents worked. Personnel often moved from the office, to a hospital, and to an educational environment within a single day. AAP felt that the size and nature of each organization were important factors that determined the degree of formality needed to help eradicate sexual harassment. This approach was included in a policy statement to be used in concert with existing procedures. The statement was used to heighten awareness and encourage reassessment of existing policies in all of its medical practice and educational settings.

It is reasonable to assume that even the most comprehensive sexual harassment policies and procedures will probably fail if a company does not enforce them quickly, consistently, and aggressively. For policies to be effective, companies must view sexual harassment seriously. Designated personnel must be made responsible for enforcement, documentation, and investigations of all complaints. A number of findings reveal that it is essential that employers regularly monitor managers' and supervisors' adherence to sexual harassment policies and procedures. This requires strategies that can include posted rules, written policies, monthly meetings, unscheduled spot checks, and periodic sexual harassment training sessions. Businesses that utilize surveys about sexual harassment issues can often gauge supervisor and other employee attitudes concerning the problem. It has been found that when companies screen annual data on hiring, firing, promotions, and compensation packages, overt patterns of sexual harassment may be discerned.

Regardless of the situation, reasonable and necessary actions need to be quickly taken that are designed to end the sexual harassment. Action steps may include verbal warnings, written warnings, job transfers, suspension of employment, and, if necessary, termination.

Most prefer a pragmatic solution that would stop the harassment and prevent future contact with the harasser, rather than turning to the police. More about the difficulty in turning an offence into a legal act can be found in Felstiner, Abel, and Sarat's (1981) study, which describes three steps a victim (of any dispute) must go through before turning to the justice system: naming (giving the assault a definition); blaming (understanding who is responsible for the violation of rights and facing them); and finally, claiming (turning to the authorities).

Boxes 4.1 and 4.2 summarize some further suggestions adopted from guidelines entitled "Sexual Harassment in the Workplace: A Primer", developed by Roberts and Mann (2012) to address sexual harassment. All companies should consider these guidelines in establishing and implementing their sexual harassment policy.

Box 4.1 Guidelines For a Sexual Harassment Policy

- Appreciate that you and your company can be held liable if your employees engage in sexual harassment.
- Know that any unwelcomed sexual activity tied to employment decisions or benefits is sexual harassment.
- Recognize that sexual harassment may include jokes, vulgar language, sexual innuendoes, pornographic pictures, sexual gestures, physical grabbing or pinching, and other unwelcomed or offensive physical touching or contact.
- Remember that every sexual harassment charge is extremely serious.
- Comprehend that employees who comply with unwelcomed sexual advances can still be victims of sexual harassment.
- Realize that men as well as women may be sexually harassed.
- Understand that employees may wait a while before lodging sexual harassment charges.

Communicate Policy

- Issue a strong policy from the CEO against sexual harassment.
- Provide a clear definition of sexual harassment, using examples of inappropriate behavior.
- Review the policy with your employees on a regular basis.
- Discuss the policy with all new employees.
- Ensure that third-party suppliers and customers are aware of your sexual harassment policy.

Establish Procedures

- Appoint a senior corporate official to oversee the implementation of the policy.
- Train your supervisors and managers to recognize and prevent sexual harassment.
- Outline procedures to use in reporting sexual harassment.
- Designate a personnel officer or other appropriate manager, rather than a direct supervisor, to receive sexual harassment complaints.
- Provide alternative routes for filing complaints.
- Keep all sexual harassment charges confidential.

Enforce Policy

- Make sure employees who bring charges do not face retaliation.
- Safeguard the rights of the accused.
- Investigate all sexual harassment charges quickly and thoroughly.
- Maintain accurate records of the investigation and the findings.
- Take immediate action when sexual harassment is discovered or suspected.
- Discipline appropriately any employee found to have engaged in sexual harassment.
- Safeguard your employees from third-party work-related sexual harassment.

Source: Roberts and Mann (2012).

Box 4.2 Guidance from the American Association of University Women

Studies by the American Association of University Women (AAUW) (2005) were very clear that sexual harassment in the academic workplace is unwanted and not to be tolerated. This organization provides an extensive and practical framework on ways that victims can address the physical and psychological effects of workplace sexual harassment. It also describes how they can maintain or return to normal socialization, regain personal relationships, and regain social approval. From an emotional perspective it suggests how they may reduce trauma, and concentrate on a successful quality of life and the work environment. The AAUW report explains the importance of organizations providing immediate psychological and legal counseling when a sexual harassment event occurs. Considerable evidence supports the idea that self-treatment may not release stress or remove the trauma of sexual harassment adequately.

The following principles provide additional suggestions for decreasing the incidence of sexual harassment in the educational workplace.

- Encourage supervisors and administrators to set an example by serving as positive role models.
- Investigate all complaints promptly and confidentially.
- Follow-up on all complaints.
- Sensitize employees through interactive training.
- Treat all complaints as serious matters.

In addition, once a complaint has been adjudicated, efforts must be taken to ensure a smooth transition for the employees coming back into the workplace. Follow-up counseling and/or periodic meetings individually with the party or parties involved should be provided as warranted.

SUMMARY

This chapter examines how organizations, businesses, workers, and victims can enhance the prevention and treatment of sexual harassment in the workplace. We begin by describing the background, scope, and severity of the sexual harassment problem. Secondly, we present some employer-related issues regarding sexual harassment in the workplace during the economic downturn. Finally, we suggest policies and approaches for the establishment and implementation of more-positive sexual harassment policy and treatment.

A good deal of the literature provides guidance regarding the scope of protection, liabilities, and remedies for sexual harassment. It is essential that all employees have a workplace in which they are treated with appropriate respect. It is necessary for employers to establish affirmative tools and methods for combating sexual harassment in the workplace. Companies should sensitize employees through interactive training and treat all complaints as serious matters. Appropriate discipline for offenders, and steps to prevent subsequent offenses, should be the rule. Once a complaint has been adjudicated, efforts must be taken to ensure a smooth and retaliation-free transition for the employees coming back into the workplace. Follow-up counseling and/or periodic meetings individually with the party or parties involved should be provided as warranted. Sexual harassment policies are recommended that support ethics programs and ethical modeling by leaders and supervisors and that link key values such as respect and trust.

REFERENCES

American Association of University Women (2005). *Drawing the line: Sexual harassment on campus.* Washington, DC: American Association of University Women Educational Foundation.

Benson, K. (1984). Comments on Crocker's an analysis of university definitions of sexual harassment. *Signs, 9,* 516–519.

Bernstein, A. (1994). Law, culture and harassment. *University of Pennsylvania Law Review, 142,* 1227–1311.

Boland, M. L. (2002). *Sexual harassment: Your guide to legal action.* Naperville, IL: Sphinx Publishing.

Bowers, T., & Hook, B. (2002). *Hostile work environment: A manager's legal liability,* Retrieved from <http://www.techrepublic.com/article/hostile-work-environment-a-managers-legal-liability/5035282>.

Brownmiller, S. (1999). *Two kinds of unknowing.* Thousand Oaks, CA: Sage.

Bureau of Labor Statistics (2012). *Worker displacement: 2009-2011.* Retrieved from <http://www.bls.gov/news.release/pdf/disp.pdf>.

Burgess, D., & Borgida, E. (1997). Sexual harassment: An experimental test of sex-role spillover theory. *Personality and Social Psychology Bulletin, 21,* 63–75.

Calvasina G. E., Calvasina R. V., & Calvasina E. J. (2011). Are men entitled to Title VII protection from a sexually hostile work environment. *Proceeding of the Academy for Studies in Business, 3*(1), 7–12.

Cole, L. L., Grubb, P. L., Sauter, S. L., Swanson, N. G., & Lawless, P. (1997). Psychosocial correlates of harassment, threats and fear of violence in the workplace. *Scandinavian Journal of Work and Environmental Health, 23,* 450–457.

Dziech, B. W., & Weiner, L. (1990). *The lecherous professor: Sexual harassment on campus.* Chicago IL: University of Illinois Press.

Ebeid, F., Kaul, T., Newman, K., & Shane, H. (2003). Workplace abuse: Problems and consequences. *International Business & Economics Research Journal, 2,* 75–86.

Felstiner, W. L., Abel, R. L., & Sarat, A. (1981). The emergence and transformation of dispute: Naming, blaming, claiming.... *Law & Society Review, 15,* 631–654.

Fitzgerald, L. F. (2003). Sexual harassment and social justice: Reflections on the distance yet to go. *American Psychologist, 58,* 915–924.

Fitzgerald, L. F, & Ormerod., A. J. (1993). Breaking silence: The sexual harassment of women in academia and the workplace. In F. I. Denmark, & M. A. Paludi (Eds.), *Psychology of women: A handbook of issues and theories* (pp. 553–581). Westport, CT: Greenwood.

Grauerholz, E. (1989). Sexual harassment of women professors by students: Exploring the dynamics of power, authority, and gender in a university setting. *Sex Roles, 21,* 789–801.

Gutek, B. (1985). *Sex and the workplace.* San Francisco: Jossey-Bass.

Hersch, J. (2011). *Compensating differentials for sexual harassment.* American Economic Review Papers and Proceedings, May 2011; Vanderbilt Law and Economics Research Paper No. 11-06. Retrieved from SSRN: <http://ssrn.com/abstract = 1743691>.

Heyman, R. (1994). *Why didn't you say that in the first place?* San Francisco: Jossey-Bass Publishers.

Joseph, J. (2000). *Ethics in the workplace.* Retrieved from <http://www.asaecenter.org/Resources/articledetail.cfm?ItemNumber = 13073>.

Kauppinen-Toropainen., K, & Gruber, J. (1993). Antecedents and outcomes of woman-unfriendly experiences: A study of Scandinavian, former Soviet, and American women. *Psychology of Women Quarterly, 17,* 431–456.

Kim, H. & Fiske, S. T. (1999, June). *Are the motives of men who sexually harass women misunderstood?: An investigation linking ambivalent sexism and sexual harassment.* Poster presented at the 11th Annual Conference of the American Psychological Society, Denver, CO.

Koss, M. P. (1990). Changed lives: The psychological impact of sexual harassment. In M. A. Paludi (Ed.), *Ivory power: Sexual harassment on campus* (pp. 73–92). Albany, NY: State University of New York Press.

Langelan, M. J. (1993). *Back off: How to confront and stop sexual harassment and harassers.* New York: Fireside.

Legalzoom (2012). *Five biggest sexual harassment cases.* Retrieved from <http://www.legalzoom.com/legal-headlines/corporate-lawsuits/five-biggest-sexual-harassment-cases> .

MacKinnon, C. A. (1979). *Sexual harassment of working women: A case of sex discrimination.* New Haven, CT: Yale University Press.

Matchen, J., & DeSouza, E. (2000). The sexual harassment of faculty members by students. *Sex Roles, 42,* 296–306.

Mattioli, D. (2010, March 23). More men make harassment claims. *Wall Street Journal.* <Retrieved from http://online.wsj.com/article/SB10001424052748704117304575137881438719028.html>.

Ms. Foundation for Women (2012a). 2011 *Community Voices on the Economy survey.* Retrieved from <http://ms.foundation.org/our_work/broad-change-areas/economic-justice/2011-community-voices-on-the-economy-survey>.

Ms. Foundation for Women (2012b). *Anika Rahman: Fighting the womancession [GRITtv].* Retrieved from <http://ms.foundation.org/newsroom/in-the-news/anika-rahman-fighting-the-womancession>.

Piotrkowski, C. S. (1998). Gender harassment, job satisfaction, and distress among employed White and minority women. *Journal of Occupational Health Psychology, 3,* 33–43.

Reichers, A. E., & Schneider, B. (1990). Climate and cultures: An evolution of constructs. In B. Schneider (Ed.), *Organizational Climate and Culture* (pp. 5–39). San Francisco: Jossey-Bass.

Roberts, B., & Mann, R. (2012). *Sexual harassment in the workplace: A primer.* Retrieved from <http://www3.uakron.edu/lawrev/robert1.html>.

Rowe, M. (1996). Dealing with harassment: A systems approach. In M. Stockdale (Ed.), *Sexual harassment: perspectives, frontiers, and response strategies, women & work* (*Vol. 5,* pp. 241–271). Sage Publications.

Schickman, M. I. (1996). Sexual harassment: the employer's role in prevention. *The Compleat Lawyer, 13*, 24–28.
Tangri, S. S., Burt, M. R., & Johnson, L. B. (1982). Sexual harassment at work: Three explanatory models. *Journal of Social Issues, 38*, 33–54.
US Equal Employment Opportunity Commission (1990, March 19). *Policy guidance No. N-915-050:Current issues of sexual harassment.* Washington, DC: EEOC.
US Equal Employment Opportunity Commission (2012a). *Sexual harassment.* Retrieved from <http://www1.eeoc.gov/laws/types/sexual_harassment.cfm>.
US Equal Employment Opportunity Commission (2012b). *Sexual harassment charges EEOC & FEPAs combined: FY 1997 – FY 2011.* Retrieved from <http://www1.eeoc.gov/eeoc/statistics/enforcement/sexual_harassment.cfm>.
Waldo, C. R., Berdahl, J. L., & Fitzgerald, L. F. (1998). Are men sexually harassed? If so by whom? *Law and Human Behavior, 22*, 59–79.
Zippel, K. (2006). *The politics of sexual harassment: A comparative study of the United States, the European Union, and Germany.* Cambridge: Cambridge University Press.

FURTHER READING

Gruber, J. E. (1998). The impact of male work environment and organizational policies on women's experiences of sexual harassment. *Gender and Society, 12*(*3*), 301–320.
Hill, C., & Silva, E. (2005). *Drawing the line: Sexual harassment on campus.* American Association of University Women Educational Foundation, 1111 Sixteenth St. N.W., Washington, DC 20036. Tel: 202-728-7602; Fax: 202-463-7169; TDD: 202-785-7777; e-mail: foundation@aauw.org; Website: <www.aauw.org>.
Howard, S. (1991). Organizational resources for addressing sexual harassment. *Journal of Counseling and Development, 69*(6), 507–511.
Huhman, H. (2011). *How to recognize sexual harassment in the workplace.* U.S. News and World Report. Retrieved February 16, 2012 from <http://money.usnews.com/money/blogs/outside-voices-careers/2011/11/11/>.
Moynihan, M. C. (2002). Avoiding sexual harassment claims: a primer. *RiskVue*, Retrieved January 28, 2012 from <http://www.riskvue.com/articles/rb/rb0208c.htm>.
O'Brien, G. (2011). *American Apparel and the ethics of a sexually charged workplace.* Business Ethics (Retrieved March 27, 2012 from <http://business-ethics.com/2011/03/15/0852-american-apparel-and-the-ethics-of-a-sexually-charged-workplace/>).

CHAPTER 5

Workplace Diversity and Discrimination

BACKGROUND OF DIVERSITY IN THE WORKPLACE

Diversity is a broad concept that can be difficult to comprehend, since there is no clear understanding about how different groups or individuals directly contribute to diversity at a given place or time (Marsiglia & Kulis, 2009). Workplace diversity has long been considered an important aspect of diversity and is projected to become even more important for several reasons. Because of the history of unfair work experiences in America and the increasing changes in US population demographics and the economy, companies will need to focus differently on diversity. They will have to find ways to become much more inclusive organizations, since diversity has the potential of yielding greater productivity and competitive advantages (Society for Human Resource Management, 2010). Stephen G. Butler, co-chair of the Business–Higher Education Forum, believes that diversity is ultimately a competitive asset that organizations cannot afford to ignore (Robinson, 2002).

Managing and valuing diversity are key components for accomplishing an organization's desired goals and objectives in order to improve workplace fairness and equality. Esty, Griffin, and Schorr (1995) suggested that people are bringing greater diversity to the workplace and that it is encompassing a wider variety of challenges. The concept of workplace diversity is an idea of acknowledging and accepting the value and contributions of all people. It further means understanding that each person is unique and important, while recognizing their individual differences. Differences among people can include the dimensions of race, ethnicity, gender, sexual orientation, socioeconomic status, age, physical abilities, religious beliefs, political beliefs, and various other factors. Having an opportunity to explore differences in a safe, positive, and nurturing workplace environment facilitates the achievement of a host of beneficial outcomes. Embracing workplace diversity is about understanding others and moving beyond mere tolerance to truly celebrating the rich dimensions of individual differences.

Treating Worker Dissatisfaction During Economic Change
DOI: http://dx.doi.org/10.1016/B978-0-12-397006-0.00005-1

Workplace diversity also encompasses a much wider variety of related individual differences, such as military experience, marital status, educational background, job training, and geographic location (Church, 1995). According to Parvis (2003), positive benefits of workforce diversity are achieved through reaching long- and short-term goals that reflect the characteristics and circumstances of the relevant population. Although the concept of workplace diversity highlights differences, its real value is that it creates an entity that is far more dynamic and greater than the sum of its individual parts. It is important for employers to reassess their concept of diversity and how it impacts their workplace during the recent economic downturn, and its implications for future changes in the economy.

Diversity is an important factor in this chapter for several reasons. First, it is directly connected to the issue of discrimination in the workplace and its negative effects related to race, gender, class, culture, and other factors. A number of studies and reports have found that workplace diversity has presented new concerns as a result of the recent economic downturn. Much of the data describe how discrimination in the workplace has risen during the downturn and how women, racial and ethnic groups, and other marginalized people have been hit hardest (Blank & Slipp, 1994). Although discrimination in the workplace can be a very challenging problem, it is not a recent phenomenon.

Workplace discrimination has existed within the whole range and continuum of history in America. Briefly stated, it was present during the European colonization of North America in the 1600s (Takaki, 1987), and various historians and social scientists have reported how groups were first brought to the western hemisphere from Africa to work as slaves. European indentured servants came in the capacity of cheap, temporary labor. Native Americans, who had resided on the continent for centuries, were exploited for the use of their labor and land. Europeans and Asian ethnic groups and others were exploited by class, religion, ethnicity, or cultural identity and experienced workplace discrimination. Many contemporary groups experience various degrees of workplace discrimination, based upon sexual orientation, gender, age, race, physical appearance, and disabilities.

The social, economic, and historical development of the United States has often been subject to ambiguity concerning the principles of fairness and equity (Hacker, 1992). As it is related to diversity in the workplace, the history can be described as an especially difficult and ongoing challenge. The problems related to obtaining equal rights and justice for people who are viewed as different from the social and political elite has been daunting (Kluegel & Smith, 1986; Takaki, 1993). This was demonstrated by the example of discrimination related to rural farming, described as "sharecropping," and the exploitation of the industrial workforce. The discrimination of African Americans and mistreatment of Hispanic immigrant labor is a more contemporary example (Burns & Ali, 2012; Marsigilia & Kulis, 2009).

Although there are a number of perspectives related to workplace diversity, this chapter will primarily focus on workplace discrimination. It will also address circumstances and experiences of discrimination in the context of a serious US economic downturn. Parallel to the overall history of diversity and discrimination in the workplace, there are the related laws and policies that protect and defend workers against challenges to their diversity. Workplace discrimination is broadly viewed as including diverse groups or individuals who are not specifically defined by equal opportunity, affirmative action, and non-discrimination laws. The provisions of the federal Equal Employment Opportunities (EEO) Laws prohibiting job discrimination are as follows:

- Title VII of the Civil Rights Act of 1964 (Title VII), which prohibits employment discrimination based on race, color, religion, sex, or national origin;
- The Equal Pay Act of 1963 (EPA), which protects men and women who perform substantially equal work in the same establishment from sex-based wage discrimination;
- The Age Discrimination in Employment Act of 1967 (ADEA), which protects individuals who are 40 years of age or older;
- Title I and Title V of the Americans with Disabilities Act (ADA) of 1990, as amended, which prohibit employment discrimination against qualified individuals with disabilities in the private sector, and in state and local governments;
- Sections 501 and 505 of the Rehabilitation Act of 1973, which prohibit discrimination against qualified individuals with disabilities who work in the federal government;
- Title II of the Genetic Information Nondiscrimination Act of 2008 (GINA), which prohibits employment discrimination based on genetic information about an applicant, employee, or former employee;
- The Civil Rights Act of 1991, which, among other things, provides monetary damages in cases of intentional employment discrimination.

The US Equal Employment Opportunity Commission (EEOC) enforces these laws and provides oversight and coordination of all federal equal employment opportunity regulations, practices, and policies, often with great difficulty.

Managing diversity in the workplace goes far beyond the limits of equal employment opportunity and affirmative action laws. Officials in charge of diversity, and other managers in companies, recognize the limitations of discrimination laws. Therefore, through strategic and policy planning, they must incorporate policies and programs that ensure fairness and equality in a challenging and diverse workforce. Progressive employers provide continuous learning opportunities and sensitivity training to address discriminatory practices. Managers and staff are encouraged to consciously work towards preventing and eliminating discrimination in an organization. This is necessary in order to establish and successfully carry out an unbiased culture of diversity based upon the mission, vision, and values set forth by the leadership of an organization.

Cox (1991) describes three organization models that address different organizational aspects of cultural diversity in the workplace. The models apply to monolithic, plural, and multicultural organizations, which are described by Cox as follows.

- In the monolithic organization, the amount of structural integration or the presence of persons from different cultural groups in a single organization is minimal, with obvious white advantages in the U.S. workplace. This type of organization may have women and marginalized members within the workforce but not in positions of leadership and power.
- The plural organization has a more heterogeneous membership than the monolithic organization and is more inclusive of persons from cultural backgrounds different from that of the dominant group. This type of organization seeks to empower those from marginalized circumstances, to encourage opportunities for promotion and positions of leadership.
- The multicultural organization contains many different cultural groups, and values diversity. It also encourages healthy conflict as a way of promoting creative thinking.

A number of employment indicators reveal that racial and ethnic minorities are particularly hard hit during economic downturns, but they don't explain some of the other important implications. The US Department of Labor recorded claims of discrimination during 2009 that were almost twice as high for African Americans than for the white population in the United States. Simply describing the increased numbers of claims alone may not reflect a realistic understanding of the degree of the impact that discrimination has had on minorities.

One way in which workplace discrimination is addressed requires trust in the impartiality and understanding of the judiciary or other redress systems. Courts and regulatory agencies may not always reflect the full significance of discrimination findings (White, 2004).

Since reliable hard data on racial and ethnic discrimination is very difficult to acquire, it often comes down to uncertain anecdotal evidence. These data may be indicative of underlying trends but rely very heavily on individual interpretations of what is occurring. Many of the factors that account for racial discrimination and socioeconomic exclusion are well understood, but monitoring them is not easy (International Labour Office, 2011).

SIGNIFICANCE OF DIVERSITY DURING THE ECONOMIC DOWNTURN

Vinokur, Van Ryn, Gramlish, and Price (1991) saw a relationship between the type of people who become unemployed at various periods of the US economy and its cycles of expansion and contraction. They determined that, at any given time, the largest segment of the unemployed population, usually 50–65%, consists of workers who have lost their jobs. Unemployment is an increasingly serious problem for minorities and youth. Their unemployment rates were roughly two to three times higher than that of the general population in 1994 (US Department of Labor, 1994). Overall unemployment during the current economic downturn beginning in 2007 has inflicted a much greater hardship on youth and on women seeking to return to gainful employment after raising their children.

Reidenbach and Weller (2010) described how the economic downturn that began at the end of 2007 produced enormous difficulties for a large part of the overall diverse workforce and a greater impact upon specific groups across the country. The downturn exacerbated longstanding employment problems for minorities. The labor market became decidedly more brutal, with job displacement disproportionally affecting African Americans and Hispanics.

Existing disparities between minorities and white Americans persisted and expanded during the recent economic downturn. A large part of the economic gains made by minorities was disproportionately erased during the downturn. White Americans have been in a much better economic situation than minorities during any period, on almost all indicators. Minorities have not enjoyed equality in work-related benefits obtained during the period of economic growth prior to 2007. Asian Americans also saw declining workplace benefits during the recent recession, despite historically faring much better than other minorities in the labor market. Paucity of data makes it difficult to measure the specific effects of the recession on the Asian American community. However, existing data provide general evidence of the effects of discrimination on minorities across the American workforce, with mixed findings during the recent economic decline.

The US Department of Labor (2011) reported data for a period prior to the economic recession, indicating that:

- Between 2001 and 2007 the unemployment rate for whites was 3.7% in 2001 and 4.2% in March 2007.
- The respective rate for Hispanics was 5.8% in 2001 and 6.0% in 2007.
- For African Americans it was 8.1% in 2001 and 8.6% in 2007.
- For Asian Americans the rate was 3.4% in 2001 and 3.7% in 2007.

Structural differences in unemployment rates by race and ethnicity persisted through the entire 2001–2007 period and exploded in 2009 (US Department of Labor, 2011). The US Department of Labor (DOL) statistics on unemployment rates constitutes the most widely used gauge of economic well-being related to the labor market. Starting at the beginning of the recession in 2007, the DOL data revealed the following.

- The unemployment rate for African Americans was 8.6% in 2007. By 2009 it had risen 7.2 percentage points to 15.8%.
- The rate of increase was essentially the same for Hispanics, with unemployment rising from 5.8% in 2007 to 12.9% in 2009.
- The unemployment rate for white Americans was 9.2% at the end of 2009, up 5 percentage points from December 2007—also more than doubling.
- Asian Americans saw their unemployment rate rise from 3.7% percent to 7.7%, increasing twofold during the recession.

The data also revealed that unemployment increased at a faster annual rate for African Americans and Hispanics than for all other major groups during the economic downturn. Based upon age, African Americans and Hispanics experienced much greater unemployment rates than the rest of the population as described in the following summaries.

- African Americans and Hispanics aged 20 to 24 had a higher unemployment rate than people between the ages of 25 and 54.
- Younger African Americans' unemployment rate rose 4.8 percentage points each year since 2007, reaching 26.4% in 2009.
- Unemployment among young Hispanics increased by 4.7% to 17.2% between 2007 and 2009.

President Obama (2006) described these circumstances in graphic terms. He stated that "in spite of all the progress that has been made in the past four decades, a continuous gap remains between the overall living standards of Black, Latino, and white workers".

The DOL data in 2009 revealed that:

- The average wage for black workers is 75% of the average white wage.
- The average Latino wage is 71% of the average white wage.
- Black median net worth is about $6,000.
- Latino median net worth is about $8,000.
- The median net worth is about $88,000 for whites.

When laid off from work or experiencing an emergency, blacks and Latinos have lower reserve savings to draw on than do white workers. Middle-class blacks and Latinos also pay more for insurance, are less likely to own their own homes, and suffer poorer health than Americans as a whole.

In relation to the workplace, White (2003) reported that, during harder economic times, some employers will treat their employees with a much more cavalier attitude. For example, if an employee doesn't like their treatment, some employers believe that they can find another employee to replace them. Some employers assume that workers that are feeling discriminated against during bad times will tend to hang on longer and endure that treatment. Another example of disparate treatment is that, in good economic times, people assume they are supposed to support diversity, and they are often inclined to hire a minority candidate to get affirmative action credit; but when times are hard, employers tend to look out for their own group and isolate outsiders, and that's when discrimination related to diversity can begin to clearly reveal itself.

THE COST TO WORKERS OF DISCRIMINATION IN THE WORKPLACE

When addressing the cost of workplace discrimination, it is important to determine what concerns and barriers to fairness are most critical to the employer and to the workers. Although specific internal barriers, which include unfair compensation and advancement, will vary from one company to another, the overall effect of discrimination is to diminish many opportunities for the workforce in general. External barriers also continue to restrict the opportunities of diverse groups of workers. These barriers may include stereotyping and prejudice, lack of career support, or inadequate skill preparation. Barriers that affect employers, such as the downturn in the US and global economy, can also be detrimental to the advancement of a diverse group of workers. Internal barriers often emerge as a result of the occurrence of external barriers, and both types of barrier can negatively affect each other (Blank & Slipp, 1994).

The social cost of workplace discrimination can occur as a result of unfair hiring, promotion, job assignment, termination, or compensation. Discrimination can create social costs that are not only monetary but often have other serious consequences. Employees sometimes suffer retaliation for opposing workplace discrimination or reporting violations to authorities. Social cost can be related to employment discrimination that might occur intentionally or unintentionally due to prejudice or ignorance. Gender discrimination, a subset of sex discrimination, refers to behaviors that are considered appropriate or inappropriate, depending on whether a person is male or female. Gender discrimination may be nonsexual in the workplace, but is directed at expected roles that are associated with masculinity by employers. In the workplace women often bear the cost of being placed into submissive roles and encouraged not to question the privileges of male counterparts.

An example of the cost of discrimination is when an employer might ask whether an employment candidate is married or plans to have children. Refusing to hire a man in what is defined as a "woman's job" or vice versa is another example. Income levels vary by gender and race, with women's median income levels considerably below the national median for men with similar skills, training, and qualifications. Women often must consider factors other than salary, such as childcare, when looking for employment. On average, women are less willing or able to travel and relocate. Women are also more likely to work for government or non-profit organizations that pay less than the private sector.

As a result of discrimination in the workplace, ethnic and racial minorities, women, and other groups receive relatively fewer promotions and opportunities for economic advancement. Women are sometimes described as reaching the "glass ceiling," or simply being prevented from reaching certain heights on the occupational ladder. In regards to racial discrimination, numerous findings have shown that African American workers are less likely to be hired and more likely to be the first fired than white Americans with the same qualifications.

The continued prevalence of traditional gender role bias and ethnic prejudice may partially account for the high cost of discrimination during economic downturns. In 2005, median income levels were highest among Asian and white males and lowest among females of all races, especially those identifying as African American or Hispanic. Despite closing gender and racial gaps, considerable discrepancies remain or have increased among some of the racial and gender demographics during the recent economic downturn.

Bennet, Martin, Bies, and Brockner (1995) described how downsizing, layoffs, re-engineering, reduction in workforce, mergers, early retirement, and outplacement can create future job uncertainty. Fine (1996) indicated that individuals who are required to accept conditions as they are, can sometimes be denied the opportunity to express their true ability in the workplace and may experience ambivalence. When workers are forced to repress important aspects of their ability, it can create further lack of confidence about being successful in the workplace. This also suggests that people who spend significant amounts of energy coping in an ambiguous discriminatory environment, have less energy left to do their best work. Ambiguity not only creates uncertainty and the likelihood of failure for employees who are different, but also decreases the productivity of the total organization.

Most people depend on employment income to provide for the necessities of life and to sustain their standard of living (Vinocur et al., 1991). The mean duration of unemployment, in the United States for example, varies between 16 and 20 weeks, with a median between 8 and 10 weeks reported by the US Department of Labor (USDOL) in 1995. The duration of unemployment has been significantly higher during the recent economic downturn. Nearly 11% of unemployed persons had been looking for work for about 2 years or more in the fourth quarter of 2010. Due to this increase, in 2011 the Bureau of Labor Statistics (BLS) and the Census Bureau updated to 5 years the duration for which unemployment benefits are payable. Costs associated with unemployment would most likely persist for all workers after unemployment benefits are exhausted. Unemployed workers who also experience discrimination are at risk of facing even greater financial and social cost during an economic downturn. That crisis could play itself out in a serious cascade of stressful events that may include the loss of an automobile, repossession of personal property, foreclosure on a house, loss of medical care, and food shortages.

An abundance of research finds that economic hardship is the most consistent outcome of unemployment (Fryer & Payne, 1986). An additional impact of discrimination is the often hidden cost on many other aspects of life. This includes a greater possibility for the deterioration of mental health (Kessler, Turner, & House, 1988). The most common mental health costs related to job loss are increases in anxiety, somatic symptoms, and depression (Dooley, Catalano, & Wilson, 1994). In addition to the adverse effects of unemployment on mental health, research implicates the cost of workplace discrimination as a contributing factor to other related outcomes. These outcomes include suicide, separation and divorce, alcohol abuse, and violence in the workplace (Liem & Liem, 1988; Stack, 1981).

Racial and ethnic groups are more likely to be exposed to hazardous work conditions than are their white counterparts, as a result of discrimination. Bullard and Wright (1987) noted this propensity and indicated that injuries are likely to vary with the type of work that one is engaged in. One of the most likely reasons, they noted, was that occupational injuries are highly dependent on the type of job and industry, and minorities tend to work in more hazardous occupations. Tough economic times have definitely impacted a great number of workers. It has made it even more difficult for women and other minorities to find and keep any job, without also having to endure the additional cost of workplace discrimination.

EMPLOYERS' COSTS RELATED TO DIVERSITY AND DISCRIMINATION IN THE WORKPLACE

The consequences of employers' ignoring diversity in the workplace will ultimately be costs of time, money, and efficiency. Some of the other consequences include: loss of productivity, due to increased conflict; inability to attract and retain a range of talented people; and legal actions. Ignoring diversity can lead to discrimination, which can result in lost investment in recruitment and training. A study by Robinson and Dechant (1997) found that the cost of workplace discrimination in the United States has been conservatively estimated to exceed 64 billion dollars. These costs arise from losing and replacing over 2 million workers annually because of unfairness and workplace discrimination. Much of the data confirm that a business that discriminates based upon characteristics such as race, ethnicity, gender, age, disability, and sexual orientation will be put at a competitive disadvantage. Businesses that discriminate lose when compared with those that evaluate workers primarily on their job qualifications and abilities.

Employers that refuse to hire workers because of irrelevant discriminatory characteristics such as race and gender will eventually create a substandard workforce. Depending upon the industry, this can result in otherwise qualified workers being forced into the ranks of the unemployed. Employers would also face the additional cost of having to recruit, employ, and retrain new workers as a result of laying off previously qualified employees.

According to a study by Burns (2012), the cost of replacing dismissed workers falls within the range $5,000 to $10,000 for hourly workers. The cost increases to between $75,000 and $211,000 for executive-level employees earning $100,000 or more annually. Discrimination in the workplace can lead to even more costly expenses in the form of legal claims and potential lawsuits. It was found in the Biliski v. Kappos Supreme Court case of 2010 that, during the current recession, the top ten private-plaintiff discrimination lawsuits cost companies more than $346 million. In January 2010, the Outback restaurant chain was forced to pay out $19 million in a sex discrimination case. In this case, a female employee filed a successful legal claim when she was denied opportunity for advancement, promotion, and favorable work assignments. Major companies, including Fox News, Goldman Sachs, Morgan Stanley, Bank of America, and Merrill Lynch, have all been sued for sexual discrimination during this recent economic recession.

Barbee (2010) reported that, in Texas, workers were awarded $28.9 million in compensation for workplace discrimination that included sexual harassment, religious intolerance, and discrimination on grounds of age, ethnicity, and race. This came to $2.7 million more than the previous year. In Texas, sexual discrimination was found to be the most common reason for complaints, followed by race, age, and disability grievances, according to the US Equal Employment Opportunity Commission (EEOC) (2010). The number of complaints dipped minimally in 2009 from the previous year. Overall, for the fiscal year that ended in 2010, 9,310 Texas workers alleged discrimination based on their gender, disability, national origin, race, religion, or other reason, according to EEOC statistics.

During the recent economic downturn businesses have competed even more aggressively for the most qualified and skilled labor to improve their competiveness. In order to increase competiveness, employers have had the opportunity to selectively hire workers from the largest and most qualified labor pool. Discriminatory practices against former, existing, and future employees can adversely impact a company's competitive efforts. Current and former employees who have been victimized as a result of discrimination will often discourage potential qualified applicants from seeking employment with the offending employer. The Level Playing Field Institute (2003) discovered that approximately one in four workers who experienced unfairness on the job indicated that they would be hesitant to recommend their employer to potential employees.

Faculty at the Arizona State A.S.P. Carey School of Business reported various studies between 2008 and 2011 that estimated the cost of replacing a displaced worker to be between 93% and 200% of the displaced worker's salary. It was further noted that companies who fail to keep qualified workers, as a result of discriminatory practices, experience a considerable loss on the investment that had been made in the departing worker. The data support previous findings that training and accommodating a new employee to reach the same level of skills and knowledge of the displaced one will incur a considerable cost in time and money.

An extensive longitudinal study entitled National Study of Employers (NSE), reported by Matos and Galinsky (2012) for the Family Work Institute, examined employer workplace flexibility and effectiveness between 2005 and 2012. The study addressed the degree to which employers encouraged workplace benefits that promoted flexibility before and during the current economic downturn in the United States. Findings revealed that there were substantial cutbacks during the economic downturn in the investment of benefits that involved a direct cost to companies. This included health care, pension plans, and paid leave options. Companies, on the other hand, demonstrated a greater willingness to offer flexibility in choices of work locations, flexible working hours, and time off for personal needs.

The study also found that, where racial minorities represented more than 50% of the employees of an organization, it suggests a negative effect and was more likely to demonstrate a lower level of flexibility and effectiveness. When women made up less than 25% percent of the employees, the organization was more likely to be less flexible and effective. This study also revealed that when there was greater diversity in management, an organization was a more flexible and effective workplace. This finding was also influenced by the degree to which employees experienced job challenges, learning opportunities, job autonomy, supervisory support, and a climate of respect, trust, and economic security.

Employees in organizations that offered more flexibility and diversity were found to exhibit:

- Greater engagement in jobs;
- Higher levels of job satisfaction;
- Stronger intention to remain with the employer;
- Less negative spillover from job to home;
- Less negative spillover from home to job;
- Better mental health;
- Better physical health;
- Low general stress level;
- Less indication of depression.

The study concluded that employers with the most diverse top leadership and non-profit organizations provided the most flexibility and concern for the well-being of both employees and employers. The study suggests that there is a better chance for effectiveness when employees are allowed more flexibility and diversity in the workplace.

Matos and Galinsky's study demonstrated that when workers do not experience flexibility and employers do not promote diversity in the workplace, a number of costs can occur. These costs include an increase in the rates of absenteeism along with physical and mental health problems. The employer completes this negative cycle by awarding fewer raises and promotions. As a result, businesses will find it increasingly difficult to operate at their full potential. During this recent economic downturn, lack of support for diversity and the avoidance of discrimination can seriously impair an organization's financial growth, vitality, and competiveness.

HARMFUL MANAGEMENT PRACTICES IN A DIVERSE WORKPLACE

The findings cited above suggest that companies are likely to lose a competitive advantage as well as harm workers when they fail to signal to their employees that they promote a fair, safe, and welcoming workplace culture. Failure to provide a positive and non-discriminatory climate in the workplace can impact an organization's competitive edge in the following areas:

- Recruitment and retention of employees;
- Productivity and job performance;
- Competing for consumer and supplier markets;
- Exposure to costly litigation.

Diversity is an important element of business strategy in order to support innovation, creativity, and effective problem-solving. Blank and Slipp (1994) suggested that homogeneous workplaces have been found to be less adept at innovating than heterogeneous ones. When employees do not represent a variety of backgrounds they provide businesses with fewer opportunities to appeal to an increasingly diverse consumer market. Employees who work in an unfair or negative environment are not always able to focus their optimum effort in performing their responsibilities. In today's economy, government bodies at all levels should enact necessary policy reforms to help businesses revise harmful management practices in the workplace.

It was mentioned earlier that workplace discrimination increases when employers feel threatened by economic downturns. In good economic times, employers realize that they are supposed to support diversity and would be inclined to hire a minority candidate to get affirmative action credits. But when times are hard, decision makers in organizations will often look out for their preferred group and cut off workers considered as outsiders. Although an employer's discriminatory behavior may often appear justified by business economics, it is toxic for profit margins. When companies elect to downsize, minorities and women are often the least experienced workers with less tenure and will usually be dismissed first. Paula Brantner, executive director of Workplace Fairness, noted that, when times are good, workers can more easily replace the income and benefits they have lost. In good times, if employees experience a negative or discriminatory workplace environment, they might leave with the prospect of soon getting another job (Walker, 2010).

The local Cleveland EEOC settled a $400,000 race discrimination and retaliation class settlement case against Mineral Met Inc., a division of the Chemalloy Company and cited the following claims.

- Black employees were disciplined for having facial hair while white employees were not.
- A white supervisor at that company placed a hangman's noose on a piece of machinery.

In another harmful management practice example, The EEOC sued DHL Express (USA) Inc., alleging the following.

- DHL discriminated against black Chicago-area employees by giving them worse assignments than their white counterparts.
- DHL assigned more-difficult and dangerous work to black employees than to white employees, violating federal civil rights laws.

An EEOC attorney in Arizona stated:

> *We often see discrimination when economic times are tough. Many employers get rid of people of color, they get rid of people with disabilities and they get rid of people who are pregnant.*

To foster a more diverse workplace, an organization has to do more than simply acknowledge differences in people. It is acknowledged in debate on the subject that a workplace which is highly diverse can also be difficult to motivate and manage for a variety of complex reasons. A major obstacle to effective management is miscommunication within an organization. Necessary communication competencies may be lacking in diverse organizational environments subject to poor management practices. Such skills include self-monitoring, empathy, and strategic decision-making. Brownell (2003) defined these skills as follows.

- Self-monitoring refers to a communicator's awareness of how his/her behavior affects another person, along with his/her willingness to modify this behavior based on knowledge of its impact.
- Empathy enables the receiver to go beyond the literal meaning of a message and consider the communicator's feelings, values, assumptions, and needs.
- Strategic decision-making implies that the communication sources and channels used to reach organization members, as well as the substance of the messages conveyed, are mindfully selected.

Brownell (2003) further explains that communication is a skill that is often difficult to master because the full meaning of a message can never be completely understood or transmitted. This can occur because people rarely experience events in exactly the same way. Even when people from the same background and culture are exposed to the same messages, they may often interpret the information differently. It is bad management practice to interpret messages and discern meaning based on a unique point of view, without a willingness to accept differing perspectives.

A poor management practice is the creation of a workplace environment where marginalized groups have little or no voice. Vaughn (2006) describes challenges to communication that diverse organizations face in maintaining a culture which supports the idea of concern for both the organization and employee's voice. When the organizational environment is not supportive of dissenting viewpoints, employees may choose to remain silent for fear of repercussions. Employees may also seek alternative or safe avenues to express their concerns and frustrations through online forums, informal gatherings, and affinity group meetings.

A process that does not take into account the diverse levels of language and reading proficiency among the staff would represent bad management practice. This might also include not taking extra time to be sure that information is understood regardless of the medium through which it is transmitted in a diverse workplace. In spite of best efforts, poor management practices continue to exist. These practices include conformity to discriminatory customer preferences, allowing prohibited stereotypes about jobs, and racially targeted recruitment procedures. Bad management practices that are particularly pernicious are those aimed at only attracting certain preferred or national origin group employees.

BEST MANAGEMENT PRACTICES IN A DIVERSE WORKPLACE

When addressing the problems of job displacement and workplace diversity, organizations have numerous alternatives to downsizing, layoffs, and reduction in force. Displaying compassion that clearly shows management realizes the hardships that job loss and future job insecurity poses for workers is an important management responsibility. During good economic times workforce practices such as reduced work weeks, across-the-board salary rises, attractive early retirement packages, retraining existing employees, and voluntary layoff programs can be implemented (Wexley & Silverman, 1993). As additional information becomes available during the recent economic downturn, managers need training to become more open-minded about attempting to help workers cope with job insecurity and layoffs. Redefining the way that workplace job displacement is organized and executed will require alternatives to traditional job design and management methods. Managers have a greater responsibility to:

- Identify and attempt to alleviate sources of job insecurity among workers;
- Encourage feelings of being in control and of empowerment in the workforce;
- Show compassion when workers express feelings of job insecurity.

A poll by the Society for Human Resource Management (SHRM) (2010) described how diversity in the workplace has continued with some positive trends, despite an economic downturn that forced drastic cuts in many human-resource practices. The poll surveyed 402 randomly selected HR professionals and compared diversity practices of 2010 with those of 2005, showing the following changes.

- The percentage of companies that provide training on diversity issues increased to 71% in 2010 from 67% in 2005.
- The number of organizations that have a diverse board of directors increased to 66% in 2010 from 53% in 2005.
- The percentage of organizations that said their diversity practices were very or somewhat effective increased to 84% in 2010, up slightly from 83% in 2005.
- However, the percentage of organizations that have workplace diversity practices, such as recruiting and retention strategies and community outreach, declined to 68% in 2010 from 76% in 2005.

The SHRM poll (2010) indicated that companies invested in building human capital during the economic downturn that began in late 2007. Larger organizations, government agencies, and multinational organizations were more likely to address workplace diversity. Some diversity practices have been put on hold during the recent recession. For example, diversity hiring programs may be suspended when there is no hiring. The findings clearly show that organizations are still making significant investments in diversity programs and that these programs are paying off for those organizations. The poll also showed that 68% of organizations continue to mandate diversity training for top-level executives.

At its Diversity and Inclusion Conference, SHRM announced that it was creating standards for diversity practices within the next 2 years that include:

- A description of the top diversity professional position;
- The essential elements of diversity;
- Inclusion programs;
- Metrics that measure an effective program.

The SHRM poll identified three sets of best management practices recommendations, concerning (a) how to better manage diversity, (b) the benefits experienced from diversity, and (c) maintaining a positive workplace environment. The three areas are described in Box 5.1.

Managing diversity effectively in any setting means acknowledging workers' differences and recognizing those differences as valuable. It enhances good management practices by preventing discrimination and promoting inclusiveness in all settings. Good management alone will not necessarily work effectively with a diverse workforce. It is often difficult to see what part diversity plays in a specific area of management in the

Box 5.1 Recommendations for Best Management Practices in Relation to Diversity, from the Society for Human Resource Management

Managing diversity

Organizations are beginning to recognize the impact of a diverse work force, and the following recommendations by Performance Resources, Inc. have been made on how to better manage diversity.

- Be flexible; try to adapt to the style of the person with whom you are communicating.
- Understand that cultural differences exist.
- Acknowledge your stereotypes and assumptions.
- Develop consciousness and acceptance of your own cultural background and style.
- Learn about other cultures.
- Provide employees who are different with what they need to succeed: access to information and meaningful relationships with people in power.
- Treat people equitably but not uniformly.
- Encourage constructive communication about differences.

Benefits of diversity

Performance Resources Inc. described how organizations who value diversity and learned to manage diversity effectively have experienced the following benefits.

- Diversity brings a variety of ideas and viewpoints to the organization, especially when creative problem-solving is required.
- Diversity increases productivity and makes work fun and interesting.
- Employees take risks, play to win rather than not to lose, and, as a result, creativity, leadership, and innovation are enhanced.
- Employees are empowered and have a sense of their potential and value to the company.

Maintaining a positive workplace environment

The following steps have been recommended by Performance Resources Inc. when organizations are attempting to maintain a positive work environment in a continually changing and diverse workplace.

- Understand that communication is the key to breaking down the cultural barriers between people.
- Be clear, concise and avoid slang, especially with those for whom English may be a second language.
- When a conflict arises, consider the possibility that the root cause may be cultural in origin.
- Be especially alert for the non-verbal language of those whose cultural background is different from your own.

- Learn to accept that different cultures have different though equally valid perspectives.
- While you are learning about the culture of others, also take the time to explain your organization's culture.

Source: Society for Human Resource Management (2012).

workplace. Organizational culture and practices that present barriers to different aspects of diversity should be examined, challenged, and removed when necessary. A good example of a starting-point for addressing diversity in different settings is the University of California San Francisco's university system Non-Discrimination Statement, extracted from UCSF's Principles of a University Community:

- Recognize, value, and affirm that social diversity contributes richness to the University community and enhances the quality of campus life for individuals and groups.
- Take pride in various achievements and celebrate differences.

As these principles suggest, workplace diversity in a university setting can provide tremendous benefits in terms of improved morale, outside-the-box thinking, greater teamwork, and an atmosphere of mutual understanding and respect.

Cox (1991) defines guiding principles for managing diversity in a university setting as "planning and implementing organizational systems and practices to manage people so that the potential advantages of diversity are maximized while its potential disadvantages are minimized." These principles are expanded as follows.

- Managing diversity well provides a distinct advantage in an era when flexibility and creativity are keys to competitiveness.
- An organization needs to be flexible and adaptable to meet new customer needs.
- Heterogeneity promotes creativity, and heterogeneous groups have been shown to produce better solutions to problems and a higher level of critical analysis. This can be a vital asset at a time when the campus is undergoing tremendous change and self-examination to find new and more-effective ways to operate.
- With effective management of diversity, the campus develops a reputation as an employer of choice. Not only will you have the ability to attract the best talent from a shrinking labor pool, you can save time and money in recruitment and turnover costs.

- The campus will fulfill its role as a public institution by reflecting the diversity of the state as well as meeting the increasing demand to provide informed services to an increasingly diverse customer base.

Some of the skills needed to transform the organizational culture so that it more closely reflects the values of a diverse workforce are:

- An understanding and acceptance of managing diversity concepts;
- Recognition that diversity is threaded through every aspect of management;
- Self-awareness, in terms of understanding one's own culture, identity, biases, prejudices, and stereotypes;
- Willingness to challenge and change institutional practices that present barriers to different groups.

The following are examples of best management practices in hiring strategies, in relation to diversity.

- Specify the need for skills to work effectively in a diverse work environment.
- Make sure that good-faith efforts are made to recruit a diverse applicant pool.
- Focus on the job requirements in the interview, and assess experience, but also
  - Consider transferable skills and demonstrated competencies, such as analytical, organizational, communication, coordination.
  - Remember that prior experience does not necessarily mean effectiveness or success on the job.
- Use a panel interview format.
- Ensure that the committee is diverse with respect to unit affiliation, job classification, length of service, variety of life experiences, etc. to represent different perspectives and eliminate bias from the selection process.
- Ensure that appropriate accommodations are made for disabled applicants.
- Know your own biases and stereotypes.

CASE EXAMPLES

Disparate treatment in hiring remains a major problem. The Equal Employment Opportunity Commission (EEOC) reported that employers are still barring large groups of people from jobs based on race, sex, age, and other prohibited reasons that are described in the following case examples.

- EEOC lawyers recounted a hiring case that was litigated against WalMart. The case arose out of a charge by two deaf applicants who were expressly denied employment by the company because they were deaf. As part of a negotiated settlement, the company aired a commercial on Arizona television stations featuring the two, telling viewers in sign language, with a voiceover, their story and educating the public about the nation's equal employment laws. A video of that commercial was shown at the meeting.
- Other EEOC officials cited recent agency lawsuits. An EEOC attorney detailed the EEOC's suit against Area Temps, a northeast Ohio temporary labor agency, which agreed to pay $650,000 in July 2010 for its systematic practice of considering and assigning (or rejecting) job applicants by race, sex, Hispanic national origin, and age. The EEOC said that Area Temps used code words to describe its clients and applicants for discriminatory purposes, such as "chocolate cupcake" for young African American women, "hockey player" for young white males, "figure skater" for white females, "basketball player" for black males, and "small hands" for women in general.
- An employee, who worked for Area Temps, told the Commission that the company fired her for refusing to help it conceal evidence from the EEOC. Lopez-Rodriguez said she had left demographically coded cards, which the company used to discriminate, in her Rolodex, instead of cooperating with the company's request to destroy them prior to the EEOC investigator's visit.
- A company which provides janitorial services to Chicago's O'Hare Airport, agreed to pay $3 million after the EEOC sued the company for failing to recruit and hire African Americans. An EEOC supervisory trial attorney in Chicago who handled the Scrub case said an economist's report showed that "the statistical disparity in hiring rates between African-American applicants and non-African-American applicants was so high that there is effectively zero probability that Scrub's failure to hire African-Americans occurred by chance."
- A job applicant, who was one of several African American discrimination victims in the Scrub case, told the panel how she tried to apply for a job at Scrub. Despite janitorial experience and 15 advertised openings, she said she was told she would be contacted if the company was interested. By contrast, a Hispanic woman who applied at the same time was asked to stay for an interview. An African American friend "went to Scrub's office later that same day. She told me that she

had a similar experience. The receptionist took her application and told her that someone would call her if Scrub was interested in her. While she was there, there were four Hispanic women and one Hispanic man filling out applications. All five of the other applicants were asked to stay for an interview," but she was not.

IMPLICATIONS FOR THE FUTURE OF A DIVERSE WORKPLACE

Vaughn (2006) reported that one of the future challenges faced by organizations striving to foster a more diverse workforce is simply acknowledging the differences in people. A major challenge is miscommunication within organizations. Better competencies will need to be developed to improve effective communication in diverse organizational workplaces. Future challenges to communication that need to be addressed by employers and employees include self-awareness, empathy, strategic planning and decision-making. Self-awareness refers to how one's behavior affects another person and the willingness to modify this behavior based on understanding how it is understood by the recipient. Empathy enables the receiver to see beyond the literal meaning of a message and consider the communicator's feelings, values, assumptions, and needs. The important aspect of strategic planning and decision-making is that communication is understood by all members of the workforce.

It is equally important that the substance of the messages is clearly conveyed and carefully selected. Brownell (2003) indicated that, by having opportunities to express dissent, individuals can begin to gather collective support and create a voice for the marginalized members so they can have a collective voice to maximize their potential and opportunities. As diversity issues change over time, government agencies and businesses will be facing rapid and continuing demographic changes in consumer markets and labor pools. The future success of the workplace will depend upon helping people to work and understand each other better (Harvey & Allard, 2012).

Best practice examples demonstrated by organizations that have successfully created inclusive environments supporting and championing diversity, will need to be emulated. MentorNet is a good example of a company that has successfully created diversity by using mentors in the workplace. This online mentoring organization focuses on women and under-represented minorities in the future-oriented STEM (Science, Technology, Engineering, and Mathematics) fields. The organization is unique in that it provides women and under-represented minorities the chance to seek mentors to discuss how to overcome diversity obstacles in their fields and eventually their workplace.

Workers can be effectively involved in downsizing efforts by, for example, choosing to reduce working hours in order to prevent drastic reductions in the workforce. Employees and employers can agree to fair reductions in wages to minimize the hardships of massive layoffs. Employers could take the initiative to retrain and/or relocate workers to take new jobs or to initiate creative workplace assignments.

There are opportunities for employers to facilitate the implementation of fair and effective strategic plans that support the initiatives and programs described earlier. This has a special importance to workers who are at immediate risk of being laid off. It will be necessary to develop comprehensive government policies to enable flexible downsizing strategies. Any successful policy will need the support of business, industry, and community-based programs to help mitigate the adverse consequences of the economic downturn that will continue to affect the lives of people for years to come. It is necessary to make clear distinctions about the special challenges that ethnic minorities and other diverse groups face. This requires a clear understanding of the demographic characteristics related to their culture, language, disparities and socioeconomic status. Failure to address issues of diversity ignores many of the problems that minorities and other marginalized individuals experience that are related to ongoing life situations such as poverty, inadequate housing, crime, and discrimination.

SUMMARY

The recent economic downturn has had a direct impact on diversity in the workplace. It is obvious that the issue is too complex for a simplistic effort to be capable of addressing all of the factors related to diversity in the workplace. A diverse workforce is a direct reflection of a rapidly changing society and unstable economy. Respecting and promoting individual differences brings great benefit to organizations. A diverse workplace can benefit both the employee and the employer. It has been demonstrated that a diverse workplace will create a competitive edge and increased work productivity. Positive diversity management benefits employees by creating a fair and non-discriminatory environment where everyone has access to opportunities and challenges. Organizations with a diverse workforce must use effective management tools to educate employees and managers concerning the value of diversity. This will include fairness based upon laws, policies, and regulations.

In the economic downturn, with the accompanying tendency to downsize, companies, organizations, and industries must resist the temptation to employ radical and unfair job displacement methods. By devising creative and equitable ways to involve workers in the decision-making process, management can lessen the pain of economic downsizing. Many businesses have experienced these difficulties in dealing with an increasingly diverse workforce during normal economic cycles. The economic downturn has created even greater concerns that require addressing different approaches in motivating and communicating with workers who have different backgrounds and lifestyles. It is understandable that the financial implications have been particularily devastating for many diverse groups such as minorities. The long-term outlook for their quality of life for diverse employees is even more dire. This chapter has suggested a number of ways to address the long-term needs and implications of a diverse workforce.

REFERENCES

Barbee, D. (2010). *Workplace discrimination complaints are up in Texas, U.S.* Retrieved from <http://www.mcclatchydc.com/2010/01/12/82104/workplace-discrimination-complaints.html>.

Bennett, N., Martin, C., Bies, R. J., & Brockner, J. (1995). Coping with a layoff: A longitudinal study of victims. *Journal of Management, 21*, 1025–1040.

Blank, R., & Slipp, S. (1994). *Voices of diversity: Real people talk about problems and solutions in a workplace where everyone is not alike.* New York: American Management Association.

Brownell, J. (2003). Developing receiver-centered communication in diverse organizations. *Listening Professional, 2*(*1*), 5–25.

Bullard, R. D., & Wright, B. H. (1987). Blacks and the environment. *Humboldt Journal of Social Relations, 14*(*1,2*), 165–184.

Burns, C., & Ali, S. (2012). Equality and diversity in the health service: Evidenced-led culture change. *Journal of Psychological Issues in Organizational Culture, 3*(*1*), 41–60.

Church, T. (1995). *Cultural Diversity in Organizations.* San Francisco, CA: Berrett-Koehler Publishers.

Cox, T. (1991). The multicultural organization. *Academy of Management Executives, 5*(*2*), 34–47.

Dooley, D., Catalano, R., & Wilson, G. (1994). The Epidemiologic Catchment Area Study. *American Journal of Community Psychology, 22*(*6*), 745–765.

Esty, K., Griffin, R., & Schorr, M. (1995). *Workplace diversity: A manager's guide to solving problems and turning diversity into competitive advantage.* Avon, MA: Adams Media Corporation.

Fine, M. G. (1996). Cultural diversity in the workplace: the state of the field. *Journal of Business Communication, 33*(*4*), 485–502.

Fryer, D., & Payne, R. (1986). Being unemployed. In C. L. Cooper, & I. Robertson (Eds.), *Review of industrial and organizational psychology*. Chichester: Wiley.

Hacker, A. (1992). *Two nations: black and white, separate, hostile, unequal*. New York: Charles Scribner's Sons.

Harvey, C. P., & Allard, M. J. (2012). *Understanding and managing diversity: readings, cases, and exercises* (5th ed.). Boston: Pearson.

International Labour Office (2011). *Racial discrimination and the global economic downturn*. Retrieved from <http://www.ilo.org/global/publications/magazines-and-journals/world-of-work-magazine/articles/WCMS_165284/lang–en/index.htm>.

Kessler, R. C., Turner, J. B., & House, J. S. (1988). Effects of unemployment on workers and their families. *Journal of Social Issues*, *44*(4), 69–85.

Kluegel, J. R., & Smith, E. R. (1986). *Beliefs about inequality: Americans' views of what is and what ought to be*. New York: Aldine De Gruyter.

Level Playing Field Institute (2003). *The how-fair study 2003: How opportunities in the workplace and fairness affect intergroup relations*. Retrieved from <http://www.lpfi.org/sites/default/files/howfairreport.pdf>.

Liem, & Liem (1988). Psychological effects of unemployment on workers and their families. *Journal of Social Issues*, *44*(4), 87–105.

Marsiglia, F. F., & Kulis, S. (2009). *Diversity, oppression, and change*. Chicago: Lyceum.

Matos, K., & Galinsky, E. (2012). 2012 *National Study of Employers*. <http://familiesandwork.org/site/research/reports/NSE_2012.pdf>.

Obama, B. (2006). *The audacity of hope*. New York: Crown Publishers.

Parvis, L (2003). Diversity and effective leadership in multicultural workplaces. *Journal of Environmental Health*, *65*, 37–38.

Reidenbach, L., & Weller, C. (2010). *The state of minorities in 2010: Minorities are suffering disproportionately in the recession*. Washington, DC: Center for American Progress.

Robinson, G., & Dechant, K. (1997). Building a case for diversity. *The Academy of Management Executives*, *11*(3), 21–31.

Robinson, K.-S. (2002). *U.S. must focus on diversity or face decline in competiveness. The Society for Human Resource Management (SHRM)*. Retrieved from <http://www.shrm.org>.

Society for Human Resource Management (2010). *Workplace diversity practices: How has diversity and inclusion changed over time? SHRM poll*. Retrieved from <http://www.shrm.org/Research/SurveyFindings/Articles/Pages/WorkplaceDiversityPractices.aspx>.

Stack, S. (1981). Divorce and suicide: A time series analysis, 1933-1970. *Journal of Family Issues*, *2*, 77–90.

Takaki, R. (1987). *From different shores: Perspectives on race and ethnicity in America*. New York: Oxford University Press.

Takaki, R. (1993). *A different mirror: A history of multicultural America* (*First Edition*). Boston, MA: Little, Brown and Company.

US Department of Labor (1994). *The employment situation: December 1994*. Retrieved from <http://www.bls.gov/news.release/history/empsit_010695.txt>.

US Department of Labor (2011). *Labor force characteristics by race and ethnicity, 2011*. Retrieved from <http://www.bls.gov/cps/cpsrace2011.pdf>.

US Equal Employment Opportunity Commission (2010). *EEOC charge receipts by state (includes U.S. territories) and basis for 2010*. Retrieved from <http://www1.eeoc.gov/eeoc/statistics/enforcement/state_10.cfm>.

Vaughn, B. (2006). *High impact diversity consulting*. San Francisco, CA: Diversity Training University International Publications Division.

Vinokur, A., Van Ryn, R., Gramlish, E. M., & Price, R. H. (1991). *Journal of Psychology*, *756*, 710–730.

Walker, D. (2010). *Is it the recession or Obama backlash? Something is fueling workplace discrimination*. Retrieved from <http://www.alternet.org/speakeasy/2010/10/06/is-it-the-recession-or-obama-backlash-something-is-fueling-workplace-discrimination?page = entire%2C1>.
Wexley, K. N., & Silverman, S. B. (1993). *Working scared*. Retrieved from <http://ia701208.us.archive.org/8/items/WorkingScared/WexleyKennethN.-WorkingScared.pdf>.
White, R. H. (2004). Affirmative action in the workplace: The signficance of Grutter?. *Scholarly Works*. Paper 305. Retrieved from <http://digitalcommons.law.uga.edu/fac_artchop/305>.

FURTHER READING

Civil Rights Organization Staff. (2002). *Affirmative action*. Available at <http://www.civilrights.org/library/permanent_collection/resources/glossary.html>.
Kenyon, A. (n.d.). The importance of diversity in the workplace. *WeLead Online Magazine*. <http://www.leadingtoday.org/Onmag/2005%20Archives/may05/ak-may05.html>.
Nuttman-Shwartz, O., & Gadot, L. (2012). Social factors and mental health symptoms among women who have experienced involuntary job loss. *Anxiety, Stress & Coping*, *25*(3), 275–290.
Raber, M. J., & Conrad, A. P. (1999). Distributive justice in the workplace. *Social Thought*, *19*(1), 15–28.
Santana, J. (2003). *Learn to harness the full potential of a diverse workforce*. TechRepublic website. Retrieved August 16, 2012 from <http://www.techrepublic.com/article/learn-to-harness-the-full-potential-of-a-diverse-workforce/5054005?tag = content;siu-container>.

CHAPTER 6

Workaholics: Understanding and Changing Work-Addicted Behavior[1]

INTRODUCTION

Americans are among the most work-obsessed people in the world. American workers use 2 days less of annual vacation time than they are given, often feeling, with considerable evidence, that taking a vacation gives a negative message to employers. American workers have less vacation time and far less maternity leave and sick leave than their European counterparts. They also work a longer week than Europeans, where the average is 35 hours per week compared with 40 in the US. The pressure on workers to produce, to put in an increasing number of hours, and to stay late in a pressure cooker atmosphere of produce or be downsized, has resulted in an increasing number of workaholics, often not by their own choice.

Linn (2009) reports that a combination of good health, inability to deal with spare time, continued interest in their jobs, economic necessity, and the other rewards of work are pushing some Americans to stay in the workforce long past traditional retirement age. Approximately 7% of people age 75 or older were in the labor force as of June, 2009—up from 5% a decade ago. That translates into more than 1.1 million people working past age 74—up from 750,000 a decade ago.

UNDERSTANDING THE CONCEPT OF WORK ADDICTIONS

Griffiths (2005) writes that "the most obvious sign that someone is a workaholic is when work and work-related concerns preoccupy a person's life to the neglect of everything else in it. What starts out as love of work

[1] Portions of this chapter first appeared in the senior author's book on workaholics in retirement (Glicken, 2010).

Treating Worker Dissatisfaction During Economic Change
DOI: http://dx.doi.org/10.1016/B978-0-12-397006-0.00006-3

can often end up with the person developing perfectionist, then obsessional traits" (p. 97).

Machlowitz (1980) reports that workaholics share the following six traits: They are intense, energetic, competitive, and driven; they have self-doubts; they prefer work to leisure; they work anytime, anywhere; they make the most of their time; and, they blur the distinctions between business and pleasure. As a consequence, it is not uncommon for workaholics to have major health problems including stress-induced illnesses, chronic fatigue, and increased anxiety levels.

Perhaps it would be useful to clarify the difference between positive work addiction and unhealthy work addictions, or workaholism. Workaholism can be defined as valuing work over any other activity when, and this is important, it affects physical and emotional health, the quality of work, and family, loved ones, and friendships. There are a number of very hard-working people who put in long hours, but, when they are free, they give back to their loved ones and enjoy relationships and outside activities. When work becomes all-consuming and someone goes well beyond what is necessary to do the job well and has no other interests or activities beyond work, we might call it a negative addiction to work. Without constant work, a true workaholic becomes anxious and depressed. A negative work addiction is a recurring obsession with joyless work.

It is true that many aspects of work are joyless and unpleasant but we put up with them by getting pleasure from other aspects of the job and from our outside activities and loved ones. And certainly, in this down economy, many people work hard just to keep their jobs. It's not a work addiction when someone is trying to survive. Real workaholics have few, if any, outside interests. They let family life fall apart. They often have health problems and suffer from depression and deep insecurities. Like any addiction, they repeat behaviors that are destructive, even though they know better and find it difficult or impossible to change.

It's important to keep in mind that work addicts should not be confused with people who are simply hard workers, love their work, and go the extra mile to finish a project. By contrast, workaholics constantly think about work and, without work, feel anxious and depressed. They're often difficult to get along with and push others as hard as they push themselves. Saul (2009, p. 1) suggests the following differences between hard workers and workaholics:

1. Hard workers think of work as a required and, at times, a pleasurable obligation. Workaholics see work as a way to distance themselves from unwanted feelings and relationships.
2. Hard workers keep work in check so that they can be available to their family and friends. Workaholics believe that work is more important than anything else in their lives, including family and friends.
3. Workaholics get excitement from meeting impossible demands. Hard workers don't.
4. Hard workers can take breaks from work whereas workaholics can't and think about work regardless of what they're doing or who they're with.

An interesting way of understanding the difference between hard workers and workaholics is found in research by Douglas and Morris (2006), who argue that what we typically call a workaholic, with its negative connotations, may more correctly be understood when we look at that person's motivation to work. The researchers found that people work hard for four reasons:

1. Because they want the financial rewards of hard work—Douglas and Morris call these people hard workers who are "material goal seekers;"
2. Because they find little enjoyment from leisure activities—they might better be called "low leisure" hard workers;
3. Because they love the perks and might more reasonably be called "perkaholics" than workaholics—perks are the intangibles of work and might include friendships, an easy commute to work, great working conditions, good health plans, etc.
4. Finally, there are those who work long hours for its own sake—these might properly be called workaholics.

We would add a fifth type of motivation: people who work a great deal because they simply love what they're doing. We know many university professors who can't wait to work on projects when they get up in the morning. They have a love affair with the work they do and consider it a blessing to have the time and support to work on special projects in addition to their teaching responsibilities. This isn't to say that some of them aren't workaholics. Most of them are like everyone else but they love their jobs and work for salaries far below what they could make in the business world. Many of them continue to work full-time or part-time well beyond normal retirement age, not for the money or because they need to stay busy, but because they love what they're doing and leaving the academic life would be unthinkable.

TEN TYPES OF WORKAHOLICS

Robinson (2001) suggests four types of workaholics:

- **Type 1: The Relentless Workaholic**. Relentless workaholics work all the time. They believe that work is more important than relationships or anything else in life. According to Robinson they are perfectionists who demand perfectionism in others, have many projects going at once, and are admired for their hard work and competence by others outside of their families.
- **Type 2: The Procrastinating Workaholic**. The procrastinating workaholic waits until the last possible minute, goes into a panic, and then works frantically to finish a task. Unlike relentless workaholics whose productivity is usually quite high, procrastinating workaholics go through long periods where they do not work. Robinson believes that the reason they go through long periods of non-activity is that they are so preoccupied with perfection that they cannot start a project.
- **Type 3: The High Stimulus-Seeking Workaholic**. A third type is the workaholic who is easily bored and constantly seeks stimulation and excitement. Robinson believes that some workaholics seek excitement in a relatively safe way by "creating tight work deadlines, keeping many projects going at one time, taking on big challenges at work, and having the chronic inability to relax without intense stimulation. Others live on the edge and engage in high-risk jobs or activities, such as playing the stock market, parachute jumping, or working triage in a hospital emergency room" (p. 43). High stimulus-seeking workaholics are easily bored with detail, have difficulty following through, and get their satisfaction by creating new projects.
- **Type 4: The Bureaupathic Workaholic**. Bureaupathic Workaholics are the folks we all hate to be on committees with. There isn't a rule, policy, standard, or ploy they won't use to control projects, committee meetings, or work assignments. Their primary function is to set up road blocks to the completion of projects. They think they bring order and rationality to the process but what they really bring is chaos and disruption, and they make easy projects impossible. The term

"bureaupathic" is used to imply the worst qualities of top-down organizations: that they are slow to change, illogical in the way decisions are made, primarily concerned with the quality of life of those who work in the organization and not the customers and clients supposedly served by a company or agency, and are endlessly rule and policy driven with little sense of the need to change even when the organization is in deep trouble. Bureaupathic workaholics prolong assignments and create additional work. Others may be ready to move on, but these workaholics hold everything up by overanalyzing, tearing ideas apart, and getting bogged down in minute detail. They drive everyone a little crazy.

The following six additional types of workaholics are suggested by Glicken (2010):

- **Type 5: The Loner Workaholic**. Type 5 is the withdrawn workaholic, who prefers to work alone. They work hard and want to be needed and approved of as well, but they do not want to be controlled or dominated. They prefer to keep their emotional distance from others. The loner workaholic prefers to be left alone to do their work.
- **Type 6: The Frightened Workaholic**. This type of workaholic is afraid of losing their job and, rather than having clear ideas of how to complete a task, worry constantly that the task isn't going to be done correctly or completed on time. While they work very hard it takes them much longer to do the job because much of their energy is spent being anxious and fearful about their work.
- **Type 7: The Burned-Out Workaholic**. This type of workaholic is so burned out they can hardly muster the energy to do the job but, out of a lack of other interests and activities or a dismal or nonexistent personal life, they keep working hard at jobs that give them no satisfaction and which they may actually dislike to the extent of becoming physically ill while they work. Without help, these people often develop depressions and anxiety-related problems that make work exceedingly difficult.
- **Type 8: The Incompetent Workaholic**. We like to think of workaholics as hard working and super productive but some workaholics have to work that much harder because, truth be told, they just don't have the ability to do the job. We've all known workaholics like this. They never take lunch breaks, stay late, come in over the weekend, but never seem to get much done. Rather than looking for psychological reasons for their work addiction, it might be better to think of

them as lacking competence. Moving into a less-demanding job would probably minimize their work addictions.

- **Type 9: The Dictatorial Workaholic.** This type of workaholic gets sadistic pleasure out of working others to death and uses insults and threats to get others to work more than is necessary. They use intimidation and put downs to eliminate rewards and never give positive feedback. While they thrive on the pain they inflict on others, including family, they also benefit from the hard work and achievement of others. Since they never give others credit for their achievement and make it their own, they often look highly competent to outsiders. This type of workaholic often rises to the top of organizations. It comes as a surprise to others not familiar with how the dictatorial workaholic functions that they create such unhappiness and often are so disliked by others in an organization.
- **Type 10: The Manic-Depressive Workaholic.** Occasionally we find people who achieve at a very high level because they have manic episodes that last long enough for them to get incredible amounts of work done. During manic highs, they may work for days without sleep before succumbing to the inevitable low they experience as the chemical nature of their condition shifts to depression. Some people have manic highs all of the time. What distinguishes them from other types of workaholics is that there is often something very troubling about their behavior and the work they produce. They appear to be high on drugs (and sometimes they are). We've read work written by students and employees during manic phases that is often just gibberish.

THE IMPACT OF WORK ADDICTIONS ON RELATIONSHIPS AND FAMILY LIFE

The negative impact of workaholism on families and relationships has been written about at length. Oates (1971) observed that workaholics are socially inadequate in their home lives and have difficulties with personal relationships. Robinson (1989) suggested that excessive work often prevents workaholics from forming and maintaining intimate relationships. Killinger (1991) found that workaholics have limited intimacy with spouses and use work as a substitute for all other relationships. Other researchers have found that workaholism results in much higher levels of spousal dissatisfaction and divorce rates (Klaft & Kleiner, 1988), less frequent sexual intercourse (Pietropinto, 1986), and a lack of sensitivity to the feelings of others (Engstrom & Juroe, 1979). Jackson (1992) found that workaholics tend to be far more irritable at work and in their personal lives than those who were not work addicted.

In terms of the effect of the workaholism of parents on children, Oates (1971) found that children saw their parents as preoccupied with work, always in a rush to get somewhere, were often irritable and lacked a sense of humor, and seemed to be depressed about their work. Robinson (1989) found that many adult children of workaholics suffer greater depression, higher anxiety, and greater obsessive-compulsive tendencies than adult children of non-workaholics. A study comparing adult children of workaholics with adult children of alcoholics (Carroll & Robinson, 2000) indicated that adult children of workaholics had higher scores on depression than adults from alcoholic homes and adults from non-workaholic homes.

To be fair, O'Driscoll and Brady (2004) reported that, although the literature tended to suggest that workaholics have problems in their personal lives, the authors' research failed to find a great deal of difference between the personal lives of workaholics and those of non-workaholics. They point out that it's often difficult to differentiate between people who are work addicted and those who just work hard because many of us work very hard. Further, the term workaholic is often vague and may not be used correctly. Our observations of retired people who exhibit workaholic characteristics is that many of them, if asked, have satisfying personal relationships, but, when spouses and children are asked, they often talk about the negative side of trying to maintain a relationship with someone who puts all of his or her energy into work, and how little is left over for them. Because there are certainly benefits of work addictions, including affluence and status, many spouses and children put up with work addictions because there is so much to gain from the labor of the workaholic spouse and parent.

CHANGING WORKAHOLIC BEHAVIOR

Workaholics are sometimes not the best candidates for counseling and psychotherapy because they deny they have a problem. Cochran and Rabinowitz (2003) argue that people with addictive personalities have been culturally programmed to repress the emotional aspects of their problems. This pertains to all aspects of problems, including those in the workplace, in relationships, with children, with parents and siblings, and in intimate relationships.

However, people with addictive personalities often respond positively to help when it is offered in a collaborative way. Rather than being critical of their beliefs and attitudes, something they've heard throughout their lives, most people with work addictions want counselors to understand how well they've done in their lives and how successful they've been, even if the results of their success are sometimes problematic. Chapter 11 goes into more detail about additional approaches to help people with work-related problems, including the use of self-help groups, but two helping approaches are briefly outlined here: brief counseling and guided reading.

Brief Counseling

Brief counseling assumes that people are having problems now because of a number of reasons and tries to sort out the major ones and help the person resolve them in five to ten sessions. Most brief counseling uses cognitive therapy, a form of counseling that tries to get people to understand the irrational things they say to themselves that end up getting them into trouble. Some irrational ideas by workaholics to reinforce their behavior include the following:

1. **Work is the most important thing in my life.** It's true that some people involved in very important work believe their work trumps everything else, but for most of us, when it's more important than our health, our families, and the pleasures we might get out of life, it's an obsession. Making work the most important thing in our lives tends to push people away, inhibits real intimacy with others, and makes children and family secondary. When work is no longer available, as in forced early retirement or being laid off, it leaves us with nothing to take its place.
2. **I won't succeed unless I work harder than anyone else around me.** That's possible, but how do you measure working harder than anyone else? Some people don't need to work as hard, because they work smart. Others are naturals at the job or have more ability. Working harder doesn't necessarily mean that you'll be successful. The better idea is that you learn the job and work smart and hard but not to the extent that putting in more hours than anyone else will actually lead to more success.

3. **If I don't succeed I'll be a failure.** It's possible to fail but it doesn't make one a failure. Failing is part of the human experience. We all fail at some point or another but we needn't then define ourselves as failures.
4. **Unless I work very hard, everything at work will fall apart.** This irrational idea is what therapists call catastrophizing, or the idea that unless we can control everything in life by working hard and being eternally vigilant, everything will fall apart. People who try to control everything are often prone to anxiety problems or have what we've come to call OCD (Obsessive Compulsive Disorder). For many people with OCD, the work required to keep anything bad from happening often leads to more time spent in repetitive behavior than in actual work.
5. **If I can't do it the right way, there's no point in doing it at all.** This is the perfectionist's motto but, in reality, we do many things each day that we don't do well. The fact is that, whatever we do, there's always someone who does it as well or better than most of us. Demanding perfection in everything we do is a recipe for unhappiness.
6. **It's essential that everyone like me.** The reality is that most people might like us but, for reasons we can't explain, some people won't. Trying to be liked is one of those no-win approaches to life that gets many people into difficulty. While we hope we can get along with everyone and have good working relationships, we can't expect everyone to like us.
7. **Work is the only way I have of dealing with the demons that haunt my life.** Better to get some good help to rid yourself of demons from the past than to work yourself to death trying to get rid of them. Many workaholics use work to deal with feelings of insecurity and lack of self-esteem, but the workplace is only part of your life. When you get home at night, the demons are still there. Work has done nothing to drive them away.
8. **If I don't continue working very hard, I'll become bored, depressed, and anxious.** In fact you might, but the time to start dealing with fears about the future is now. What's irrational about this idea is that nothing is inevitable. If you feel that way then surely you'll experience all of the unhappiness you've been predicting for yourself.
9. **It's not *what* you know, it's *who* you know.** Of course, this is sometimes true but, for most of us, it isn't. Even if we have special relationships with people who can make things happen for us, we don't always want to ask favors for fear of alienating them. Giving

people that much power over us is also a mistake since we assume they can, and will, do us favors if we ask. Often they won't. And finally, most of us know that calling in a favor can sometimes be costly. It's not who we know, it's what we know and how we use it that impresses people and gets us the rewards we desire.

10. **It'll never get done right unless I do it myself.** This is one of the cardinal rules followed by most workaholics. It's irrational because there are many things we're not good at and other people are. Not using others means that you might do the job more poorly than they would. It's also irrational because, in any job, doing everything means that you've loaded yourself down with heaps of work because you don't trust people to do their jobs. Not being able to delegate is inconsistent with the way most organizations operate, and it tends to offend people. Further, it's an indication that you think so little of your co-workers that you dismiss their capabilities—never a good way to be, in most organizations.

An Example of Brief Counseling

Nelson Byers is a 63-year-old executive in a manufacturing company who has just been told that, because the company is facing severe financial problems, he is being giving a generous severance package but will no longer have a job. Nelson is experiencing anxiety about the future and depression over the loss of his job well before he thought it was time to retire. Nelson sought out a licensed psychologist who specializes in short-term cognitively oriented counseling.

The psychologist explained his approach to Nelson, who thought it made sense. He also said that he expected Nelson to do a good deal of reading and that, in any event, he could only provide 10 or fewer sessions. In the type of help he provided, the person receiving help had to do a lot of the work, so Nelson shouldn't expect the psychologist to do it for him. The more Nelson read and asked questions the sooner he'd stop feeling so badly.

The psychologist asked Nelson to discuss his feelings about the loss of his job. Nelson replied, "I worked my ass off for that company. I put in longer hours than anyone should ever be asked to work and look what they did to me." The following is a verbatim dialogue between Nelson and the psychologist.

The psychologist asked, "What did they do?"

Nelson (N): "They fired me, for God's sake, the S.O.Bs."

Psychologist (P): "That's really tough and I can imagine how upsetting it is after all the years you spent working for the company but isn't the company going bankrupt? I'm hearing you say they should have kept you on even though the company is going under."

N: "I was important. I was a big deal in the company. I should have been one of the last ones to go not one of the first."

P: "Why do you think you were one of the first?"

N: "Because the bastards never did appreciate my hard work."

P: "By hard work do you mean the number of hours you worked or what you achieved."

N: "Everyone knows that I worked my butt off."

P: "But you haven't answered the question."

N: "I mean I worked hard. Are you saying it didn't accomplish much?"

P: "I'm asking."

N: "Yeah, you're going to say I was a workaholic, right? Work hard but accomplish little."

P: "Are you a workaholic?"

N: "I've heard that before. Some people thought so."

P: "What did those people say?"

N: "That I worked hard but didn't do much."

P: "Is it true?"

N: "No way but you can see what they did to me. They must have thought my work wasn't so red hot."

P: "But you equate hard work with accomplishment. Might that be the way you approached the job?"

N: "I was always very cautious at work. I didn't want to make mistakes."

P: "In this helping approach I use, we try and figure out the illogical things people tell themselves that get them into trouble. It sounds like you've been telling yourself that the harder you try not to make mistakes, the more you'll control the outcome, but it doesn't lead to better work. It's just a way to protect yourself."

N: "That's what my wife says. She says I can't make decisions and that I always do the most cautious thing possible."

P: "Who taught you that caution beats risk?"

N: "My dad. He never took a risk in his life. He figured the more cautious you were, the more you had control and were vigilant, the better things would be."

P: "And did it work for him?"

N: "He was a failure at everything he ever did including being a father."

P: "And you? How would you assess yourself?"

N: "Hell, I tried but my kids hate me and my wife's been talking divorce after 35 years of marriage. I guess you could say I haven't been so successful but at least I made better money than the old man and I had higher status."

P: "That's certainly something to be proud of but as you move to this next stage in your life, might it be good to think through the strategies of caution that you've used at work with the many extra hours you put in to make certain everything was controlled for and perhaps use some different strategies, particularly as they relate to your family?"

N: "Looks like I'll have lots of time to be with my family if they'll let me. What should I tell them?"

P: "Were it me I'd explain what you did at work, and why, and how you know it pushed them away from you and that you apologize from the bottom of your heart and want to make things a lot better."

N: "You don't think they'd laugh at me?"

P: "Would you laugh knowing what you've just gone through at work?"

N: "No, I surely wouldn't."

The psychologist gave Nelson some material to read about cautious and controlling behavior as well as the type of counseling he was using—cognitive therapy. He asked Nelson to read the articles and email back his take on the material and how it applied to him. At first Nelson used excuses or gave feedback that was intelligent but didn't really apply to him. Nelson also had trouble getting into his own reasons for the job loss and kept blaming the company, but after a few sessions he got down to work and started understanding his own involvement in the problems at work. He also had a family session and, much to his amazement and surprise, his family was very understanding. Nelson broke down and cried during the family meeting. For once in a long time he felt the deep connection he once had with his children and wife. It was a very moving experience for him.

Nelson has enough money to retire early and live well but he wants to continue working. Over the years he has developed a network of colleagues and, after contacting them, found many of them were also the victims of the recession. They banded together as a cooperative and, after 6 months of working at it, he now has enough work to keep him occupied. He struggles with putting too much time into making things perfect so he won't make mistakes but he's doing better and his wife helps. They've agreed that, no matter what, Nelson will have dinner with his family every night, go to social and cultural functions together, and never ever work on Sundays, which is a designated family day.

In a follow-up meeting with his therapist, Nelson said, "You introduced me to a new way of thinking. I had a hard time with it at first because it was a lot more comfortable to keep doing what I always did. . .

throw work at any problem. I'm not sure any workaholic can ever say that they're really happy, but I keep pinching myself to make sure I'm telling myself the truth, and you know what? I'm a lot happier than I've been in a long, long time."

Guided Reading

Many people use the Internet to gather information about emotional problems. The purposes of finding information about one's problems are: (1) to provide information; (2) to gain insight; (3) to find solutions; (4) to stimulate discussion of problems; (5) to suggest new values and attitudes; and (6) to understand how others have coped with problems similar to one's own (Pardeck, 1995).

Novels, poetry, music, films and videos can also be particularly useful because they often depict issues that many of us are trying to resolve in our own lives (problems with children, problems at work, relationship problems, and problems with drinking and other addictions, for example).

When we work with clients, we help them find articles online that will give them some understanding of their problem and will also help them resolve it. We try to use articles that are written in a clear and understandable way. Many professional articles are written for other professionals and are difficult to understand if you have no background or training in the mental health profession.

Case Example

Jenny Blair is a 62-year-old accountant and a workaholic. She works 80 hours a week and sometimes more. The amount of work she gets done isn't at all in keeping with the number of hours she works, and Jenny has begun to realize that much of the time she puts into her work is wasted. She doesn't understand this at all, and the anger her long hours have produced in her husband threatens their marriage. I helped Jenny find a number of useful articles about workaholics. One in particular about perfectionism hit a core in Jenny, and she began to talk about her perfectionistic mother who was also fearful and anxious much of the time. Jenny wondered to what extent her mother's perfectionism had affected her. The more articles she found on her own the more she was able to self-diagnose and treat the problem. She told the counselor:

"I've always been able to figure out what to do when I have a problem but in the past 5 years as I get closer to retirement I've begun putting in many more hours than are needed to do the work. The articles I read suggested that this was a form

of anxiety and that letting go of work was difficult for many people as they got older. I guess many of us start wondering if we're going to be useless when we stop working. I found the articles very helpful and talking to them with my counselor sort of helped use the information in the articles to focus on my problems".

"I found many articles just using the word 'workaholic' in a Goggle search. I also used words like 'perfectionists' and 'adult anxiety.' Once I got proficient at using the Internet I was able to use my husband's website at his work which allowed me to read professional articles on a browser called 'EbsoHost,' a social science and psychology website. I also found good material on 'Psych Abstracts.' Some of the articles were a bit difficult to understand but my husband, who's a statistician, helped me out. Knowing that I was trying to do something to help myself really motivated him to help me."

"Counseling is usually just 50 minutes long once a week. That doesn't mean you can't do some work when you're away from counseling. I did and what was a really upsetting and intrusive problem began to resolve itself in less than 10 weeks. I think that's pretty good considering how nutty I was getting and how angry my husband was starting to get. I work normal hours now and enjoy my marriage and I'm actively looking forward to retiring in a few years. I've worked hard all my life and I deserve some quality time. I may work part-time or I may not. Right now it just feels good to be normal again."

SUMMARY

One of the more common workplace problems in America today is that of workaholic behavior. As the chapter notes, hardworking individuals should not be confused with workaholics, and neither should people be thought of as workaholic if their jobs are demanding and require a great deal of time spent on work. Workaholics are those individuals who work hard for reasons that are dysfunctional and often include using work to fill in lonely time rather than dealing with loneliness, perfectionism, fear of failing, and a host of other problems that are better dealt with in counseling than through long, often unproductive hours spent on work. Ten types of workaholics are noted in the chapter. Irrational ideas that often lead to workaholic behavior are also provided along with several types of counseling that have potential to reduce workaholic behavior. Several case studies are provided that demonstrate how specific types of counseling can help change workaholic behavior.

REFERENCES

Carroll, J. J., & Robinson, B. E. (2000). Depression and parentification among adults as related to paternal workaholism and alcoholism. *The Family Journal*, *8*, 33–41.

Cochran, S. V., & Rabinowitz, F. E. (2003). Gender-sensitive recommendations for assessment and treatment of depression in men. *Professional Psychology: Research and Practice, 34*, 132–140.

Douglas, E. J., & Morris, R. L. (2006). Workaholic, or just hard worker? *Career Development International, 11*(5), 394–417.

Engstrom, T. W., & Juroe, D. J (1979). *The work trap.* Old Tappan, NJ: Fleming H. Revell.

Glicken, M. D. (2010). *Retirement for workaholics. Life after work in a downsized economy.* Santa Barbara, Ca: Praeger.

Griffiths, M. (2005). Workaholism is still a useful construct. *Addiction Research and Theory, 13*(2), 97–100.

Jackson, D. L. (1992). *Correlates of physical and emotional health among male and female workaholics.* Unpublished PhD thesis, University of Oregon.

Killinger, B. (1991). *Workaholics: The respectable addicts.* New South Wales, Australia: Simon & Schuster.

Klaft, R. P., & Kleiner, B. H. (1988). Understanding workaholics. *Business, 38*(3), 37–40.

Linn, A. (July 29, 2009). *When the golden years include a commute: Some are opting to work into their 70s, 80s and beyond.* Retrieved from the Internet August 3, 2009 at http://www.msnbc.msn.com/id/32089674/ns/business-personal_finance.

Machlowitz, M. (1980). *Workaholics.* New York: Mentor.

Oates, W. E. (1971). *Confessions of a workaholic: The facts about work addiction* New York: World Publishing Company.

O'Driscoll, P., & Brady, E. C. (2004). The impact of workaholism on personal relationships. *British Journal of Guidance & Counselling, 32*(No. 2); May 2004, pp 171–186.

Pardeck, J. T. (1995). Bibliotherapy: An innovative approach for helping children. *Early Childhood Development and Care, 110*, 83–88.

Pietropinto, A. (1986). The workaholic spouse: A survey analysis. *Medical Aspects of Human Sexuality,* May, 94–98

Robinson, B. (2001). *Chained to the desk.* New York: NYU Press.

Robinson, B. E (1989). *Work addiction: Hidden legacies of adult children.* Deerfield Beach, FL: Health Communications.

Saul, T. T. (2009). *Being a hard worker vs being a workaholic.* Retrieved from the Internet Aug. 12, 2009 at: <http://www.saulandsaul.com/resources/BEING + A + HARD + WORKER +VS + BEING + A + WORKAHOLIC.pdf>.

FURTHER READING

Scott, E. S. (2012). *Type A personality traits: Characteristics and effects of a type A personality.* About.com. Retrieved August 17, 2012 from <http://stress.about.com/od/understandingstress/a/type_a_person.htm>.

Bakalar, N. (2006). *Retirement contentment in reach for unhappy men.* NewYorkTimes.com. Retrieved from <http://www.nytimes.com/2006/04/04/health/psychology/04reti.html>.

Benson, E. (2003) *The many faces of perfectionism.* American Psychological Association website. Retrieved April 30, 2012 from <http://www.apa.org/monitor/nov03/manyfaces.aspx> .

Glicken, M. D. (2012). *The truth about workaholics.* Retrieved August 17, 2012 from <http://www.careercast.com/career-news/truth-about-workaholics>.

Anon. (2009). *Treatment for workaholics.* Addiction Treatment Magazine. Retrieved August 17, 2012 from <http://www.addictiontreatmentmagazine.com/addiction/treatment-for-workaholics/>.

CHAPTER 7

Workplace Violence

INTRODUCTION

The US Department of Labor (2011) defines workplace violence as any act or threat of physical violence, harassment, intimidation, or other threatening disruptive behavior that occurs at the workplace. It ranges from threats and verbal abuse to physical assaults and even homicide. Homicide is currently the fourth-leading cause of fatal occupational injuries in the United States. Of the 4,547 fatal workplace injuries that occurred in the United States in 2010, 506 were workplace homicides. Homicide is the leading cause of death for women in the workplace. Nearly 2 million American workers report having been victims of workplace violence each year. Unfortunately, many more cases go unreported.

Romano, Levi-Minzi, Rugala, and Van Hasselt (2011) report that an average of 20 workers are murdered each week in the US, making homicide the second highest cause of workplace deaths and the leading one for females. Eighteen thousand non-fatal violent crimes such as sexual and other assaults also occur each week while the victim is working, or about a million a year. The actual figures are probably higher since many are not reported. The Institute notes that "Certain dangerous occupations like police officers understandably have higher rates of homicide and non-fatal assaults. Nevertheless, postal workers who work in a safe environment have experienced so many fatalities due to job stress that 'going postal' has crept into our language" (p. 1).

Workplace violence can strike anywhere, anytime, and no one is immune. According to the US Department of Labor (2011), research has identified factors that may increase the risk of violence for some workers, which include exchanging money with the public and working with volatile, unstable people. Working alone or in isolated areas may also contribute to the potential for violence. Providing services and care, and working where alcohol is served may also impact the likelihood of violence. Additionally, time of day and location of work, such as working late at night or in areas with high crime rates, are also risk factors that should be considered when addressing issues of workplace violence.

Treating Worker Dissatisfaction During Economic Change
DOI: http://dx.doi.org/10.1016/B978-0-12-397006-0.00007-5

Among those with higher risk are workers who exchange money with the public, delivery drivers, healthcare professionals, public service workers, customer service agents, law enforcement personnel, and those who work alone or in small groups.

WORKER TO WORKER VIOLENCE

The following indicators of potential for workplace violence by co-workers have been identified by the Federal Bureau of Investigation's National Center for the Analysis of Violent Crime, Profiling and Behavioral Assessment Unit, in its analysis of past incidents of workplace violence (Romano, Levi-Minzi, Rugala, and Van Hasselt, 2011):

- Direct or veiled threats of harm to others in the workplace.
- Intimidating, belligerent, harassing, bullying, or other inappropriate and aggressive behavior.
- Numerous conflicts with supervisors and other employees.
- Bringing a weapon to the workplace, brandishing a weapon in the workplace, making inappropriate references to guns, or fascination with weapons.
- Statements showing fascination with incidents of workplace violence, statements indicating approval of the use of violence to resolve a problem, or statements indicating identification with perpetrators of workplace homicides.
- Statements indicating desperation (over family, financial, and other personal problems) to the point of contemplating suicide.
- Drug and/or alcohol abuse.
- Very erratic behavior with serious mood swings.

Each of these behaviors is a clear sign that something is wrong, and none should be ignored. Some behaviors require immediate police or security involvement whereas others constitute misconduct and require disciplinary action or an immediate referral to an employee assistance program. It is not advisable to rely on "profiles" or "early warning signs" to predict violent behavior. "Profiles" often suggest that people with certain characteristics, such as "loners" or "men in their forties," are potentially violent. Stereotyping of this kind will not help predict violence and may lead to unfair and destructive treatment of employees. The same must be said of the use of "early warning signs" such as assuming that anyone in therapy or those experiencing marital difficulties may be at risk of workplace violence. Most of us experience emotional turmoil, but very few of us become violent.

If an employee displays a significant change in behavior or suddenly becomes hostile, it is important to find out why the change has occurred. A referral for counseling may determine the cause of the problem, and treatment may reduce the risk that symptoms will turn into workplace violence. Employees who are acutely unhappy and blame others for their problems may be at risk for workplace violence. Generally, the difference between chronic unhappiness and risk of violence occurs when an employee makes threatening comments or actually physically confronts another employee. Should this happen, an evaluation of potential violence must be made with a referral to a mental health professional. Mental health professionals may be helpful in determining potential for danger and should be used when signs of possible violence are noted.

VIOLENCE THREAT LEVELS

Workplace threats need to be taken seriously. Organizations should have written policies outlining the procedures for reporting all threats of violence. Those procedures should also describe the actions that will be taken in cases of workplace violence. Threatened employees have a right to know what an organization will do to protect them and what measures they need to take to protect themselves. Since it is impossible to know, with any certainty, whether a threat is going to be carried out, the organization should always treat threats in a serious manner and act as though the person may carry out the threat. Glicken and Ino (1997) describe the progression in the development of violent behavior in the workplace as follows.

Level 1. A preoccupation with the feeling that the worker has been mistreated and a tendency to blame others for his/her lack of success on the job and to obsessively complain about how badly he/she has been treated by someone specific or by unspecified others in the workplace. At this stage, the problem should be evaluated and an attempt should be made to try to resolve the concerns the worker has openly shared with others. If the worker's concerns are voiced irrationally or if illogical, they should be seen as problematic and needing to be dealt with in a proactive way by encouraging counseling or by trying to help the worker develop a more accurate perception of the problem. Employee assistance programs or mediators can help at this early point. If the worker is unwilling to become involved in counseling, mediation, or some other form of dispute resolution, the worker needs to be clearly told about the organization's "no-tolerance for violence" rules. There must also be an agreement from the worker to accept a "no-violence" contract so that any future concerns will be dealt with in a violence-free atmosphere. It is wise, at this point, to provide the worker with an advocate or an ombudsman to help in future disputes. The advocate represents the interests of the worker and is recognized as the worker's ally.

Level 2. Obsessive thoughts about a plan to pay others back for the way the worker believes that he/she has been treated. The plan may be diffuse and non-specific or it may be elaborate. The plan is sometimes shared with others on the job who may think that the person is just venting anger. Usually, others do not take the plan seriously. This is a considerable mistake since, at this point in time, the worker begins to obsess about revenge, and the plan they've devised becomes more firmly fixed in their minds. The reason for the progression to level two is that organizations often badly handle the worker at level one. The way the worker is dealt with initially can have significant meaning for the progression or the lack of progression of violent impulses. All threats, plans, indications of payback, obsessive thoughts and preoccupations with unfairness should be seen as problematic by the organization, and every attempt should be made to deal with the problem through the use of an EAP, mediation, or some conciliatory process to logically resolve the problem. If the worker is being laid off, it should be done with notice, with respect, and with some semblance of concern for the worker's long-term well-being. Stories of the way organizations lay people off in cruel, insensitive, and often rude and disrespectful ways suggest reasons for the development of anger in workers and dramatically increase the risk of violence.

Level 3. The plan is now articulated to those in the workplace, who need to respond. Generally, pre-violent workers will confide their plan or make specific threats to supervisors they trust or find sympathetic. At this stage, if threats are not taken seriously and if something isn't done to deal with them, the anger grows and workers become unable to control feelings and emotions that are now clearly out of control. Most perpetrators of workplace violence have discussed their plan, to the extent that it is now clear, with others in a position of authority. Some managers act on this information, but all too many others ignore it, thinking it best not to make problems for the worker, or they worry that any report of the plan might end in a legal action by the worker. For whatever reason, most workplace homicides have been articulated clearly by perpetrators, and it often doesn't come as a surprise when perpetrators actually end up killing someone. When one hears about a workplace killing, it is almost always followed by statements from co-workers saying that they didn't take the worker's threatened violence seriously or that they misjudged the degree of the anger. This is the moment in time to make formal reports to the police or to company security so that action can be taken to protect other workers.

Level 4. Actual threats are made to those directly involved in the worker's obsessional system, or they may be made to anyone who is handy. The worker's anger is now increasingly more difficult to control since they have made a decision to confront others as a release for intense feelings of anger at the organization and they have clearly lost control. Co-workers begin to complain to superiors who often do nothing to control the behavior or who may terminate the worker without necessary professional help or police involvement. The worker, at level 4, is now ready to commit an act of violence. In almost all cases of workplace violence, supervisors, personnel departments, and union stewards were forewarned about problematic employees but did nothing to ensure that help would be given or that the problem would be resolved. When threats are made, it may be necessary to bring in the police and to file charges against a violent employee. While this may end in a trial or in a prison sentence, it may also end in mandatory treatment and the safety of innocent people.

Level 5. The worker acts out his or her obsessional system and commits violent acts on the job. When workers say that they are going to kill someone or commit an act of violence to co-workers, take it seriously. Threats are more than words. They are acts about to take place and are often the worker's unconscious attempt to have the act stopped. When a threat is made and nothing constructive is done to help the worker, violence is very likely to follow. The violence may be directed at specific people but more often than not, it is random and affects people who have nothing to do with the worker's grievances against the organization.

It should not surprise us that many workers move to level 5 in the development of violence. Far too many managers and supervisors worry about lawsuits or union actions if they intervene and may withdraw from the issue when violent behavior begins to show itself. Nor should it surprise us if workers show none of the levels noted above and act-out without seeming provocation. These are the anomalies of the workplace and the individual workers within the workplace. By and large, however, workers give advanced notice of potentially dangerous behavior. When that behavior is dealt with badly by organizations, violence is likely to result.

ORGANIZATIONAL INTERVENTIONS IN WORKPLACE PROBLEMS

When problems in the workplace begin to surface, managers should meet with the worker and find out what is bothering them. If the problem is beyond their ability to resolve, professional help should be sought. Many problems, however, can be dealt with by the organization. Work assignments can be varied to prevent burnout. Promotional and salary decisions can be made equitably to ensure that all workers feel treated with dignity and respect. References of workers can be checked carefully with the added protection of having potential workers undergo careful screening and evaluation before they are hired, to identify those applicants with obvious emotional problems or histories of violent behavior on other jobs. Disputes between workers can be mediated informally before they become serious problems. Laying workers off should be done with care and concern for the individual and not in the heavy-handed and insensitive way that it is usually done. When workers feel diminished and no longer believe that the organization cares about them, the potential for workplace problems grows in severity.

When organizations are responsive to their workers, many of the problems that lead to workplace violence can often be resolved. In these companies, Employee Assistance Programs (EAPs) are used to offer workers an alternative way of resolving problems that may be difficult to resolve for managers and supervisors. Companies using EAPs offer a variety of alternatives to workers. Some EAPs are located in the organization and are readily available. In these organizations, managers, workers, and treatment personnel work closely together to resolve the problem. In other organizations, the worker might go to a social agency or counseling center with which the organization has contracted. The services provided may be time-limited and supportive, or they may be longer term and designed to meet the individual needs of the client.

Often workplace problems have their origins in the personal lives of workers. Resolving personal problems is important, but keeping the worker employed supersedes the resolution of a personal problem. Organizations often correctly complain that workers do not improve on the job after treatment is provided. This complaint is valid, but organizations also need to be made aware of how long it may take for the worker to improve. Problems such as addictions to substances are slow to respond to treatment and may take months to improve with the added possibility of a need for residential treatment. Just as employers give workers time to mend after an illness or surgery, employers need to give workers time to mend when they have emotional problems.

Robinson (1996) believes that training is a "critical" component of any prevention strategy since it permits employees to become acquainted with experts within the agency who can help them when potentially violent situations arise. Robinson suggests further that, "employees and supervisors seek assistance at a much earlier stage when they personally know the agency officials who can help them" (p. 6).

Other forms of prevention suggested by Robinson (1996) and others include a confidential background check on new employees, which at the very least would include a check on the applicant's criminal, credit, and employment history and driving records. Once an applicant is hired, it is important to track and record observable and relevant changes in behavior and take the proper steps toward intervention. Most experts suggest a "zero tolerance" for threats, intimidation, and any act of violence, which should be included in the personal policies of all organizations with assigned personnel to investigate all threats or acts of violence. This might be similar to the way many organizations handle complaints of sexual harassment. Ongoing training and education and easy access to grievance procedures are also important aspects in preventing violence.

Some organizations use ombudsman programs, facilitation, mediation, and other methods of dispute resolution to identify and prevent potential workplace violence. These strategies are often most useful before the threat of violence becomes serious enough to require a formal workplace action. The following is a short description of some preventative techniques suggested by Robinson (1996) that organizations have found useful in dealing with workplace violence problems at their beginning stages.

1. **Ombudsmen.** Ombudsmen are employed by an organization and use a variety of strategies to resolve workplace disputes, including counseling, mediation, conciliation, and fact-finding. An ombudsman may interview all the parties involved in a dispute, review the history of the problem and the organization's personnel policies to see if they've been correctly applied, and might offer suggestions and alternative ways of resolving the dispute to the workers involved in a disagreement. An ombudsman doesn't "impose" solutions but may offer alternative strategies to resolve it. Workers involved in a dispute may refuse options offered by the ombudsman and are free to pursue other remedies or strategies including legal ones.

2. **Facilitation.** The facilitator focuses on resolving the dispute and is most helpful when the level of emotions about the issues is fairly low and the people involved trust one another to develop acceptable solutions.
3. **Mediation.** Mediation uses a third party who is not a member of the organization and is free of bias in the situation. The mediator can only recommend—although some organizations accept binding mediation as a way of resolving disputes, with the mediator placed in the role of decision-maker. Mediation may be helpful when those parties involved in a dispute have reached an "impasse" and the solution is potentially dangerous. A mediator may offer advice, suggestions, and options to help resolve the problem. The authority the mediator brings to the dispute is neutrality and expertise. Care must be taken to bring someone in with a track record of fairness and lack of bias in mediating disputes.
4. **Interest-based problem solving.** Interest-based problem solving attempts to improve the working relationship between the parties in dispute by using rational and focused ways of resolving problems as well as reducing emotions among the people involved. Techniques suggested for use in interest-based problem solving include brainstorming, creative alternative solutions to a problem, and agreed-upon rules to reach a solution.
5. **Peer review.** Peer review involves the evaluation of a problem and recommendation of a possible solution by fellow employees. Because these suggestions come from peers, they may have more impact on the involved parties. However, peer reviews are fraught with concerns about objectivity, composition of the review panel, dual loyalties, and conflicts of interest and are usually only helpful if done with the complete confidence of the parties involved. Review panels in sexual harassment cases might be a good model to explain this approach. Sexual harassment review panels have a mediocre to poor record of objectivity, and recommendations to upper management are often rejected because of due process issues and concerns regarding objectivity. On the other hand, courts have been reluctant to overturn decisions made by organizations when review panels are used in sexual harassment investigations.
6. **Employee training.** All employees should understand the correct way to report potentially or actively violent and disruptive behavior observed in other workers. Robinson (1996, p. 6) suggests that the following topics be included in all workplace violence prevention training:

Discussion of the organization's workplace violence policy; a willingness of employees to report incidents; suggested approaches to preventing or coping with potentially violent and hostile behavior; conflict resolution training; training in managing stress and anger; training in the location and operation of alarm systems; personal security measures; and, understanding the various programs offered by organizations including employee assistance programs, the ombudsman, and mediation.

7. **Supervisory training.** Special attention should be paid to effective training of supervisors so that they know how to identify, evaluate, and resolve workplace problems that may lead to violence. This includes the use of personnel policies to provide accurate evaluations of performance and reports that correctly identify the worker's behavior with just and organizationally correct disciplinary actions provided. Skills necessary to prevent workplace violence by managers may include the ability to screen applicants for potential for violence, crisis management and conflict resolution skills, and encouragement of other workers supervised by the managers to share incidents of observed violence or potential violence in co-workers.
8. **Security measures.** Workers need to feel safe on the job. Organizations can increase this feeling of safety by providing weapons checks, employee identification badges or cards with pictures, immediate response by the police if threats have been made, and assurance of the safety of workers who have been threatened or assaulted by co-workers. All organizations need to have a no-tolerance policy against all forms of weapons on the premises, with immediate suspension if a weapon is found on a worker. Reports of weapons must be immediately shared with the police.
9. **Pre-employment screening.** Before a worker is officially offered a position, the HR department should be contacted to find out what pre-employment screening techniques (such as interview questions, background and reference checks, and drug testing) are permitted by federal and state laws and regulations.

COUNSELING WORKERS WITH POTENTIAL FOR WORKPLACE VIOLENCE

This discussion of treatment focuses on ways to help clients who have anger issues in the workplace and summarizes recent research on ways to reduce anger and more adequately deal with underlying reasons for anger.

In a meta-analysis of 50 studies with a total of more than 1600 subjects using cognitive-behavioral therapy (CBT) with clients experiencing abnormal levels of anger, Beck and Fernandez (1998) found that 76% of the clients treated with CBT had greater improvement in anger control than that achieved by the control groups. The authors conclude that the use of CBT has been proven to an extent that it is the primary treatment approach for use with anger issues.

Tafrate, Kassinove, and Dundin (2002) found that people with historically high levels of anger have anger reactions that are more frequent, intense, and enduring and report more physical aggression, negative verbal responses, drug use, and negative consequences of their anger. Their anger negatively affects their relationships, their health, and their jobs. Tafrate et al. found that cognitive therapy and relaxation techniques were able to reduce levels of anger in college-age drivers from the 85th percentile to normal by training clients in progressive relaxation until they can quickly use personal cues, such as words, phrases, or images to relax in situations that might normally make them angry. Tafrate et al. believe that new combinations of treatment will incorporate four stages of change:

1. Preparing for change by helping clients increase their motivation and awareness of their anger;
2. Actual change that includes assertiveness training, avoiding and escaping from situations that often create angry responses, and triggering anger and then teaching clients to relax;
3. Teaching clients to rethink what sets off their anger, forgiving others, and avoiding grudges;
4. Making long-term plans to prevent relapses because new situations may reignite anger.

WORKPLACE VIOLENCE AND PTSD

One of the primary problems that result from acts of violence is the development of PTSD. According to the DSM-IV (American Psychiatric Association [APA], 1994), the core criteria for PTSD include distressing symptoms of (a) re-experiencing a trauma through nightmares and intrusive thoughts; (b) numbing by avoiding reminders of the trauma, or feeling aloof or unable to express loving feelings for others; and (c) persistent symptoms of arousal as indicated by two or more of the following: sleep problems, irritability and angry outbursts, difficulty concentrating, hypervigilance, and exaggerated startle response, with a duration of more than a month, causing problems at work, in social interactions, and in other important areas of life (APA, 1994, pp. 427–429). The DSM-IV judges the condition to be acute if it has lasted less than 3 months, and chronic if it has lasted more than 3 months. It is possible for the symptoms to be delayed. The DSM-IV notes that a diagnosis of delayed onset is given when symptoms begin to show 6 months or more after the original trauma (p. 429).

PTSD is thought to be linked to a highly traumatic experience or life-threatening event that produces intrusive thoughts related to a very disturbing aspect of the original traumatic event. Those thoughts are difficult to dislodge once they reach conscious awareness. In many cases of PTSD, the client physically and emotionally re-experiences the original traumatic event and is frequently in a highly agitated state of arousal as a result. Symptoms of PTSD usually begin within 3 months of the original trauma. In half of the cases of PTSD, complete recovery occurs within 3 months of the onset of symptoms, but many cases last more than 12 months (APA, 1994, p. 426). Ozer, Best, Lipsey, and Weiss (2003) describe the symptoms associated with returning Vietnam veterans that led to a recognition of PTSD as a distinct diagnostic category: "Intrusive thoughts and images, nightmares, social withdrawal, numbed feelings, hypervigilance, and even frank paranoia, especially regarding the government, and vivid dissociative phenomena, such as flashbacks" (p. 54). The authors believe that the complexity of the symptoms often led to a misdiagnosis of schizophrenia.

Stein (2002) indicates that an additional symptom of PTSD is physical pain and writes, "Patients with PTSD are among the highest users of medical services in primary care settings. Ongoing chronic pain may serve as a constant reminder of the trauma that perpetuates its remembrance" (p. 922). Asmundson, Coons, Taylor, and Katz (2002) report that patients with PTSD present a combination of physical and mental health problems including increased alcohol consumption and depression. They also indicate that pain is one of the most commonly reported symptoms of patients with PTSD and write, "patients who have persistent, chronic pain associated with musculoskeletal injury, serious burn injuries, and other pathologies (such as fibromyalgia, cancer, or AIDS) frequently present with symptoms of PTSD" (p. 930). In a study by White and Faustman (1989), 20% of military veterans with PTSD developed chronic pain. McFarlane, Atchison, Rafalowicz, and Papay (1994) found that volunteer firemen who developed PTSD in response to acts of terrorism and violence developed a significant amount of pain, primarily back pain, as compared with 21% of those without symptoms of PTSD.

However, Gist and Devilly (2002) worry that PTSD is being predicted on such a wide scale for every tragedy that occurs that we've watered down its usefulness as a diagnostic category, and they write, "Progressive dilution of both stressor and duration criteria has so broadened application that it can now prove difficult to diagnostically differentiate those who have personally endured stark and prolonged threat from those who have merely heard upsetting reports of calamities striking others" (p. 741). The authors suggest that many early signs of PTSD are normal responses to stress that are often overcome with time and distance from the event. Victims often use natural healing processes to cope with traumatic events, and interference by professionals in natural healing could make the problem more severe and prolonged. In determining whether PTSD will actually develop, people must be given time to cope with the trauma on their own before we diagnose and treat PTSD. To emphasize this point, Gist and Devilly report that the immediate predictions of PTSD in victims of the World Trade Center Bombings turned out to be almost 70% higher than actually occurred 4 months after the event. Of course, symptoms of PTSD may develop much later than 4 months after a trauma. Still, the point is well taken. People often heal on their own, and a premature diagnosis of PTSD may be counterproductive.

TREATING THE VICTIMS OF WORKPLACE VIOLENCE

The following treatment approaches are used in treating PTSD and may be useful to clinicians treating the victims of workplace violence.

Exposure Therapy

Rothbaum, Olasov, and Schwartz (2002) describe a type of treatment, "Exposure Therapy," based on emotional-processing theory which is rooted in the belief that PTSD develops as a result of memories eliciting fear that trigger escape and avoidance behaviors. Since the development of a "fear network" functions as a type of obsessive condition, the client continues to increase the number of stimuli that serve to increase his or her fear. To reduce the number of stimuli that elicit fear, the client must have his or her "fear network" activated so that new information can be provided that rationally contradicts the obsessive network of emotions reinforcing the PTSD symptoms. The authors believe that the following progression of treatment activities serves to reduce the client's fear network.

1. Repeated reliving of the original trauma helps to reduce anxiety and correct a belief that anxiety will necessarily continue unless avoidance and escape mechanisms are activated.
2. Discussing the traumatic event reduces negative reinforcement of the event and helps the client see it in a logical way that corrects misperceptions of the event.
3. Speaking about the trauma helps the client realize that it's not dangerous to remember the trauma.
4. The ability of the client to speak about the trauma provides the client with a sense of mastery over his or her PTSD symptoms.

Hensley (2002, p. 338) provides the following explanation of exposure therapy as it might be applied to a client suffering from PTSD as a result of rape:

1. Memories, people, places, and activities now associated with the rape make you highly anxious, so you avoid them.
2. Each time you avoid them you do not finish the process of digesting the painful experience, and so it returns in the form of nightmares, flashbacks, and intrusive thoughts.
3. You can begin to digest the experience by gradually exposing yourself to the rape in your imagination and by holding the memory without pushing it away.
4. You will also practice facing those activities, places, and situations that currently evoke fear.
5. Eventually, you will be able to think about the rape and resume your normal activities without experiencing intense fear.

Effectiveness studies of using exposure therapy for PTSD have been quite positive. In the annual review of important findings in psychology, 12 studies found positive results using exposure therapy with PTSD. Eight of these studies received special recognition for the quality of their methodology and for the positive nature of their outcomes (Foa & Meadows, 1997). Rothbaum et al. (2002) write that, "Exposure therapy has more empirical evidence for its efficacy than any other treatment developed for the treatment of trauma-related symptoms" (p. 65).

Debriefing

A form of treatment with potential for use in work with PTSD victims following a workplace tragedy is a single-session treatment, or what has also been called "debriefing." In this approach, clients who have experienced a trauma are seen in a group for 1 to 3 hours and within a week to a month of the original traumatic event. Risk factors are evaluated and a combination of information and opportunity to discuss their experiences during and after the trauma are provided (Bisson, McFarlane, and Rose, 2000). Most debriefing groups use crisis intervention techniques in a very abbreviated form and may provide educational information to group members about typical reactions to traumas, what to look for if group members experience any of these symptoms, and where to seek professional assistance if additional help is needed. Debriefing groups may also attempt to identify group members at risk of developing PTSD.

Despite the considerable appeal of this approach, there is little evidence that debriefing works to reduce the number of people who experience PTSD, and there is some evidence that it may increase PTSD over other forms of treatment (van Emmerik, Kamphuis, Hulsbosch, & Emmelkamp, 2002). Debriefing may be less effective than no treatment at all following a trauma (van Emmerik, Arnold, Kamphuis, et al., 2002).

There are several primary reasons for the lack of effectiveness of debriefing, as follows:

- Debriefing interferes with natural healing processes and sometimes results in bypassing usual support systems such as family, friends, and religious groups.
- Upon hearing that PTSD symptoms are normal reactions to trauma, some victims of trauma actually develop the symptoms as a result of the suggestions provided in the debriefing session, particularly when the victim hasn't had time to process the various feelings he or she may have about the trauma.
- Clients seen in debriefing include both those at risk and those not at risk. Better results may be obtained by screening clients at risk through a review of past exposure to traumas that may have served as catalysts for the current development of PTSD.

Combinations of Therapy

Resick, Nisith, Weaver, Astin, and Feuer (2002) tested two forms of cognitive therapy with women who had been sexually assaulted. The researchers found that cognitive therapy using exposure techniques was very successful in treating PTSD in this sample and that the success of this approach would bode well for PTSD caused by traumas other than sexual assault and rape. Many of the women in the study who showed marked improvement had histories of other traumas and were considered to be chronically distressed. Therapy was equally effective for recent traumas (3 months previously) and prior traumas (30 years previously). In contrast, the women in the control group did not improve at all.

Case Study: Worker to Worker Violence

Robert Sanders is a 55-year-old Caucasian engineer working in a tech company making drivers for computers. Because of the poor economy and a downturn in sales Robert and his colleagues have been on pins and needles about their job security. Robert thinks he'll be one of the first to go if the company starts downsizing, because of his age and his troubled relationship with his supervisor. For the past 2 years, Robert and his supervisor have had a running battle over the quality of Robert's work. Robert thinks that his work is fine, as do his colleagues, but the supervisor believes that Robert doesn't follow directions and that his work wanders off into areas that aren't related to his assignments. On several occasions, they've almost come to blows.

Robert was referred to the company's Employee Assistance Program and was told by his supervisor that he either accept counseling or that he'd be fired. Robert has a wife who doesn't work and two children in college. His salary barely covers his expenses and, many months, he lives on credit cards and loans. Quitting isn't a realistic option since a weak business market in the computer industry limits his work opportunities. The opportunities to transfer to a different department at work are also limited since what Robert does is highly specialized. At 55, he doesn't want to ruin a very good pension plan. He feels stuck and resents going for counseling. He believes that his problems at work are the supervisor's fault and thinks the supervisor should be in treatment, not him. He is becoming surly and difficult at work. On several occasions he's written derogatory things about the supervisor in the men's rest room or on the company elevator. While no one can prove that Robert is guilty, everyone knows that he is to blame.

In the past 6 months, Robert has begun to deteriorate. He often comes to work looking haggard and unkempt. People have begun to find his body odor offensive and wonder if he bathes. His EAP counselor suspects that Robert is drinking heavily and has ordered a random alcohol test.

Robert has made several indirect threats against his supervisor that co-workers have heard but have not reported. They believe that Robert has a grievance and they feel obligated to protect him. His co-workers just feel that Robert is going through a mid-life crisis but, on closer examination, Robert is deteriorating badly. His thoughts, which he confides to his wife and family, have increasingly become violent. He purchased a gun and shoots it in the basement of his home and outside in the desert. The feel of the gun and the sound of the bullets give him a sense of power that he finds intoxicating. He has also begun to drink heavily and has a DWI charge that resulted in the removal of his license and the impounding of his car. He drives anyway, using a second car he purchased in his wife's name.

He feels invincible and doesn't think anything will happen to him. Because of his sophistication with the Internet, he has begun sending e-mail messages to everyone at work that implies violence to certain people in upper management. He never mentions the name of the supervisor he hates so much and his e-mails are untraceable. In a company with thousands of people, it's difficult to pinpoint who made the threats or how seriously they should be taken, but the messages unnerve everyone at work and there is a sense of foreboding in the company that something awful will happen.

Robert's EAP counselor believes that his deteriorating condition is reason to worry about potential violence and has warned the company that he may be at risk. The company fears a law suit if they fire Robert. They believe that he will do something serious enough, but not dangerous enough, to fire him. The EAP counselor disagrees. He sees concrete signs of potential for serious workplace violence. Those signs include a highly intelligent man who is emotionally deteriorating and who also demonstrates increasing paranoia and an obsession for getting revenge. The drinking and fondness for guns add to the counselor's sense of potential violence. If the counselor knew of the verbal threats Robert had shared with his co-workers and the fact that Robert is the one making email threats, the counselor would be absolutely certain Robert's volatile behavior will end in a violent act.

Robert has always been eccentric. His aloofness from people, his distain for others he considers to have lesser ability, his angry feelings at management for not recognizing his abilities, all provide a backdrop to his potential for workplace violence. As an unsupportive supervisor thwarts his ambitions and as he suffers the indignity of having to go for counseling, Robert has begun to have fantasies of violence. They include going into the management side of the company and randomly killing every manager in sight, starting with his own supervisor. The fantasy is so clear and appealing to him that it has almost taken on sensuous overtones. Although Robert seems troubled, he's able to do his job but is having moments of irrationality and severe emotional dysfunction that make him highly dangerous.

The EAP counselor is concerned about Robert's potential for danger and has repeatedly warned the company. Unfortunately, he cannot pinpoint a specific threat or act to concretely suggest that Robert will be violent at work. While Robert seems to be going through a rough stretch, his co-workers aren't seeing the dangerous side of his behavior and believe that, like all eccentric people, Robert has a side of him that is different from the rest of the engineers he works with. That side, aloof, uncomfortable with people, egocentric, also makes him a good engineer, probably the best engineer in the group. For these reasons, his co-workers haven't accurately evaluated his level of increasing danger.

A day after a particularly degrading and offensive meeting with his supervisor where Robert was placed on administrative leave without pay because of the deterioration in his work, Robert took his guns to work and shot and killed three managers, including his supervisor. He wounded four others including several people who had nothing to do with the company and who were just there to deliver packages. The security guards assigned to the company shot and killed Robert in a struggle, and the company is left to sort out the reasons that it took them so long to take remedial action and to correctly determine his level of violence. Everyone interviewed believed that Robert was going through a patchy time but he would snap out of it. No one felt that he was excessively dangerous or that he had potential for violence, other than the EAP counselor whose warning to the company went unheeded.

Questions from the Case

1. Do you believe that Robert's company should have taken earlier action to help Robert by suspending him with pay and referring him for counseling in a facility not connected with the company?
2. If you were the counselor, how would you have treated Robert's growing anger at the company?
3. Do you think that companies have the right to fire workers who are not violent but have the potential for violence? How do you think this determination should be made to protect the rights of all parties involved?
4. What types of behavior in Robert should the company have seen as possible predictors of violence? Do you think a program to help co-workers and colleagues identify potential for violence would reduce violence in the workplace or might it contribute to increased paranoia and dismissals for potential violence that aren't warranted?
5. As a consequence of unfair dismissals, might a proactive policy actually lead to more violence by people who had no intention of doing anything violent but who now feel so badly treated that violence is now an option they might consider?
6. What is management's role in preventing workplace violence?

SUMMARY

This chapter discusses workplace violence, a problem that may be seen as the culmination of the stressors and dissatisfaction workers may feel as a result of conflict with co-workers and managers, feelings of unfairness in work assignments and promotions, and a host of problems that fester and build and may result in deadly violence. Data suggest that workplace violence, particularly worker to worker violence, is all too common in the American workplace. The aware manager and HR professional will note many early signs of worker unhappiness coupled with anger, a combination that all too often leads to violence. Primary ways of dealing with violence by organizations and mental health workers are discussed, and suggested effective treatment is provided both for perpetrators and victims. Often victims suffer from PTSD, and several treatment approaches are suggested including exposure and cognitive therapies. Most workplace violence can be prevented by early intervention and a concern for the safety of workers but, as in all human behavior, violence may be masked by other symptoms including withdrawal, silence, and restraint—behaviors that may be mistaken for compliance or may so mask the intensity of emotions that many managers and co-workers claim they had no idea that a worker was capable of violent behavior. We think denial of awareness of potential for violence is a symptom of the lack of sensitivity to workers too often associated with the American workplace and needs to be dealt with by more training and a closer relationship with Employee Assistance Programs and other mental health services. To help practice the reader's responses to workplace violence, a case is presented with questions placing the reader in the position of a manager dealing with an increasingly angry worker.

REFERENCES

American Psychiatric Association (1994). *Diagnostic and statistical manual of mental disorders* (4th Edition). New York: American Psychiatric Association.

Asmundson, G. J. G, Coons, M. J., Taylor, S., & Katz, J. (2002). PTSD and the experience of pain: Research and clinical implications of shared vulnerability and mutual maintenance models. *Canadian Journal of Psychiatry, 47*(Issue 10), 930–938.

Beck, R., & Fernandez, E. (1998). Cognitive-behavioral therapy in the treatment of anger. *Cognitive Therapy and Research, 22*(1), 63–74.

Bisson, J. I., McFarlane, A. C., & Rose, S. (2000). Psychological debriefing. In E. B. Foa, T. M. Keane, & M. J. Friedman (Eds.), *Effective treatments for PTSD* (2000, pp. 39–59). New York: The Guilford Press.

Foa, E. B., & Meadows, E. A. (1997). Psychosocial treatments for post-traumatic stress disorder: A critical review. In J. Spence, J. M. Darley, & D. J. Foss (Eds.), *Annual review of psychology* (Vol. 48, pp. 449–480). Palo Alto, CA: Annual Reviews Inc.

Gist, R., & Devilly, G. J. (2002). Post-trauma debriefing: the road too frequently traveled. *Lancet*, *360*(Issue 9335), pp. 741–743.

Glicken, M. & Ino, S. (1997). *Workplace violence: A description of the levels of potential for violence.* Unpublished Paper.

Hensley, L. G. (2002). Treatment for survivors of rape: Issues and interventions. *Journal of Mental Health Counseling*, *24*(Issue 4), 331–348.

McFarlane, A. C., Atchison, M., Rafalowicz, E., & Papay, P. (1994). Physical symptoms in post-traumatic stress disorder. *Journal of Psychosomatic Research*, *38*, 715–726.

Ozer, E. J., Best, S. R., Lipsey, T. L., & Weiss, D. S. (2003). Predictors of posttraumatic stress disorder and symptoms in adults: A meta-analysis. *Psychological Bulletin*, *129*(1), 52–73.

Resick, P. A., Nisith, P., Weaver, T. L., Astin, M. C., & Feuer, C. A. (2002). A comparison of cognitive-processing therapy with prolonged exposure and a waiting condition for the treatment of chronic posttraumatic stress disorder in female rape victims. *Journal of Consulting and Clinical Psychology*, *70*(4), 867–879.

Robinson, J. L. (1996). *10 facts every employer and employee should know about workplace violence: It may save your life!* Retrieved March 3, 2003 at:// <www.smartbiz.com>.

Romano, S. J., Levi-Minzi, M., Rugala, E. A., & Van Hasselt, V. (January, 2011). *Workplace violence prevention.* Readiness and Response. FBI Law Enforcement Bulletin. Retrieved August 17, 2012 from <http://www.fbi.gov/stats-services/publications/law-enforcement-bulletin/january2011/workplace_violence_prevention>.

Rothbaum, B., Olasov, C., & Schwartz, A. C. (2002). Exposure therapy for posttraumatic stress disorder. *American Journal of Psychotherapy*, *56*(Issue 1), 59–75.

Stein, M. B. (2002). Taking aim at posttraumatic stress disorder: Understanding its nature and shooting down myths. *Canadian Journal of Psychiatry*, *47*(Issue 10), 921–923.

Tafrate, R. C., Kassinove, H., & Dundin, L. (2002). Anger episodes in high- and low-trait anger community adults. *Journal of Clinical Psychology*, *58*(12), 1573–1590.

US Department of Labor. (2011). *Workplace violence.* Retrieved from the Internet Dec. 13, 2011 at: <http://www.osha.gov/SLTC/workplaceviolence/index.html>.

van Emmerik, A. P., Kamphuis, J. H., Hulsbosch, A. M, & Emmelkamp, P. M. (2002). Single session debriefing after psychological trauma: a meta-analysis. *Lancet*, *360*(Issue, 9335), 766–772.

White, P, & Faustman, W. (1989). Coexisting physical conditions among inpatients with post-traumatic stress disorder. *Military Medicine*, *154*, 66–71.

FURTHER READING

Rugala, E. A. & Isaacs, A. R. (2012). *Workplace violence: Issues in response.* US Department of Justice, Federal Bureau of Investigation. Retrieved August 17, 2012 from <http://www.fbi.gov/stats-services/publications/workplace-violence>.

USDA. (1998). *The USDA Handbook on workplace violence: Prevention and response.* United States Department of Agriculture. Retrieved August 17, 2012 from <http://www.usda.gov/news/pubs/violence/wpv.htm>.

PART *Three*

Using Human Resource and Management Approaches to Prevent Work-Related Problems

CHAPTER 8

Preventing Workplace Problems through Competency-Based Management

INTRODUCTION

Throughout our book we've discussed the many reasons for workplace problems. This chapter provides our best suggestions for rectifying the many preventable problems in the workplace though a more logical approach to management using the new research-oriented management tool known as competency-based management (CBM). CBM uses many of the same tools to evaluate and apply research on best management practices as does competency-based practice in the medical and mental health fields. This chapter provides an overview of CBM and suggested ways it can be used to minimize work-related problems.

MANAGERIAL IMPERATIVES TO REDUCE WORKPLACE PROBLEMS

Given the rapid changes in the social, economic, and cultural climate of the country, the role of managers to help organize and run complex organizations and still provide cutting edge services is increasingly important. In noting the importance of management, the American Board of Examiners in Clinical Social Work (2004) indicates that when management is competent, the new worker will be transformed "from an anxious novice into an effective, contributing employee—but only if the supervisor is highly competent and capable of providing high levels of guidance, instruction, and support" (p. 1).

Scheaffer and Mano-Negrin (2003) indicate that another important aspect of middle and upper management is to anticipate and plan for the normal and the unusual crises that affect all organizations. Workplace crises may include budget cuts, loss of competent workers, difficulty in hiring competent workers, and many other usual and unusual problems that continually affect organizations. The authors call for crisis preparedness by

Treating Worker Dissatisfaction During Economic Change
DOI: http://dx.doi.org/10.1016/B978-0-12-397006-0.00008-7

middle and upper management "to foresee and effectively address internal or exogenous adversary circumstances with the potential to inflict a multidimensional crisis, by consciously recognizing and proactively preparing for its inevitable occurrence" (p. 599).

Haines and Donald (1998) urge managers in health care to use very current research findings for managing organizations. The authors write, "Research findings can influence decisions at many levels in caring for individual patients, in developing practice guidelines, in commissioning health care, in developing prevention and health promotion strategies, in developing policy, in designing educational programs, and in performing clinical audit" (p. 74). The authors argue that "Organizational change is often also necessary to implement clinical change" (p. 74) and suggest that much of what is hampering the development of good-quality services and products is the inability of organizations to change when pressing social and economic pressures demand change.

Weiss (2004) believes that a serious mistake managers make in dealing with future demands is to rely on past ways of doing their jobs without recognition that changing times require managers to stay current. To guard against obsolescence, Weiss urges managers to "Continue your education. College courses, graduate and certificate programs present the latest developments and the newest technology in your field of interest" (p. 19). Contrary to common wisdom, Russell and Petrie (1994) found that managers do not improve in their performance over time without significant preparation and continuing education and urge better training before and during the actual work assignments.

In agreeing with Weiss that managers need to be prepared for new and changing times in organizational life, Reiss and Fishel (2000) studied the preparation of managers supervising therapists. They found that almost none of the professionals surveyed had a formal course in management and that most lacked any significant management training.

ANTICIPATING AND PLANNING FOR THE FUTURE

Pina e Cunha, da Cunha, Joao Vieira, and Kamoche (1984) argue that one of the major mistakes management has made is to approach their function as if they know what is going to happen in the future. This traditional approach to managing for the future requires maintenance of external clarity and internal calm. In other words, to manage for stability with minor changes here and there in order to cope with changing organizational pressures. The authors write (p. 26),

> *[This] traditional mindset arose in an era where the pursuit of predictability and order constituted major organizational tasks. To counter chaos and disobedience, [organizations] were designed as hierarchies, emphasizing efficiency and pursuing the optimal use of resources. In an organization built on the image of the machine, planning was a critical activity. Managers contributed to the smooth functioning of organizations through authoritarian leadership.*

The authors argue that this approach to the future is detrimental to organizational life. To anticipate and deal with rapidly changing organizational pressures, or what they call the age of emergence, organizations require leadership that doesn't pre-plan a specific strategy in a changing environment, but one that allows all members of the organization to be involved in responses to a crisis. Of the new approach to the demands of the future, the authors write, "The 'age of emergence' refers to the growing acceptance that organizations cannot predict what is going to happen [in] the future" (p. 27) and must instead adapt to changing times by not holding rigidly to prior plans of action that may be completely unusable and counter-productive and argue that strategic anticipation of crises "must be complemented by mechanisms able to facilitate strategic adaptiveness" (p. 27).

In describing the elements of strategic adaptiveness, the authors urge a melding of the old with the new, suggesting that managers operate as leaders of a quiet revolution by inspiring workers to think outside of the box and to come up with new solutions that are considered, discussed, and, if they seem appropriate, utilized. This new style of management, which the authors liken to jazz, with its improvisation within a set structure, allows managers to approach the future in a creative, subjective, and open way. Rather than fearing change, this approach recognizes and encourages change because it keeps the organization youthful and energized.

Communicating effectively with workers is also a highly important aspect of middle management. Loganbill, Hardy, and Delworth (1982) describe critical communication interventions with workers that should be a strong part of any middle manager's skills and include the following:

1. Facilitative interventions are worker-centered and help workers learn and apply the necessary work skills either in face-to-face meetings or in a more indirect way (memos, telephone conversations, and emails).
2. Interventions that use confrontation are used to examine and compare work because workers are experiencing conflict in their work-related

relationships or because managers have concern about a worker's performance. This should always be done face-to-face.

3. Conceptual interventions are used when supervisors ask workers to think analytically or theoretically. In this type of interaction, group discussion, staff development, papers sent on the Internet to workers, staff meetings, and case presentations can all have positive impact on workers if resistance isn't great. If it is, a confrontation might be needed to help a worker understand his or her resistance and to soften it so that new material can be integrated into the worker's job performance.
4. Prescriptive interventions are a way of coaching workers to perform or eliminate certain behaviors. Loganbill et al. (1982) caution that prescriptive interventions lower morale when a supervisor always negates a worker's point of view in favor of that of the supervisor.
5. Catalytic interventions exist when a supervisor helps a worker understand something so significant about his or her work performance that it could lead to a substantial breakthrough in the performance of the worker. This might include watching the worker perform a task and giving on-the-spot feedback.

THE SIX COMPONENTS OF COMPETENCY-BASED MANAGEMENT

Competency-based management (CBM) is a form of evidence-based practice that applies best evidence to management practices. CBM utilizes information from well-done research studies, which provide logical reasons to assume that the best way to practice management is to objectively know what works and to determine when it should be used and the conditions under which its use will be optimal. Competency-based management (CBM) can be distinguished from more traditional forms of management because of the following:

1. Focus on Outcomes

Competency-based management focuses on work-related outcomes. Gambrill (1999) believes that the use of competency-based practice can help us "avoid fooling ourselves that we have knowledge when we do not" (p. 342). As Gambrill further notes, competency-based practice "requires an atmosphere in which critical appraisal of practice-related claims flourishes, and clients [and workers] are involved as informed participants" (p. 345). Ghoshal (2005) believes that best evidence for managers can be found in research that seeks positive outcomes. While CBM does not attempt to provide theory, it is a roadmap for managers to use best evidence of work-related practices known for their excellence and high ethical standards. The goal of CBM is to improve the quality and quantity of management practices by providing proven research evidence.

Management has often believed that unsystematic observations from one's management experience provide legitimate ways of building and maintaining an acceptable knowledge base, and that common sense and practice wisdom are valid ways to approach management. Rather than searching for best evidence, many managers who don't use a competency-based approach value traditional sources of authority, standard approaches to management that may not work, and direct contact with local experts thought to possess management-related wisdom, who often don't. Gambrill (1999) believes that, all too often, managers rely on the "opinions of others, pronouncements of authorities, unchecked intuition, anecdotal experience, and popularity or the authority of the crowd" (p. 343) and she notes that while intuition is a "vital source of guesses about what may be true, it cannot tell us what in fact is the case regarding the accuracy of assessment measures or the effectiveness of service methods" (p. 343). She also points out that "consensus, popularity, or anecdotal experience [often fail to] provide sound criteria regarding questions of effectiveness or validity of assessment measures. Experience does not necessarily result in improved performance. In fact, it may have the opposite effect" (p. 344).

In furthering the case for knowledge-guided practice, Gambrill (1999, p. 344) argues that managers too often seek knowledge and guidance from what she refers to as pseudoscience, or the tendency to seek sources that make science-like claims when none really exist. She describes pseudoscience as having the following characteristics: (1) Pseudoscience discourages objective examinations of the claims it makes. (2) It uses scientific language without the substance. (3) It relies on anecdotal experiences. (4) It isn't skeptical. (5) It doesn't try to disprove itself. (6) It uses language that is unclear. (7) It appeals to faith. (8) Its beliefs are not testable.

On the other hand, competency-based management places a much lower value on authority and the use of poorly done research or pseudoscience, believing that managers

... can make independent assessments of evidence, and thus evaluate the credibility of opinions being offered by experts. The decreased emphasis on authority does not imply a rejection of what one can learn from colleagues and teachers whose years of experience have provided them with insight. A final assumption of the new paradigm is that practice based on an understanding of the underlying evidence will provide superior practice.

American Medical Association Evidence-Based Practice Working Group (1992, p. 2421)

An example of searching for best evidence is the problem we often have in supervising workers with high degrees of education and a belief that what they do is generally well done. These workers often feel that they need considerable autonomy and that management is intrusive. How do we supervise workers who are sometimes antagonistic to the entire idea of supervision? And won't management lead to conflict with the supervisor and disenchantment with the organization? After all, turnover in the human services is no small problem.

Davenport (2005) studied more than 100 companies and 600 individual highly educated and competent workers. Davenport concluded that the old dictum of hiring smart people and leaving them alone wasn't the best way to get the most out of workers. Rather, he concluded that, while knowledge workers can't be managed in the traditional sense of the word, managers can intervene, but not in a heavy-handed or hierarchical way. Davenport's conclusion is that knowledge workers need to be handled with a light touch, but that they also need work-related rules and policies as well as behavioral expectations and measurements to evaluate performance. Not all knowledge workers are the same, and the assumption that they are, Davenport says, leads to under-management, which may result in reduced performance.

2. Use of Management Research and Best Evidence

Competency-based management emphasizes the critical role of best evidence in making supervisory decisions. Best evidence is generated by high-quality research data, but when practice wisdom exists and it has been shown to be effective over time, best evidence may also include practice wisdom. Timmermans and Angell (2001) indicate that competency-based practice has five important features, as follows.

- It is composed of both research evidence and practical experience.
- There is skill involved in reading the literature that requires an ability to synthesize the information and make judgments about the quality of the evidence available.

- The way in which information is used is a function of the supervisor's level of authority in an organization and his or her level of confidence in the effectiveness of the applied information.
- Part of the use of competency-based practice is the ability to independently evaluate the information used and to test its validity in the context of one's own practice.
- Competency-based judgments are grounded in the Western notions of professional conduct and professional roles, and are ultimately guided by a common value system.

Practice wisdom, regardless of how long it has been thought to be effective, often presents problems. O'Donnell (1997) cautions that practice wisdom is often a justification for beliefs and values that bond us together as professionals but often fail to serve workers, clients, or organizations since many of those beliefs and values may be comforting, but they may also be inherently incorrect. O'Donnell likens this process to making the same mistakes, with growing confidence, over a long number of years. Isaacs and Fitzgerald (1999) call practice wisdom "vehemence-based" practice, where one substitutes volumes of experience for evidence so that it becomes, "an effective technique for brow beating your more timorous colleagues and for convincing relatives of your ability" (p. 1).

Although we have come to value practice wisdom, all too often it has been based on what the American Medical Association Evidence-Based Practice Working Group (1992) refers to as unsystematic observations, a belief in common sense, a feeling that a management degree and experience are a way of maintaining a certain level of effective practice, and an assumption that there are wise and more experienced managers to whom we can go when we need help. All of these assumptions are grounded in a paradigm that tends to be highly subjective and is often manager-focused rather than worker- and consumer-focused.

An example of competency-based management can be seen in the research on the use of flextime. Most of us believe that flextime is a positive aid to workers who need flexibility in their work schedules that takes into consideration the needs of child rearing, care of parents or sick children, and other personal considerations that require flexibility in the hours worked. However, a review of the literature suggests that flextime has a particularly negative affect on health because it interferes with normal sleep cycles and social lives that are based on traditional work days (9–5, for example). Giebel, Janßen, Schomann, and Nachreiner (2004, p. 1015) write,

> *Recent studies on flexible working hours show at least some of these working time arrangements seem to be associated with impairing effects of health and wellbeing. Analyzing the data from our study of 15 companies and 137 service workers showed impairments in circadian controlled functions like sleep and digestion. The results thus indicate that analyzing flexible working hours seems to be a promising approach for predicting impairments which should be investigated further in the future.*

Does this mean that we shouldn't use flextime? Not necessarily, but it does suggest, along with a number of other studies the authors include in their report (almost all of which are German or European in origin and over half of which are by the authors), that flextime may have a negative impact on the health and emotional well-being of workers because workers use schedules that may force them to work during times normally used for sleep. Should we look for studies with American workers before we completely reject flextime? Absolutely. These authors are reporting on a culture that is very different from that of the United States, and service workers are a subset of workers who may have little in common with professionals and more highly skilled workers.

3. CBM Requires Managers to Understand Best Evidence

Competency-based management requires the manager to locate, read, and understand data that constitute best evidence. Hines (2000) suggests that some fundamental steps are required by managers to obtain usable information in a literature search. They are: (a) developing a well-formulated question; (b) finding the best possible answers to your questions; (c) determining the validity and reliability of the data found; and (d) testing the information with your workers and clients. Hines also notes that a well-formulated question must accurately describe the problem you wish to research, limit the interventions you think are feasible and acceptable to the worker, consumer, and agency, search for alternative approaches, and indicate the outcomes you wish to achieve. According to Hines, the advantage of this process is that it allows managers to develop quality practice guidelines that can be applied to a variety of functions of organizational life. It also identifies appropriate literature that can be shared with workers, suggesting that their ideas and input are valued.

Gambrill (1999, p. 343) indicates that a complete search for best evidence will provide the following relevant information, first suggested by Enkin, Keirse, Renfrew, & Neilson (1995):

1. Beneficial forms of [practice] demonstrated by clear evidence from controlled trials.
2. Forms of [practice] likely to be beneficial. The evidence in favor of these forms of care is not as clear as for those in category 1.
3. Forms of [practice] with a trade-off between beneficial and adverse effects. Effects must be weighed according to individual circumstances and priorities.
4. Forms of [practice] of unknown effectiveness. There are insufficient or inadequate quality data upon which to base a recommendation for practice.
5. Forms of [practice] unlikely to be beneficial. The evidence against these forms of care is not as clear as for those in category 6.
6. Forms of [practice] likely to be ineffective or harmful. Ineffectiveness or harm is demonstrated by clear evidence.

4. Commitment to Rational Practice

Competency-based management requires a commitment to objective practice. In describing the ease with which competency-based practice can be used, Bailes (2002) writes, "... [It] is not beyond your capability, even if you do not engage in research. You do not have to perform research; you can read the results of published studies [including management] research studies, meta-analyses, and systematic reviews" (p. 1). Bailes notes that the Internet permits access to various databases that allow searches to be done quickly and efficiently. In clarifying the type of data competency-based management looks for in its attempt to find best practices, Sackett, Rosenberg, Muir-Gray, Haynes, and Richardson (1996) write that it "involves tracking down the best external evidence with which to answer our practice [and management] questions" (p. 72).

In its position paper on the need for competent management in clinical social work, the American Board of Examiners in Clinical Social Work (2004) expresses its concern with the lack of research guiding practice, regardless of the discipline (i.e., clinical social workers, physicians, psychologists, psychiatric nurses, counselors, etc.). The board argues that scientific research in management is needed "to improve outcomes and to increase our knowledge of what practices are being employed in the field of clinical management, what findings are being disseminated and applied, and which techniques might be adopted to improve the quality of practice" (Harkness & Poertner, 1989; Hensley, 2002) (p. 20). The Board concludes that the social work management literature is almost completely devoid of best evidence. Even when best evidence is provided, it seems to have a limited impact on management. An example is Kadushin's (1992) research that managers fail to provide sufficient feedback to workers, often leaving them confused and frustrated about the adequacy of their work. Similarly, Kadushin found that, while managers prefer to teach new workers new skills, they spend most of their time on administrative tasks, suggesting a disconnect between what they want to do and what they have to do, a perfect situation for burnout and job unhappiness. The Board goes on to point out that "Despite this preference, managers make minimal use of the large body of educational research and theory (e.g., learning styles and theory, multiple intelligence, emotional intelligence) or of the large body of research in organizational theory" (American Board of Examiners in Clinical Social Work, 2004, p. 19). The Board continues by stating (p. 19) that

> *Even basic tenets of clinical management are untested. The supervisor's mediating or "advocacy" role (negotiator of issues between agency and supervisee), much-described as essential in the literature, is unsubstantiated for lack of any research. Similarly, the concept of "parallel process," which posits that practitioner-client processes are re-enacted at the supervisor-supervisee level, has never been verified by the evidence of research.*

5. Cooperative Management Styles

Competency-based management exists as a cooperative venture between managers, workers, the community, and consumers. CBM is cooperative in its inclusion of others. This means that managers do not function from a position of isolation. In a sense, this makes managers facilitators who believe that cooperative relationships are not only democratic and egalitarian, but that they are empowering. This shift from authoritarian approaches to cooperative ones can be difficult for managers who may believe that what is needed to run a unit is a strong, decisive hand and certainty in the way workers are managed. Without certainty, these managers believe, chaos results, when in fact the organization may seethe with discontent.

6. Managers Understand and Value Diversity

CBM respects and understands the need for culturally competent practice. Cultural competency includes not only an understanding of diversity, but an understanding of diversity within diversity (Kaiser, 1997; Shulman, 1993). This means that managers need to understand diverse populations in a way that rejects stereotyping.

For example, we know from a good deal of evidence that helping-professionals in the human services often allow their own biases to enter into assessment and treatment issues. While clients state that gender is important, parallel interviews with helping-professionals suggest that it isn't important. Gehart and Lyle (2001) believe that this "potential oversight has significant implications for the practice of ethical, gender-sensitive therapy and training" (p. 444). Laszloffy and Hardy (2000) found that a large number of African American and Latino patients were misdiagnosed as schizophrenic. Whaley (2001) is concerned that Caucasian clinicians often believe that African American clients have paranoid symptoms that are more fundamentally a cultural distrust of Caucasians because of historical experiences with racism. Whaley believes that helping-professionals discount the negative impact of racism and make judgments about African American clients suggesting that they are more disturbed than they really are, and argues that cultural stereotyping leads to "more severe diagnoses and restrictive interventions" (p. 558). Competent managers not only know a great deal about diverse groups but they have done the necessary work to eliminate personal biases in their work.

A Case Example and Discussion: Distinguishing Competency-Based Management from Common Wisdom and the Use of Authority

Jack Briscoe has been supervising a unit of health workers in a general hospital in a mid-western community. His unit has functioned well because he has a core of experienced workers who reinforce his management by mentoring and supporting newer workers. Several retirements and promotions to new positions have eliminated the more experienced workers from his unit and he now finds himself dealing with new workers who have little experience and very mediocre to poor educational experiences. He has read several management books that seem conventional and a bit dated in their advice and thinks that they fail to describe the problems many managers experience with new workers in this new era when the work ethic of younger workers may be less well defined than that of older workers. He has also sought help from his boss, but the advice seems intuitive and overly general.

In the times that he's tried the advice from the management books or his boss, the results have been poor. He has gone to meetings of managers where the suggestions made all seem like common wisdom with little evidence that any of the suggestions actually work. He's tried every suggestion with very poor results and wonders how managers can be so lacking in information about what really works. With the help of the statistician at work, he has begun to read the middle management research literature and is surprised to find that many of the studies support the very approaches that he has found not to work. The statistician has helped him separate the well done from the poorly done studies. Most of the poorly done articles, and there were many of them, were mainly anecdotal or presented common sense solutions that turned out to be, on the whole, incorrect.

The statistician found some research articles on the Internet and in the virtual library at a local university that provided some help. She indicated that the methodologies varied in sophistication, but set aside 20 articles for Jack to read on various issues that seemed relevant for the problems he has been facing. Most of the articles were very modest and made reasoned and careful suggestions that were never more than the data suggest. At first he was annoyed that the articles didn't tell him what to do, but as he read the literature reviews in each article and began to see that many other researchers had done similar studies and had come to similar conclusions, he began to see that the carefully done studies offered a wealth of information and provided, through the literature reviews, numerous other sources for him to consult.

As he read the literature, many of the things he has been taught about management and the common wisdom in his field about how best to supervise workers were discounted by the research. To begin with, he discovered that his way of orienting workers, leaving them pretty much on their own to read and then ask questions, was not supported by the research. He also failed to use the Internet and email to help workers resolve problems quickly and when they were most pressing. He had failed to set a clear standard for work, one which he holds all workers to, believing instead that one must individualize workers and accept each worker's strengths and weaknesses and the uneven work that results. His management was much too clinical with little actual mentoring or teaching. He almost never saw actual examples of direct work with patients and used the worker's case notes or reports to determine effectiveness, both of which, according to the research, are often misleading or just plain incorrect. He tried to be a buddy to everyone, thinking that it would ease the power differential between him and his workers when all it did was reduce his authority. He didn't use team work correctly and, rather than the workers' feeling cooperative togetherness, they felt in competition with one another.

With the statistician's help, Jack has begun doing systematic reviews that allow him to find articles providing an overview of the latest research. He has also begun taking courses in management that emphasize an objective, competency-based approach. Like all fields, there seems to be a good deal of extraneous and incorrect theory in the management literature. There is also a great deal of cheerleading, or what Jack considers to be fairly innocuous homilies. For example, an article on developing team work ends, "Making teams requires recognizing that it is our nature to belong—that we want to be part of something larger than ourselves. Thriving in teams requires acknowledging the essential humanness of each member. It all begins with choice and voice" (Axelrod, 2002, p. 12). Jack could not find a shred of evidence that anything in the article had been proven and decided the article consisted of statements made that sounded good but had no support and could have been completely wrong.

In another example from the management literature, the reasons given for low morale in organizations were that "Rumor, negativity, gossip, and quiet character assassination kill organizations, kill productivity, kill morale and crush the spirit" (Schuler, 2004, p. 2). While that may be true, the author failed to offer data to support this statement and failed to provide best evidence about how to rectify low morale. Like so many articles he has read, Jack finds that these articles just add to his confusion and lack of direction.

With the help of several instructors and a friend with a good research background, he has been able to separate the evidence that provides best practices from platitudes that seem overly general and prescriptive. What he failed to realize was that it takes time and practice to apply best evidence and that not all workers enjoy such an objective, results-oriented approach to management. Several of his workers argued that the process of helping patients had become too rational and objective and that the fun they used to have was gone. Others said that the use of best evidence didn't individualize them and that they felt like cogs in a machine. And yet others complained that what they did in practice was very subjective. Bottom line expectations failed to consider that some patients, while not seeming better on objective measures, really were better.

Jack thinks these are all good concerns and has begun meeting with workers individually and as a group to respond to their concerns. But the effort to institute best evidence has begun to have a positive impact on the overall performance of the unit and is self-reinforcing. Additionally, Jack is feeling much more comfortable about his supervisory skills and has begun to realize that one must provide humane, supportive management that reinforces positive behavior, helps change negative behavior, and melds various personalities into a cohesive working unit. And much to his surprise, Jack has begun to realize that some of the practice wisdom and common sense suggestions he at first rejected because they failed to have a research base, actually did seem to work. It's made him much more respectful of his colleagues and more willing to listen to the past experiences of others that actually work. And finally, he has begun to understand and use the supervisory approaches that work for him. What works for him is a complex mix of his personal skills, best evidence, and suggestions from workers and other managers. Jack thinks that this is the way it should be and believes that he is becoming the sort of supervisor he always wanted to be: wise, knowledgeable, and creative, with improving patients and workers more satisfied with their jobs.

SUMMARY

This chapter discusses the basic characteristics of competency-based management (CBM) and how it differs from managerial wisdom. It also provides arguments for and against the use of best evidence and notes that the positive arguments outweigh the negatives. Nonetheless, there are some concerns about the use of best evidence in management. These include the lack of well-done studies showing that competency-based management is superior to less research-oriented approaches and the resistance of managers to use research findings as a management tool. Managers often make the argument that every work situation is different and generalizing from studies to a specific workplace or a specific worker will lead to serious mistakes. A case example is provided to show how managers can use CBM in their own practice with common managerial problems that, left unresolved, may morph into serious problems for workers, individually and collectively.

REFERENCES

American Board of Examiners in Clinical Social Work (2004). *Clinical management: A practice specialty of clinical social work. A position statement of the American Board of Examiners in Clinical Social Work.* Retrieved on the Internet, May 12, 2006 at <www. abecsw.org>.

American Medical Association Evidence-Based Practice Working Group (1992). Evidence-based practice: A new approach to teaching the practice of medicine. *Journal of the American Medical Association, 268*, 2420–2425.

Axelrod, R. (2002). Making teams work. *Journal for Quality & Participation, 25*(1), 10–12.

Bailes B. K. (2002) Evidence-based practice guidelines: One way to enhance clinical practice. *AORN Journal, 12(6),* 1–8.

Davenport, T. (2005). *Thinking for a living: how to get better performance and results from knowledge workers.* Cambridge, MA: Harvard Business School Press.
Enkin, M., Keirse, M. J. N., Renfrew, M., & Neilson, J. (1995). *A guide to effective care in pregnancy and childbirth* (2nd Ed.). New York: Oxford University Press.
Gambrill, E. (1999). Evidence-based practice: An alternative to authority-based practice. *Journal of Contemporary Human Services, 80*(4), 341–350.
Gehart, D. H., & Lyle, R. D. (2001). Client experience of gender in therapeutic relationships: An interpretive ethnography. *Family Process, 40*, 433–458.
Ghoshal, S. (2005). Bad management theories are destroying good management practices. *Academy of Management Learning & Education, 4*(Issue 1), 75–92.
Giebel, O., Janßen, D., Schomann, C, & Nachreiner, F. (2004). A new approach for evaluating flexible working hours. *Chronobiology International, 21*(6), 1015–1024.
Haines, A., & Donald, A. (1998). Getting research findings into practice: Making better use of research findings. *British Medical Journal, 317*, 72–75.
Harkness, D., & Poertner, J. (1989). Research and social work management: A conceptual review. *Social Work, 34*, 115–119.
Hensley, P. H. (2002). The value of management. *The Clinical Supervisor, 21*(1), 97–110.
Hines, S. E. (2000). Enhance your practice with evidence-based medicine. *Patient Care, 60*(2), 36–45.
Isaacs, D., & Fitzgerald, D. (1999). Seven alternatives to evidence based medicine. *British Medical Journal, 319*, 1619.
Kadushin, A. (1992). *Management in social work* (3rd ed.). New York: Columbia University Press.
Kaiser, T. L. (1997). *Supervisory relationships: Exploring the human element.* Pacific Grove, CA: Brooks/Cole.
Laszloffy, T. A., & Hardy, C. B. (2000). Uncommon strategies for a common problem: Addressing racism in family therapy. *Family Process, 39*, 35–50.
Loganbill, C, Hardy, E, & Delworth, U. (1982). Supervision: A conceptual model. *Counseling Psychologist, 10*, 3–42.
O'Donnell, M. (1997). *A skeptic's medical dictionary.* London: BMJ Books.
Pina e Cunha, M., da Cunha, J. V., & Kamoche, K. (1984). The age of emergency: Toward a new organizational mindset. *SAM Advanced Management Journal, 66*(3), 25–30.
Reiss, H., & Fishel, A. K. (2000). New ideas: The necessity of continuing education for psychotherapy supervisors. *Academic Psychiatry, 24*(147), 155.
Russell, R. K., & Petrie, T. (1994). Issues in training effective supervisors. *Applied and Preventive Psychology, 3*, 27–42.
Sackett, D. L., Rosenberg, W. M. C., Muir Gray, J. A., Haynes, R. B., & Richardson, W. S. (1996). Evidence based medicine: What it is and what it isn't. *British Medical Journal, 312*, 71–72.
Scheaffer, Z., & Mano-Negrin, R. (2003). Executives' orientations as indicators of crisis management policies and practices. *Journal of Management Studies, 40*(2)573, 606.
Schuler, A. J. (2004). Turning around low morale. *Chronobiology International, 21*(6), 1015–1024.
Shulman, L. (1993). *Interactional management.* Washington, DC: NASW Press.
Timmermans, S., & Angell, A. (2001). Evidence-based medicine, clinical uncertainty, and learning to doctor. *Journal of Health & Social Behavior, 42*(4), 342.
Weiss, W. H. (2004). Managing effectively and efficiently. *Supervision, 65*(12), 17–20.
Whaley, A. L. (2001). Cultural mistrust: An Important psychological construct for diagnosis and treatment of African Americans. *Psychology: Research and Practice, 32*(6), 555–562.

FURTHER READING

Lai, H. F. (n.d.). *An analytic framework for developing the key performance indicator of knowledge management systems*. Retrieved August 17, 2012 from <www.ehow.com/...competency_based-performance-management-system.html>.

Pulakos, E. D. (2012). *Performance management: A roadmap for developing, implementing and evaluating performance management systems*. Retrieved August 17, 2012 from <http://www.shrm.org/about/foundation/research/Documents/1104Pulakos.pdf>.

Spenser, L. & Spencer, S. (1993). *Competency-based management: What, why and how.* Adapted from: Competence At Work by Lyle Spencer and Signe Spencer, 1993, John Wiley & Sons. Retrieved August 17, 2012 from <http://www.workitect.com/pdf/PM_Article.pdf>.

CHAPTER 9

Three Primary Human Resource Functions: Hiring, In-Service Training, and Termination

INTRODUCTION

The mistakes made when we hire workers are mistakes that can haunt us for a good deal of time, but the mistakes made in terminating a worker can have long-term legal ramifications. This chapter is about hiring and terminating workers in the most effective and legally correct ways. One of the most important aspects of hiring and keeping the best people for the job is the use of an evaluation process that takes subjectivity out of the mix. Chapter 10 discusses the how and why of behavioral worker evaluations that set organizational standards and measure a worker's performance based on those standards rather than a subjective evaluation process that will not hold up if there are legal challenges. Key to keeping good workers is the degree to which organizations provide staff development and in-service training. Both issues are discussed in the chapter. Additionally provided are addresses of five Internet sites which may be useful in better understanding best practices in hiring and termination, and a case with questions that puts you in an actual organizational setting experiencing difficult worker problems.

HIRING

Fernandez-Araoz (1999) notes that, two thousand years ago, officials in the Han dynasty tried to make hiring scientific by developing detailed job descriptions for civil servants, but discovered that even with the job descriptions and an attempt to make the process objective, few new hires worked out as well as expected. Today, according to Fernandez-Araoz, we tend to use many of the same approaches utilized by early management researchers, with the same unhappy results: between 30% and 40% of all hires end in terminations or resignations.

Treating Worker Dissatisfaction During Economic Change
DOI: http://dx.doi.org/10.1016/B978-0-12-397006-0.00009-9

McCarter (2003) believes that hiring is the single most important function of HR and argues that "the roots of unhappy employment situations often go back to the original hiring" (p. 20). The author believes that many problems can be avoided by using some of the following steps, which I've elaborated and augmented: (1) develop a clear and concise job description and keep the hiring interview focused on the person's ability to do the job as described in the job description. Only bring in applicants whose paperwork and references suggest that they will be able to do the job at a high level. (2) Use a checklist with the important job variables to compare applicants. (3) Look for relevant past experiences and how they might be helpful, or hurtful, to the organization. (4) Carefully check references.

McCarter thinks that applicants are often careless about references and use people who might say negative things about them. It's important to get the applicant's permission to call references and listen carefully to what they say. Ask the tough questions and follow up on anything that sounds problematic. It's also a very good idea to get the worker's permission to contact employers or others not listed as references. This should be done with the written consent of the worker. If the worker refuses to give permission it probably tells you they have employers in their work histories who might say unflattering things about them. As Steingold (2000) notes, checking references is "especially important if you're hiring someone who will be interacting closely with people. You don't want to hire a worker with drug and alcohol problems or a worker with a history of violence or sexual aggression" (p. 14).

In further concerns about references, Cherne (1999) says that it's important to read between the lines and to learn to translate politically correct or safe language. An applicant can be described as independent. Independent can be a positive and safe descriptor, but the reference may also mean the applicant cannot work in a team effort. Another safe descriptor is the individual "has a lot of potential," which usually means they didn't live up to that potential yet. "She's a real go getter" can also mean "she wants to move up the ladder, and she doesn't care who she steps on." The information is still there in the references, you just have to look for the underlying meaning (Cherne, 1999, p. 12).

Cherne (1999) cautions that hiring should be an objective process. When it becomes emotional, as in hiring someone because they appeal to you or because you like them, you've hired someone who may be a good person to talk to but not necessarily a good worker. "If you really liked the applicant and felt you could talk to him or her indefinitely," she writes, "unfortunately, once hired that is exactly what you will do—talk for hours and get very little done" (p. 9). Good employees are the center of any organization. When bad workers are terminated, Cherne says that it costs an organization the equivalent of one year's salary to find and train a replacement, because new workers underperform until they learn the job. That's another reason why it's so important to hire the right person the first time.

Mistakes Made in Hiring

Fernandez-Araoz (1999) suggests that hiring often goes badly because managers attempt to look for someone different from past hired workers who failed but, in reality, tend to hire the same type of person again, based on their pleasing personalities or affective differences rather than on whether or not they can do the job. This always happens when there are very unclear specifications for the job. What, for example, does the following mean in behavioral terms? "Applicant must have high energy, be a team player, be creative and spontaneous, be able to accept feedback and criticism, and change with the changing expectations of the job." This comes from an actual job announcement the authors found. How could anyone evaluate whether the applicant has those attributes? Questions to applicants about their strengths and weaknesses or where do they expect to be in 5 years are all vague and have different meaning for everyone asking and answering the question. Applicants find them annoying and useless.

Accepting what people say or write in an application at face value is another mistake. While we would like to think that people are painfully honest, and most workers are, it's also natural to edit resumes and to provide what the applicant thinks is the right answer rather than the honest one. For this reason, never take what an applicant says or writes as fully truthful. And the same goes for references. We know that applicants tend to use only those people who will write good references, but what we should also know is that many references, fearing law suits, write vague or mildly positive references for workers they actually believe did a poor job. Fernandez-Araoz (1999) reports that a recent survey conducted by the Society of Human Resource Management found that only 19% of 850 managers surveyed would reveal to reference-seekers why an applicant left their organization, and that only 13% would discuss an applicant's work habits, all because they were afraid of law suits. This tendency to shy away from saying anything negative is reinforced by the ability, in many settings, for applicants to have access to their references.

Another common mistake is the use of unstructured interviews. Fernandez-Araoz (1999) reports that the research since World War I shows that interviews that are logical, have a set of relevant questions, and are used in the same way with all applicants, get the best results. Be sure, however, to consider the applicant's emotional intelligence: self-awareness, self-regulation, motivation, empathy, and social skills. These are key areas for all work requiring interaction with customers, clients, and co-workers. The use of stress interviews (discussed in more detail later in this chapter), where applicants are brought in as a group with 2–3 facilitators who judge the communication skills of applicants, is one way to evaluate emotional intelligence when you use real-life work problems and ask each group member to offer solutions.

Using Structured and Stress Interviews in Hiring

Buhler (2005) states that a structured interview should use standard questions that have been determined in advance. The questions are asked of all candidates. Buhler suggests two types of structured interviews, both of which should be employed in the interview: behavior description interviews, where an interviewer asks about an actual situation that was encountered in the past, and situational interviews where candidates are asked how they would deal with hypothetical but relevant job-related issues. Many search committees videotape the structured interview so it can be seen by others who may not be able to attend the interview. A videotape can also be analyzed objectively, after the interview, rather than relying on memory alone. Interviewers always need to know which questions cannot be asked by law, including age, marital status or living arrangements, gender orientations, whether someone is pregnant or has physical or emotional problems, religious orientations, or number of children. Amazingly enough, these questions keep being asked and form the basis for a large number of discrimination suits.

The Structured Interview

In the structured interview, the potential worker is asked a series of relevant questions. The questions are the same for all workers. This is very important. Interviews where different questions are asked can be subject to grievance procedures by workers who didn't get the job, but follow-up questions to get clarity or to expand your understanding of a statement made by the worker are fair game if they are done objectively; that is, the follow-up question does not show bias, disagreement, or an opinion, and is only meant to clarify what the interviewee said. The interview is usually done in a group by a small committee of people. Perhaps 3–5 people are optimum. Some questions one might ask in a structured interview are as follows:

1. You've read the job description. Please respond to the competencies required in the description and tell the committee whether you possess those competencies and at what level.
2. Tell us about your reasons for wanting to work in this agency.
3. Tell us about your past work and educational experiences.
4. Our agency works with a very diverse population. Could you tell us how you might help a (gay male, a Hispanic client, a Black client experiencing anxiety/depression, or any number of diverse clients the agency might treat).
5. Why did you become a (mention the profession or type of work performed)?
6. How can you contribute to the agency?
7. Do you prefer working with a team or alone?
8. If you saw something unethical happening in the agency, would you report it and to whom?
9. Describe your notion of the function of a supervisor.
10. What areas of the work are you most excited about?

Once the interview is completed, members of the committee should score the interviewee on a 10-point scale for answers to each question. It's important that each member of the committee understands and correctly uses the scoring system. Some discussion of how it works should be done before the actual interviews begin, perhaps using a videotaped role-played interview. Colleagues who score Advanced Placement exams (a program to provide college credit for courses taken in high school taught at the college level) using a 5-point scale assure me that, with discussion and practice, inter-judge reliability is very high. Comments, if relevant, should also be written down. The scores and comments should be used to choose the best candidate. If this is not done, there is ample room for other workers who were not hired to raise grievances on the selection. Notes and scores are routinely subject to scrutiny, particularly in large bureaucracies where such proceedings have a quasi-legal status.

Be aware that some interviewees lie and they do it well. A recent study by the University of Southern California reported by Hotz

(2005, p. A16) indicates that lying is often a function of the structure of the brain. The study reports that a group of compulsive liars was found to have 26% more white matter and 14% less gray matter in the frontal cortex of the brain. "Lying is congenitally complex. It is not easy to lie. It is certainly more difficult than telling the truth. Some people have a biological advantage in lying. It gives them an edge" (Hotz, 2005, p. 16A).

Gladwell (2005) discusses the instant decisions we make and the biases behind them. The author points out that some of us are able to read faces and determine whether someone is lying at a very high level of accuracy. It's always a good idea to include these people in search committees. It's also important to know that instant judgments about applicants can often be based on an unconscious bias. The bias might include people of color, gay and lesbian candidates, or applicants whose appearance is pleasing or displeasing to us, and it can dangerously skew perceptions and result in dismissing very good applicants. Gladwell cautions against instant judgments and suggests that we take time in forming opinions so that an immediate perception of an applicant doesn't bias our judgment of the applicant's potential performance as a new worker.

The Stress Interview

I (Glicken) was asked to develop a group "stress interview" to help select graduate social work students during a period when applications were insanely high and we were having trouble choosing students for admission purely on the basis of their paperwork (grades, application letter, and references). A small committee made up of faculty and field instructors conducted the interviews, which were to last 3 hours and included 15 students in each group. We first agreed on what we were looking for in applicants: good eye contact; a willingness to participate; a focus on the student being a helper and not a victim; a realistic and positive helping philosophy and a good reason to become a social worker (to help people help themselves, for instance); good body language (no slouching or other indications of boredom or anxiety); intelligent responses and a willingness to give honest answers, even if they took some luster away from the person's chances.

We did use the paperwork as well but, with the addition of the independent rating and evaluations of the three raters, we had over a 90% agreement rate among raters regarding who did well in the interviews and who should be admitted. When all three raters agreed at a high level, the success rate of the students was phenomenal. Our highest-rated students in the interview, regardless of their paperwork, constituted the top 5% of the class in grades as well as in field performance. This approach, which combined structured and non-structured questions with awareness of behavior in the group led to a high degree of confidence among the raters about emotional intelligence. The top-rated students appeared much more at ease with themselves than others and were able, for 3 hours, to not show signs of undue anxiety. They didn't avoid questions and gave honest answers. They seemed comfortable with who they were and appeared as energetic at the end of the interview as they were at the beginning. And they had very good reasons for wanting to be social workers, reasons that weren't unrealistically idealistic such as "to change the world. All of it? Yes!" or self-serving answers such as "to find out more about myself or to get a promotion at work". Instead, they spoke about helping others because they thought they had the skills and motivation, and they were very interested in the work. Or they said that a social worker helped their family and it motivated them to do the same thing for others.

STAFF DEVELOPMENT AND IN-SERVICE TRAINING

Joyce and Showers (1983) believe that effective staff development for new and more experienced workers requires sustained, ongoing efforts with proper funding. Joyce calls the primary purpose of staff development a "problem of transfer." As workers learn new knowledge, skills, and values, they need to cope with the obstacles to make new learning work with clients. One of the functions of staff development is to help workers practice new skills and values in a safe setting until they have some degree of mastery, which is then advanced through coaching and mentoring by supervisors and co-workers (Joyce and Showers, 1983, pp. 15–22). Hunt (1971) believes that staff development deals largely with two issues: changes in competence, and the value system and knowledge that support the development of new skills. Such training requires immersion in the subject and must build matches between the way people learn new material and their willingness to use it in practice, quite different tasks for staff development and one of the reasons workers stick with practice approaches that may not work but feel comfortable.

McKenzie (1991) reports that the following elements must be present for effective staff development: (1) Change requires time and immersion in the subject and includes time to reflect and think through how new material tracks with old beliefs and practices. (2) Staff development must be inspirational and must create motivation to change. (3) Staff development must be experiential and allow workers to practice new skills until they achieve mastery. A worker's fears and anxieties about change should be dealt with. Instruction must take into consideration the worker's perspective of practice. All workers, regardless of their stage of professional development, must be engaged in the learning else the group dynamic changes from one of excitement for new knowledge to resistance and cynicism. There must be long-range planning, sufficient funding, and a desire on the part of the organization to implement change for specific objective reasons. Those reasons might include new research evidence of the effectiveness of a new approach, a changing client culture, new treatment issues, diminishing numbers of qualified staff, reliance on short-term treatment, and others realistic reasons for providing funding for education and change.

Schramm (2005) notes that severe labor shortages in the human services will produce a need to retrain the existing labor pool in more efficient and effective approaches to practice with client groups. She reports a survey by the Society for Human Resource Management (SHRM) showing that finding ways to tap existing talent through new forms of employee development will be critical in addressing skills shortages that may develop, and she writes, "The survey exposes a large disconnect between the number of women and minorities in management roles and the number in executive positions. This may indicate that current approaches to employee development are not working at an optimal level for a large and growing-proportion of the workforce" (p. 144). Because supervisors are primarily responsible for staff development, greater emphasis needs to be placed on the ways workers learn (learning curves) so that staff development not only leads to being able to perform jobs better but encourages growth and, ultimately, promotion.

Because computers offer so many varied ways of presenting material, many staff development programs have gone from formal presentations to giving workers DVDs to view in their spare time (or time made available by the supervisor). This can also be done online using a website. The benefit of staff development done online is that workers can review material that may not be clear, and the style of learning best suited to the worker can be included on the DVD. While some learners respond well to formal lectures without audiovisual assistance, others don't and may need more time to achieve mastery of the material. It's also a very good idea to test workers after they've been involved in staff development presentations to see if learning has been achieved and at what level. This gives the supervisor who developed the training program a way of knowing whether the program is doing what it was intended to do.

TERMINATION

With official unemployment rates at over 8% and some analysts saying that, when you add the underemployed and those who have given up looking for work, it's over 18% of the workforce, many workers have begun to anticipate that dreaded feeling of being told that their services are no longer needed. Anyone who has experienced a termination knows it has severe emotional and physical consequences including depression and small to large persistent physical ailments. How can you terminate someone, especially someone you've known for a long time, and help them retain their dignity and optimism for the future?

McCarter (2003) believes that a mistake new manager's make is that they anguish too long over terminating a poorly functioning worker because they realize that firing anyone is bound to have a depressing impact on the morale of the other workers who might worry that the same thing will happen to them. As a way to avoid this, she suggests that supervisors make every effort to assure well-performing workers that they have nothing to worry about. Frost (2001) suggests that frequent performance appraisals need to be done so that a running record of job performance can be used. Often, organizations have no clear policy about absenteeism or tardiness and while it constitutes a serious problem, the organization doesn't have a specific consequence.

Doyle (2012) reports that over 250,000 workers are wrongly terminated each year. Even if a job is considered "employment at will" where the employer can fire a worker without a reason, workers still have rights if discrimination is involved, public policy is violated, or if an organization's guidelines for termination are incorrectly followed. They also have rights if a company terminates them because they are a whistle blower or refuse to commit an illegal act when asked to do so by an employer. If you question whether a termination will be done correctly, immediately check with your state and federal departments of labor to see if a possible termination violates state or federal law. If it does, workers have a legal case against the employer and it may lead to reinstatement or a very nice settlement that tides him or her over while they look for work.

Three Legal Reasons for Terminating an Employee

1. **The employee violated a known company rule or rules.** Erickson (2005, p. 1) says that before this rule can be used and legally upheld, an employer will need to prove that: "(1) the rule actually exists; (2) the employee knew that it existed; (3) the rule was violated; (4) other employees were terminated for the same infraction; and (5) the termination was reasonable punishment for the infraction." Documentation is very important. To make certain that an employee has all the organization's policies and rules you should have them sign a statement that they have received, read, understand, and intend to abide by all policies and rules.
2. **The employee is unable to perform the job adequately.** Erickson (2005) indicates that to prove incompetence an employer must document that they tried to improve a worker's performance several times before they terminated the employee. They must also show that the expectations were reasonable and that other employees showing the same degree of incompetence were fired. All of this requires proof of policies setting out levels of competence required to maintain the position and clear indications of when evaluations will take place and how unacceptable work will be handled.
3. **The organization is reducing its workforce for economic reasons.** The final legal reason for terminating an employee is if it is in the best economic interest of the company in question. Layoffs are common reasons for terminations, especially in larger corporations that are downsizing or restructuring. Here, courtesy is expected, and employees who are involved in a large-scale layoff need to be given at least 60 days notice of the layoff. This courtesy is required by the Worker Adjustment and Retraining Notification Act (WARN).

The Importance of Documentation

To make sure that you have all of the documentation you need in case of a grievance or law suit (this is particularly important in civil service and public employee termination), Erickson (2005, p. 6) says that you should have the following in your personal files:

- Critical incident reports;
- Employee evaluations (at least one a year. I would recommend evaluations every 6 months, especially for new employees for the first 3 years.). See Chapter 10 for a discussion and example of how to do a competency-based evaluation;

- Job analysis of all jobs. (Conduct job analyses at least every 2 or 3 years.);
- Job descriptions for every job. (Update job descriptions at least every 2 or 3 years.);
- History of how infractions have been handled in the past;
- Supervisor's employee log documenting good and bad incidents;
- Customer or client evaluations and feedback forms;
- Work samples;
- List of rules, signed by each employee;
- List of progressive disciplinary actions signed by each employee;
- Employment-at-will doctrine signed by each employee.

The Termination Meeting

Villano (2005) believes there is no easy way to dismiss a worker and that, while TV reality shows make it look easy, most supervisors report that it is a thoroughly unpleasant experience marked by the guilt of the supervisor and the pain of the worker. Villano suggests brevity in the process (no more than 15 minutes) and that the actual dismissal should come within the first 75 to 120 seconds using sentences such as "I'm sorry to notify you that your employment with us has been terminated." He also suggests that supervisors practice what they intend to say before the actual meeting. Villano believes that explaining the reasons for the dismissal often leads to mistakes in facts that may prove problematic later on if a worker decides to litigate. Since prior work evaluation should let the worker know he or she is in deep trouble, the termination interview should focus on the termination and not the reasons. While most workers take the news calmly, but with obvious emotional pain, the interview usually doesn't end in a confrontation. Sometimes it does, however, and for this reason you may want to have someone nearby or notify security that you may need them. And beware! Termination is one of the primary reasons for later workplace violence, so do it with great respect for the worker, maintaining his or her dignity in the process.

Erickson (2005, p. 8) suggests the following guidelines to the termination meeting:

- Go over all documentation making certain it's all there and it's correct. Be gentle and kind. One of the primary reasons for workplace violence is a termination process that's been done insensitively and with no concern over how the worker feels.

- If the worker agrees to a severance package, and one should always be given, have the worker sign a waiver agreeing not to sue over their termination. As Erickson notes, "This may be a necessary evil if the termination is expected to be controversial or combative in nature" (2005, p. 9) as it almost always is in the public sector.
- Don't try to sugar coat the reasons for the termination but be professional at all times.
- Thank them for their efforts and mean it.
- Take care of administrative duties like collecting keys and company property, and hand the employee his or her final check.

A Dialogue of a Termination for Cause Meeting

Supervisor (S): Jason, because of ongoing problems with your job performance and the agency's policy regarding unacceptable work, I must inform you that the agency is terminating you effective immediately. As our policy manual and your letter of termination note, you will have 2 weeks separation benefits and salary.

Jason (J): I don't understand this at all. I haven't done anything to deserve to be fired.

S: From our point of view, you have, Jason, and I'd encourage you to read your performance reviews.

J: But they didn't say anything about being fired.

S: I'm afraid they did, Jason, and perhaps you might want to read them closely to see the reasons why.

J: How can you do this to me, Sam? You know I've been going through hell in my marriage.

S: Yes, but this is about the work, Jason, and your performance reviews have spelled out the serious concerns we've had.

J: Like what?

S: I'd encourage you to read the periodic reviews over again, Jason, and the termination document I'm giving you now and which I'm also sending by certified mail to your home.

J: This is really crappy of you, Sam. You're a therapist for God's sake; I'd think you'd be more caring.

S: I can understand why you would feel that way but our decision is final, Jason.

J: Is this about me mouthing off to the secretary?

S: It's quite a bit more than that, Jason. By reading the many evaluation reviews noting problems on the job and your termination notice, I think you'll have enough information to understand the agency's decision.

J: What am I gonna tell my wife? Now for sure our marriage is over. Can I empty my desk?

S: Of course you can and, as you will see after reading the termination letter, you can come by and talk to me, but only if you've read the letter and all the material we've noted in the letter that determined your status with the agency.

J: Will you at least write me a reference, Sam? How am I going to get a job without a decent reference?

S: I'm afraid I just couldn't do that. It wouldn't be right for me to terminate you and then recommend you to another agency.

J: I'm really upset, Sam. You know I'd never hurt anyone. I didn't mean it when I told the secretary to watch her backside.

S: It's just one of many things we spell out in your evaluations and termination letter. Please take the time to read everything and do come by and chat if you'd like. Good luck, Jason.

Discussion

There is no easy way to break the news of termination, particularly when a worker is in complete denial, but the supervisor stuck to the task. He didn't get into an argument but correctly kept referring Jason back to his many poor evaluations. You can tell that part of the reason for the termination had to do with anger and potential workplace violence, so this is not an easy task for the supervisor. One would assume that Jason will get up a full head of steam when it all sinks in and consider some retaliatory measure. We hope it's not violence, but it happens, even among human service professionals. You need to forewarn security when you fire someone and unless they have an appointment to see someone in the agency, they should not be allowed back. You should give them enough time to pack their desk and belongings and leave the building, but someone should supervise what is taken. You certainly don't want a terminated employee to take confidential client files. If a worker refuses to leave or causes a commotion that's upsetting to others, unfortunately, they'll have to be escorted out of the building. One never wants that to happen but it does happen and it may increase the potential for workplace violence.

For Therapists Working with Clients Facing Possible Termination

Anyone reading the financial news understands the precarious economic position the country is in and will likely be in for a long time to come. Encourage your clients not to wait passively for termination to take place but to be aware of the often subtle signs that an organization is in trouble and begin looking for other jobs while they're still employed. Those signs are clear enough in the public sector where newspaper articles carry stories of budget cuts every day. In the private sector, earnings reports, office gossip, abrupt changes in leadership, frequent mission changes, and emergency meetings to reorganize are all signs of trouble. It may be a good time to encourage clients to read the financial news if the company they work for is large enough to be written about. At the very least, specific work sectors (airline, energy, etc.) are almost always covered, and the coverage may give the client advanced notice of problems in the sector to come.

It's a sad fact that employers would rather hire currently employed workers than workers who are unemployed. The reason is the belief, however true or not, that employed worker's skills are more up to date and that their work ethic is still intact. Rather than waiting until they've been terminated, encourage clients to begin looking for work, while they are still employed, in organizations that have stronger financials and seem clear of future layoffs. Other good advice is the following.

- Stay up to date and get as much training as possible. The more a client has to offer an employer the more likely they are to get another job. Dr Nan Carle, Director of Community Initiatives at Arizona State University and a longtime public sector manager, encourages her workers to gain new knowledge and skill for this very reason. Out of her limited budget, she provides opportunities for workers to receive added education along a spectrum of activities that will not only help in a current job but will expand a worker's employability if budget constraints require her to downsize staff.
- Network. Any number of possibilities open up to workers when they keep in touch with others. They can do this by joining local organizations in their field, volunteering to help out when there are charitable events, speaking on subjects they have expertise in at workshops and conferences, and just the day to day niceties that help people remember who they are and why they might want to be added to their staff. Dr Carle says that networking involves reaching out to others, connecting with old and new friends, and seeking advice, support, and encouragement from others, when needed. In any given field, there are people of wisdom who many of us go to when we need help. These folks are often well connected and know the job market well. In fact, many of us get jobs because of people we know, including former teachers, bosses, and mentors who often go to bat for us. Keep in touch, because you never know when you might need their help.

Forced Early Retirement

Older workers often have little choice about whether they continue working full-time. Mor-Barak and Tynan (1993) point out that "older workers are more likely to lose their jobs than younger workers in instances such as plant closings and corporate mergers" (p. 45). The authors note that many businesses can't or won't deal with life events faced by older workers such as "widowhood and caring for ailing spouses, and as a result many older workers are forced to retire earlier than planned" (p. 45).

De Vaus and Wells (2007) found that sudden forced retirement significantly increased negative feelings and decreased positive feelings and marital cohesion. Retirees who were forced out of work and did not regain employment over 3 years appeared to miss out on the retirement 'honeymoon,' and were less likely to report benefits after 3 years.

Writing about the loss of work and its impact on older men, Levant (1997) says that, as men lose their good-provider roles, the experience results in "severe gender role strain" (p. 221), which affects relationships and can be disruptive to the point of ending otherwise strong marriages. Because older adults are more likely to lose high-level jobs because of downsizing and age discrimination, social contacts decrease and many otherwise healthy and motivated workers must deal with increased levels of isolation and loneliness in retirement. Schneider (1998) points out that many of us are workaholics and that, when work is taken away or jobs are diminished in complexity and creativity, many older adults experience a decrease in physical and mental health. And while early retirement is touted as a way to achieve the good life while still young, the experience is a complex and even wrenching one in which older adults who are financially able to retire often have little ability to handle extra time, have failed to make sound retirement plans, and find out quickly that not working takes away social contacts, status, and a way to organize time. For many healthy, work-oriented, and motivated older adults, volunteer and civic roles are not at all what they are looking for. They want to continue to work, to contribute, and to receive the financial and social status and benefits related to work.

Early retirement is a complex issue for many older adults who may feel unappreciated and mistreated at work and see retirement as a way of coping with low morale and stress. Often it isn't a solution, since many early retirees haven't thought through retirement as a life style change and may still desire to work in new organizations but may believe that their age makes new employment unlikely. Financial incentive plans for early retirement that seem lucrative may in fact offer a person less financial security in the long run and reduce social security and pension benefits. Work is important to most people because it offers status and a daily schedule. When those two factors are taken away, many early retirees feel unimportant and confused about how to spend their day.

A troubled economy and the loss of investments and equity in housing suggest that the American workplace will see many older workers continue to work well into their 70s and beyond. The fact that social security has a benefit scale based on birth date will make it unlikely for many workers currently in their forties and fifties to retire early. But a longer work-life also has negative ramifications for workers who have worked at physically and emotionally demanding jobs and have seen their bodies wear out.

In an analysis of the impact of paid work and formal volunteerism, Zedlewski and Butrica (2007) found that numerous studies support the finding that work and formal volunteering improve health, reduce the risk of serious illness and emotional difficulties such as depression, and improve strength and cognitive functioning, while full retirement without work and early loss of jobs increased the probability of illness and emotional difficulties. Having something of value to do after retirement helps keep older adults healthy and emotionally engaged with the world around them.

Competency-Based Management Applied to a Poorly Functioning Work Unit: Strategic Terminations and Fallout

Laura Levine is the supervisor of a unit of 15 workers, 3 students, and 2 volunteers providing services in a community mental health agency serving adults with varying degrees and forms of chronic mental illness. The unit is a dysfunctional mess with workers failing to come to work on time, missing work much too often, failing to do needed reports, providing services that are so poorly done that clients and their families have complained, and the all too pervasive sense that everything in the unit is in chaos. Whenever Laura gets tough with workers, they quit. She has tried everything she can think of but nothing seems to work. In desperation, she took a course on competency-based management from the author and applied the following CBM practices.

1. She reviewed the research literature on management in a number of different professions to find out ways of better understanding the problems she was having with the unit. She hadn't realized that research on middle management was common in fields other than management

and was pleasantly surprised to find a number of very helpful and decidedly sympathetic studies in the human services. All the articles confirmed her belief that being a supervisor in an era of reduced budgets and increased workplace litigation was not easy. It was clear to her, after doing some reading, that she was inconsistent in her management by allowing some workers to get away with poor performance while placing others in severe jeopardy if they didn't change. She decided to treat all workers equally. Two pieces of research she found in the public health literature gave strong research evidence that treating all workers in a fair and equitable way created a sense of unity in workers and increased productivity.

2. She decided to hold weekly meetings and involve all the people she supervised in developing solutions. She found eight articles on team work in the management literature to validate this approach. The initial reaction to these meetings was a great deal of grousing about taking time away from clients, but in subsequent weeks the unit began to value the meetings because they focused on problems that everyone was experiencing.
3. She found evidence in three well-done social work studies that setting reasonable work rules improved morale, and she proceeded, with the help of the workers, to develop clear and reasonable work rules for all workers to follow.
4. She found four studies on firing people and determined that two workers were undermining the functioning of the unit. Using the CBM evaluations discussed in Chapter 10, she kept a log of incompetent practice and rule breaking and was able to terminate both workers with little difficulty.
5. Using eight articles on CBM hiring practices, she hired two very positive and well-trained workers to take the place of the fired workers. They are working out fine and have set a much more professional tone on the unit.
6. Believing that many of her workers were developing symptoms of burnout, she read studies with very good research designs and methodologies that gave reasons for burnout and suggested remedies. She began to provide workers with different assignments and offered much more supportive management in recognition of expanding workloads with limited financial rewards or incentives. She also went to bat for several outstanding workers by providing references for promotions and, in one case, arguing that the agency should help pay some of the expenses related to attending graduate school in counseling.
7. Laura began reading about evidence-based practice (Glicken, 2004) and asked her workers to begin basing their practice on best evidence.

She hired a speaker to explain EBP and a consultant to help workers find best evidence. The process of basing their treatment on best evidence had a decidedly positive impact on the workers, who now feel that what they're doing has a scientific base. There is also clear evidence that the clients are doing better.

8. Having been promoted directly from practice with no training in management, Laura took a series of courses offered in the schools of business, counseling, education, public health, and social work on middle management and management. She is developing a level of expertise she didn't have before she took an initial workshop on CBM. She now realizes that being a good therapist doesn't ensure that she'll be a good supervisor and has decided to hire a management consultant to act as a mentor, just as she hired a consultant to help her with practice. This has not only resulted in better supervisory skills, but it has given her needed support to do her job.

A meeting with her unit to find out how things were going indicated that Laura was surer of herself, which translated into less stress for the workers. They liked the meetings they'd had to resolve problems and the fact that Laura was treating them as equals. They thought firing the two workers was needed, but that it had a negative effect initially since it made many people worried that they'd be next. They also felt that Laura had begun acting like a boss, albeit a warm and effective one, rather than a therapist providing therapy to workers. One of the workers said, "It's pretty difficult to take a supervisor seriously who thinks that the best way to get you to do good work is to analyze your behavior and help you develop insight. We need someone who helps us to do our best work, and that's someone who has knowledge and can communicate it effectively to others. We're all reading the research on best practice evidence now, and if Laura did one thing that has made a difference, it's to force us to think in rational ways and not to use treatment approaches just because they feel good. And it's prompted a lot of healthy discussion and interaction we never had before when there was only one way to do things and, whether or not it made sense or worked, that was that."

Questions

1. Isn't it difficult to be creative when we're expected to use treatment protocols and manuals and don't most of us use our own ways of doing things, regardless of the evidence? If that's true, why go through all the time and trouble to do reviews of the research?
2. Laura is saint-like in her ability to work with others who resist change. Do you think most of us would be able to control our emotions and be as rational as Laura is when faced with a poorly functioning unit of workers?

3. Laura held group meetings where there was a good deal of complaining initially. Don't you think complaining often leads to conflict and divisiveness as members of the unit pair off with one another and form camps that lead to more divisiveness and conflict?
4. Laura hired a mentor to help her with her management and to keep her from, one assumes, burning out or becoming overly angry. Do you think this is a wise practice and, if so, who should pay for the service—Laura, or the agency?
5. Firing the bad actors in her unit created a good deal of anxiety among workers. Do you think Laura should have met with the unit after she fired the workers and explained her reasons, assuring them it would not happen again without extreme provocation, or do you think this might have created a confidentiality problem that could lead to legal action by the fired workers against Laura and the agency?

SUMMARY

This chapter on hiring, in-service training, and termination presents practical information on the importance of correct ways of hiring and terminating workers for cause. Because of the bad economy where employers have used lack of money in an organization to terminate workers, it's wise to remember that workers have rights and that, even if money isn't as available as it has been in the past, termination must be done in a way that can be justified if a worker files a grievance or law suit. Up to 200,000 workers each year are terminated and have had their legal rights violated. Similarly, hiring can be an arduous process if it is done badly; practical information from the literature is provided to make hiring as scientific and accurate as it can ever be, realizing that there are limits even in the best hiring process. An example of a termination meeting with a worker is provided along with a case study of a badly functioning work unit with examples of how the manager is able to deal with the many problems in her unit. Material is also presented on the importance of in-service training. Chapter 10 shows how behavioral worker evaluations are done and how they afford organizations more protection from law suits and grievances if workers don't meet standards and are terminated for cause.

REFERENCES

Buhler, P. M. (2005). Interviewing basics: A critical competency for all managers. *Supervision*, *66*(3), 20–22.

Cherne, F. (1999). Hiring so you won't be firing. *Supervision*, *60*(7), 9–11.

De Vaus, D., & Wells, Y. (2007). Does gradual retirement have better outcomes than abrupt retirement? Results from an Australian panel study. *Ageing & Society, 27*, 667–682.

Doyle, A. (2012). *Wrongful termination*. Retrieved August 23, 2012 from <http://jobsearch.about.com/od/jobloss/g/wrongfultermination.htm>.

Erickson, R. (2005). *How to legally terminate an employee*. GoogoBits.com website. Retrieved April, 30, 2012 from <http://www.googobits.com/articles/2259-how-to-legally-terminate-an-employee.html>.

Fernandez-Araoz, C. (1999). Hiring without firing. *Harvard Business Review*, 77(4), 14–22.

Frost, M. (2001). The hiring and firing question and answer book. *HR Magazine*, *46*(11), 132–133.

Gladwell, M. (2005). *Blink: The power of thinking without thinking*. New York: Little Brown.

Glicken, M. D. (2004). *Improving the effectiveness of the helping professions: An evidence-based practice approach to treatment*. Thousand Oaks, CA: Sage Publications.

Hotz, R. E. (2005). Some minds appear wired to lie. *Los Angeles Times*, A 16.

Hunt, D. (1971). *Matching models in education*. Toronto, Ontario: Ontario Institute for Studies in Education.

Joyce, B., & Showers, B. (1983). *Power in staff development through research in training*. Alexandria, Virginia: ASCD.

Levant, R. F (1997). The masculinity issue. *The Journal of Men's Studies*, *5*(3), 221–229.

McCarter, J. (2003). The fine art of hiring and firing. *National Public Accountant*, 20–21.

McKenzie, J. (Ed.), (1991). *The Educational Technology Journal, 1*(No. 4), 24–36.

Mor-Barak, M. E., & Tynan, M. (1993). Older workers and the workplace: A new challenge for occupational social work. *Social Work*, *38*(1), 45–55.

Schneider, K. J. (1998). Toward a science of the heart: Romanticism and the revival of psychology. *American Psychologist*, *53*(3), 277–289.

Schramm, J. (2005). Learning curves. *HR Magazine*, *50*(Issue 2), 144.

Steingold, F. (2000). Hiring without fear: Tips for avoiding legal trouble. *Grounds Maintenance*, *35*(2), 1–30.

Villano, M. (2005). Career couch: Dismiss, yes. *Demoralize*, no. *New York Times,* August 14, 2005, p. BU 9.

Zedlewski, S. R., & Butrica, B. A. (2007). *Are we taking full advantage of older adults' potential? The retirement project: Perspectives of productive aging* (9, 1–8). The Urban Institute.

FURTHER READING

Anon. (n.d.). *74 interview questions and answers*. HumanResources.Hrvinet.com website. Retrieved April 29, 2012 from <http://www.humanresources.hrvinet.com/74-interview-questions-and-answers/>.

Erickson, R. (2005). *How to legally terminate an employee*. GoogoBits.com website. Retrieved April, 30, 2012 from <http://www.googobits.com/articles/2259-how-to-legally-terminate-an-employee.html>.

Heathfield, S. M. (n.d.) *Hiring employees: A checklist for success in hiring employees*. About.com website. Retrieved April 30, 2012 from <http://humanresources.about.com/cs/selectionstaffing/a/hiringchecklist.htm>.

CHAPTER 10

Competency-Based Evaluations

INTRODUCTION

In this chapter, we discuss the evaluation of work done by human service workers (social workers, psychologists, counselors, etc.). Their work often uses vague treatment techniques and often vaguer goals; hence, managers often use attendance, completion of paperwork, and other readily measurable work behaviors in evaluation, rather than attempting to determine the degree to which people are helped with problems that affect their social functioning (the ability to work, for example). Readers in other fields may understand from the content of this chapter that it is possible to measure more-significant work-related behaviors that really cut to what workers are hired to do with clients and consumers.

The human services have generally not done a good job of behaviorally defining expectation for workers. Some authors argue that what we do is often difficult to quantify and that, other than agency expectations regarding easily measurable behaviors such as attendance and report deadlines, the clinical work we do is too complex to measure. Witkin and Harrison (2001) point out that what human service professionals do may not be open to the same level or type of evaluation used in medicine because we often act as cultural bridges between systems, individualize clients in ways that may defy classification and evaluation, and work with oppressed people whose problems may not allow use of more traditional evaluative strategies.

We sympathize with this concern, but we don't agree. If we can't explain the impact of our work to the public at large, our clients, and to policy makers, how can we expect continued support? If we argue that what we do is too complex to measure, then we exist outside the definitions traditionally used to define professions. And more to the point, we ignore the progress made in finding evaluation strategies that actually *do* help us measure client change.

This chapter will take a very behavioral approach, one that argues that if you can't set worker standards for performance and measure how well workers achieve or surpass those standards, you can't really evaluate

Treating Worker Dissatisfaction During Economic Change
DOI: http://dx.doi.org/10.1016/B978-0-12-397006-0.00010-5

workers. We should always be able to know how many clients a worker should see each week, how much improvement they should achieve, how many reports a worker should write and when they are due, and how long it takes, on average, to achieve desired results.

One of the reasons we have difficulty evaluating workers is that many work-related behaviors in the human services are stated in the vague and unhelpful language that policy makers find upsetting and courts find unhelpful whenever law suits are filed because a worker believes he or she has been mistreated. To better show what this means, consider the American Board of Examiners in Clinical Social Work (2008) statements regarding the skills, knowledge, and values that social work clinical supervisors should possess. The following was chosen at random: "The clinical supervisor is aware of how client outcomes can be affected by supervisor/supervisee bias about social work modalities when formulating treatment interventions" (p. 31). That certainly sounds good, but how could we possibly *know* if the supervisor is aware of biasing factors without some measurement? Being aware isn't an active behavior. Supervisors might be aware but not change their behavior or that of the worker. Is there a connection between knowing something and doing something? Often there isn't, but in competency-based evaluation, the relationship between expectations and the actual achievement of those expectations is the primary way to accurately evaluate a worker.

Similar vague language is used in agency practice to describe expectations of workers, which are equally difficult to measure. I can recall being on a tenure and promotion committee where we were asked to make decisions, important decisions, about people's career without specific standards of productivity. How many refereed journals were required for tenure to associate professor level? We would ask our dean. He'd shrug and say, "That's your decision to make. If I don't agree with you, you'll know it." How many committees should a faculty member be on to suggest acceptable university service? "That's up to you." If a professor has evening courses should we cut them some slack on student evaluations? Are student evaluations even relevant? "That's your decision," he said "although I might not agree."

And let's remember that caught in the middle is the client who expects to be better as a result of the service we offer. How can he or she expect to be better if we have no way of knowing ourselves? To help give worker evaluation a more rational base, this chapter will argue that if it can't be measured, it doesn't belong. If it isn't related to client improvement and good agency citizenship, it must be irrelevant. Does coming to work on time affect the client? Yes, of course it does. Does getting reports in on time affect the client? Very often it does. Is being a good team player good for the agency? I think so, but what does that mean? Is knowing agency polices and procedures good for the client? Maybe, but do we have evidence that not knowing them very well is bad for clients? I don't know, but I'd certainly want to find out if I were a supervisor.

And finally, let's be clear about wrongful termination suits and worker grievances against supervisors. The best defense against wrongful termination charges are well-done evaluations that spell out how the worker's performance compares with the agency's standards of performance. If a worker isn't performing and the standards are realistic, you have vital protection against a possible law suit if you terminate a worker.

EXAMPLES OF COMPETENCY-BASED STANDARDS THAT MATTER AND ARE MEASURABLE

Attendance

We expect workers to come to work on time, be on time for client interviews, stay through the entire day, and not take extended coffee or lunch breaks. We can measure all of these behaviors by using time cards or check-in procedures. We should not tolerate attendance problems unless, of course, we use flextime, which is the best way to take care of individual reasons for coming late (taking children to school, elderly parents to care for, etc.). I'm in favor of focusing on getting the work done and allowing wide variations including flextime and working from home. This assumes that the work will get done and that productivity won't suffer. If it doesn't, I'm all in favor of either alternative. But assume that for good reasons, you need workers to work from the office (I can think of child protective workers who worry about security problems, for example), then simple rules are always the best.

Attendance Objectives "All workers must be to work on time unless other arrangements have been made and approved by the worker's supervisor in advance and in writing. Workers who come late will be docked in pay proportionate to the time they've missed. Staying late does not offset the late fee. The same can be said of workers who leave early.

Their pay will be docked. If lateness happens twice in a week, or more than four times in a month, the worker will be placed on probation. If the worker continues to be late the month of probation, he or she will be terminated." Too tough? Maybe. Good for clients and others trying to contact workers? You bet.

Reports

Some agencies aren't funded if worker reports are late. It's a very important matter, particularly when there are late night or weekend emergencies that on-call workers have to cover. Reports are important when workers are on vacation and others have to cover cases, and when workers resign and leave the agency. It is also important that workers use the report format expected by the agency. That format represents the agency's legal representation of what has been done in a case and the rationale for services provided. Reports should be constructed in ways that permit outside readers to understand what took place in the case and why. Hiding botched cases from legal scrutiny by indicating client confidentiality provides the worst message to the public. Often case records are so badly done and so full of errors and missing data that it would be highly embarrassing to the agency were they made public. Supervisors have the responsibility to ensure that records are up to date and accurate. The following competency-based evaluative standard for report writing might serve as an example.

Report Writing Objectives "Workers must complete all written work on cases actively seen during the week by the end of every week. Workers are required to use the agency's format for report writing. Failure to have all reports completed and up to date each week will result in the docking of pay at the rate of 2 hours per late report. If five reports are late during the probationary period, the worker will be terminated from the position. If the worker has achieved more permanent status, the same pay-docking system will be used and the agency will move to terminate the worker for cause. Report writing is vital and the agency takes seriously the lack of up-to-date, accurately written reports. Reports represent our contract to provide a service to clients and the public's expectation that we provide that service in a timely and effective way."

Ethical Conduct

Good work is work that is ethical. Workers who are unethical in their practice can't possibly be providing the client with a positive service. For that reason, knowing, understanding, and practicing the ethics of the agency and the profession are absolute musts. Ethical conduct means that we don't manipulate the truth to make ourselves look better as workers. It means that we function in a way that models the highest ethical standards for clients. It assumes knowledge and agreement with the ethics of the agency and the profession. In matters of ethical conduct, competency-based objectives might read as in the following paragraph.

Ethics Objectives "The agency expects workers to know the policies of the agency and to abide by them. Those policies that deal with ethical issues are particularly important. A set of rules spelling out unethical behavior are provided in the policy manual of the agency and have been developed because of past problems encountered by the agency. For that reason, workers who conduct social and/or sexual relationships with clients will be terminated immediately. Workers who sexually harass other workers, clients, staff, or supervisors, if found responsible for that conduct by a sexual harassment committee of the agency, will face disciplinary actions which might include termination. Workers who share confidential material with non-professionals, unaffiliated members of the agency, or others who have no right to know the information, will be terminated. Workers who take files out of the agency without permission will be terminated. Workers who take agency property or make unauthorized long-distance calls must pay the agency back and will be subject to other disciplinary actions described in the policy manual. The agency accepts the ethical policies of the professions employed by the agency and expects workers at all times to abide by the ethical standards of their profession. If the standards of the agency conflict with those of the worker's profession, the worker should discuss those conflicts with their supervisor and seek acceptable resolution."

Competent Practice

While competent practice can be affected by many variables including the seriousness of the client's problem, client motivation, and worker preparation to work with certain types of psychosocial problems, agencies need to have expectations of competent practice. If they don't, how can anyone judge the quality of the service provided? For this reason use of a measure to determine whether the primary goals of treatment have been achieved in a timely manner is suggested. Goal attainment scales with single subject designs or common psychological instruments to measure client improvement might also be used. Client satisfaction is also an important indicator, although when clients are required to get help from agencies when drug and alcohol treatment is required because of a DUI (Driving Under the Influence of Substances) or in sexual harassment or workplace violence cases, you can expect clients to be generally unhappy about the entire situation. Still, clients who are satisfied and believe that they've been helped provide strong support for workers who correctly believe they are doing a good job and that they should therefore be rewarded accordingly. Finally, evidence of improved social functioning is vital. To do this the worker must verify that change has actually occurred by going to primary sources such as employers and teachers to verify the extent of the change. Let's consider the way this might be stated in an objective.

Objectives to Measure Competent Practice "Workers are expected to provide competent service to clients and to do it in a timely manner. Over the years the agency has developed norms regarding the definition of competent practice. They are as follows: Workers are expected to develop contracts for service by the end of the first client session. Those contracts spell out the goals to be achieved, how long it will take to achieve those goals, the inclusion of the standard client satisfaction survey administered by the secretarial staff after every session, and weekly contact with primary people in the client's life to determine actual changes in social functioning. Contracts must be approved by a worker's supervisor in writing. Workers who achieve the norm can expect average evaluations. Workers who achieve above the norm can expect superior evaluations and compensation using the agency's merit pay system. Workers below the norm will be placed on 6 months of probation. If the service they provide by the end of the 6-month probationary period is not at the norm for the agency, they will be terminated."

Good Agency Citizenship

You may think this is of secondary importance in evaluations, but agencies that have internal squabbling and loose standards of acceptable behavior are often troubled agencies who are not serving clients well. For that reason we expect agency personnel to get along, to treat one another with kindness and respect, and to support the agency in the community. We expect people to be supportive and encouraging in group meetings and to help mentor one another. We would react strongly to workers who berate one another or to workers who hold supervisors in low regard by continually ridiculing them or negating their role publicly. There are humane and professional ways to handle disagreements and they typically aren't in public gatherings where others experience embarrassment and lose of respect. For those reasons, good agency citizenship is important. Let's consider how this can be outlined in the standards for evaluation of workers.

Objectives for Good Agency Citizenship "Workers are expected to act in a professional manner. That includes treating others with respect, consideration, and dignity. Workers who openly disagree with others and cause discomfort to agency personnel and who fail to work differences out with other workers, staff, and supervisors will have this undesirable behavior identified in written evaluations. If the identified behavior is not resolved in a 6-month period, with help and assistance from the agency, the worker will be terminated. Undesirable behavior includes frequent public arguments with others, using derogatory names or terms with others either publicly or privately, shouting at others, and the use of words suggesting racial, religious, or gender bias. Problems with other employees are to be worked out using the supervisor as the mediator. If he or she is unavailable, the agency will provide mediators to help work out legitimate professional and work-related problems. If the problems causing the unacceptable behavior are personal, the agency expects the worker to seek assistance from the agency's EAP or from a professional provider."

Community Involvement

The human services are part of a broad community effort to help people. Involvement in community efforts and professional organizations should be an expectation of all human service agencies since it adds to the strength of our helping efforts and creates a helping community that may be a substantial force for change. I suggest released time to be a part of community efforts and that supervisors might even be proactive and suggest ways workers can be involved in community efforts. As Saleebey (1996, p. 297) writes in his discussion of the importance of healthy community life,

> *Membership [in a community] means that people need to be citizens—responsible and valued members in a viable group or community. To be without membership is to be alienated, and to be at risk of marginalization and oppression, the enemies of civic and moral strength (Walzer, 1983). As people begin to realize*

and use their assets and abilities, collectively and individually, as they begin to discover the pride in having survived and overcome their difficulties, more and more of their capacities come into the work and play of daily life.

Objectives for Community Involvement "Workers are expected to be involved in community or professional groups that directly lead to stronger community life and better assistance for our clients. The agency will provide up to 2 hours a week of released time for workers to attend community and professional meetings that are acceptable to the agency and supported by the worker's supervisor. We particularly encourage workers to take leadership roles on community boards."

Attaining New Knowledge

Agencies change and improve as workers gain knowledge of the many new approaches available in the helping professions. We hope that what they learn will be passed on to others and the investment made by the agency to offer workers paid opportunities to attend workshops, conferences, or to receive special training will pay off in cutting-edge services to clients that keep the agency competitive.

Objectives for Gaining Knowledge "Workers are encouraged to learn new work-related behaviors that will assist our clients and help the organization. We will provide workers up to $1,000 a year for attendance at approved conferences, workshops, courses, or tutorials on subjects of special need to the agency. Workers are expected to give formal presentations about what they've learned and to mentor other workers. Released time will be given for approved mentoring activities."

PROVIDING FEEDBACK TO WORKERS

Glicken (2008) notes that there are four types of evaluative feedback: positive, negative, evaluative, and developmental.

- Positive feedback recognizes aspects of the worker's performance that are well done and provides reasons the work is exceptional.
- Negative feedback focuses on aspects of a worker's performance that are inadequate, insufficient, or inappropriate.
- Evaluative feedback compares a worker's performance with agency standards and expectations. In competency-based supervision the appraisal involves objective facts and not merely judgment.

- Developmental feedback helps workers understand why they did well or badly, confirms behaviors that should be retained, and identifies behaviors that should be changed.

Glicken indicates that, for feedback to be effective, it must be: useful; frequent; timed so that the worker is listening and receptive to the feedback; directed to the specific problem without a preamble; helpful to the worker in doing the job more effectively and efficiently; understood by the worker as a behavior that needs to be reinforced or changed; and clearly understood by confirming that workers know what you mean and that they understand the reasons for the feedback.

In competency-based supervision, to be effective, feedback must be clearly tied to established expectations of practice; come from trusted and accurate means of monitoring performance; be based on information that is accurate and can be verified; be presented in a logical, helpful, and persuasive manner; be given in the context of a good worker–supervisor relationship; and be given in a way that supports the mission of the agency, benefits clients, and helps resolve relationship problems between the worker and other workers.

PAY FOR PERFORMANCE: MERIT PAY

Many human service organizations have decided that they no longer want to pay for mediocre work and believe that employees should be rewarded for the quality of their work and their value to the agency, including the new skills and competencies they've learned over the years. In merit systems, the better a worker's performance, the higher their pay. Performance is determined by competency-based evaluations which are always behavioral and which focus, to the extent possible, on behaviors that are objective in nature and can be measured.

In Opposition to Merit Pay

This rational-sounding system has been widely criticized *and* widely touted as the solution to improving worker performance, reducing turnover, and improving morale. For those opposed to merit pay, the arguments are that merit pay creates tensions among workers because it stresses competition rather than teamwork and cooperation; merit pay decisions are usually reduced to whomever the supervisor likes best and are subjective and biased in nature; merit pay actually reduces productivity; the indicators of meritorious work are so easily manipulated by workers that the real issue, the quality of their work with clients, often gets pushed back and other less important indicators are used to determine merit pay; it is not unusual for workers to argue for more merit pay for those aspects of the work for which they are most effective even though they may be of secondary importance; and that accountability-driven workplaces that focus on measuring effectiveness are real turnoffs to professionals. As Kohn (2003, p. 48) notes in discussing the reasons why new teachers leave education,

> *In 2000,* Public Agenda *questioned more than 900 new teachers and almost as many college graduates who* didn't *choose a career in education. The report concluded that, while "teachers do believe that they are underpaid," higher salaries would probably be of limited effectiveness in alleviating teacher shortages because considerations other than money are "significantly more important to most teachers and would-be teachers." Two years later, 44 percent of administrators reported, in another* Public Agenda *poll, that talented colleagues were being driven out of the field because of "unreasonable standards and accountability."*

Kohn (2003, p. 51) believes that the following reasons explain why merit pay does not work.

1. **Control.** People with more power usually set the goals, establish the criteria, and generally set about trying to change the behavior of those below them. If merit pay feels manipulative and patronizing, that's probably because it is.
2. **Strained relationships.** In its most destructive form, merit pay is set up as a competition, where the point is to best one's colleagues. It creates terrible tensions and leads to lowered morale and job turnover.
3. **Reasons and motives.** The premise of merit pay, and indeed of all rewards, is that people *could* be doing a better job but for some reason have decided to wait until it's bribed out of them. This is as insulting as it is inaccurate. Dangling a reward in front of workers does nothing to address the complex, systemic factors that are actually responsible for poor service to clients.
4. **Measurement issues.** It's an illusion to think we can specify and quantify all the components of good client services, much less establish criteria for receiving a bonus that will eliminate the perception of arbitrariness.
5. **Manipulating outcome measurements.** One of the sad facts of merit systems is that certain behaviors on the part of the person being evaluated can improve scores on effectiveness ratings even though

those scores aren't deserved. In academia, for example, high grades on examinations are a prime way to increase students' satisfaction scores, one of the significant ways in which merit is determined in academia. Another way is to have a party or to say excessively nice things about a class before the survey is given. I've known instructors who even tell stories about the personal problems they have to gain sympathy from students and improve satisfaction scores. As one might guess, these devices cause great unhappiness among workers who eschew them and who feel that they thereby miss out on valuable raises and promotions.

In Support of Merit Pay

On the other hand, it is demoralizing to good workers to see poorly performing workers receive the same salary increases. It tends to lower the quality of their work. Why work so hard if the rewards aren't there? Applying the same salary increases to everyone fails to encourage the acquisition of new skills. As one of the participants in a workshop I gave recently said about merit pay, "We have a merit pay system. You get a 2% raise if you're outstanding and a 1% raise if you're terrible. What kind of merit system is that? I'm leaving social work because, hard as I try at work and much as I am told I do a terrific job, I'm not rewarded for my work. My husband who works in business got a 15% merit salary increase this year. Some of his co-workers got nothing. It's a tough world out there. The ones who perform should get the rewards."

Another student said, "I've been at my agency for 5 years. During that time I got a total of a 5% salary increase. It's nothing. Before I came they had a merit system that increases a person's salary for really good work up to 10% a year, but the workers rebelled and they bagged the program. The good workers left because they wanted to feel rewarded for their work. We're left with mediocre to poor workers. I just took a new job and the response from the agency was, too bad, we'll miss you. They didn't even bother to ask why I was leaving."

Recognizing the impact of inequitable salaries for exceptional workers, Van Ark (2002) reports that "dissatisfaction with performance appraisal systems is another of the most common complaints heard among human service workers" (p. 10). The options for workers are either to move into administration, where the rewards are better even though the work itself may not be satisfying, or to "continue their excellent service delivery without any tangible recognition, which only contributes to poor morale" (p. 11). Clive (2004) says that when standard salary increases are given that do not factor in merit, "The message to the outstanding performers is that their efforts are not valued and they should either perform at an 'average' level or find an employer who is willing to pay for their skills" (p. 2), while the message to marginal workers "is that their performance is acceptable and no significant increase in performance is required" (p. 2).

There is evidence that merit pay has a positive impact on worker performance. Dee and Keys (2004) report that

> *Despite widespread pessimism among educators about whether merit pay systems can effectively reward good teachers, most of the limited empirical evidence has been surprisingly positive. For example, two studies (in 1992 and 1997) found that the math and reading test scores of students in South Carolina improved significantly when the students were taught by teachers receiving merit pay. Similarly, related and more recent literature suggests that mathematics students learn more when their teachers have certification in mathematics.*

The Center for the Study of Social Policy (2002) reports that, in organizations using competency-based measurement tools to evaluate workers' performance, satisfaction of workers with the system was 97% while dissatisfaction with the old system of evaluating performance was 93%. The new system linked performance to pay while the old system gave everyone the same increase regardless of their performance.

Setting Up a Merit Pay System

In a merit system, the total amount available for raises is placed in a merit pool. Below you will see how points are given. Let's say the pool is 3% of the agency's budget for salaries for the year, or $100,000. Rather than giving the 3% out to everyone, based on their salaries and regardless of their performance, merit pay is based on each worker's individual performance across several indicators. I'm using the following as an example. (1) Client improvement is worth up to 14 points while good agency citizenship is worth up to 6 points. A perfect score would be 20. The points are totaled and then each point is given a dollar worth. Let's say that there are 500 points given out and that each point is worth $200. This is accomplished by dividing the total points (500) into the merit pool ($100,000). The worker who scores 20 points on their evaluation would get a raise of $4,000 while the worker who scores 5 points would get an increase of $1,000. This is irrespective of their salary. For a salary of

$30,000 the merit increase for 20 points would be over 13%, while 5 points would be a salary increase of 3%. There would be no raises given out at all for workers who receive fewer than 5 points since their work is considered unsatisfactory. By not giving out points for unsatisfactory work, the worth of each point increases.

A COMPETENCY-BASED EVALUATION SCALE

The following guide is tied to the above merit pay scheme. Each point will equal a certain amount of money, and raises will be based on point totals. In this approach it's possible that workers will receive no increase at all if their work is at an unsatisfactory level. This is a very behaviorally oriented approach which requires accurate evaluation of work.

A. Points for practice (total points available: 0–14)

1. Client satisfaction score based on a 0–5 point scale with 5 the highest possible rating (4 total points possible):
   - **a.** On a 0–5 point scale, an average score of 4.50–5.00 (4 points)
   - **b.** On a 0–5 point scale, an average score of 4.0–4.49 (3 points)
   - **c.** On a 0–5 point scale, an average score of 3.50–3.99 (2 points)
   - **d.** On a 0–5 point scale, an average score of 3.00–3.49 (1 point)
   - **e.** Below 3.0 (0 points).
2. Achievement of contracted-for goals (5 total points possible):
   - **a.** 95%–100% of the goals achieved in the time contracted for (5 points)
   - **b.** 90%–94% of the goals achieved in the time contracted for (4 points)
   - **c.** 85–89% of the goals achieved in the time contracted for (3 points)
   - **d.** 80–84% of the goals achieved in the time contracted for (2 points)
   - **e.** 75–79% of the goals achieved in the time contracted for (1 point)
   - **f.** Below 75% (0 points).
3. Better psychosocial functioning (5 total points possible):
   - **a.** A 95–100% improvement over first client session (5 points)
   - **b.** A 90–94% improvement over first client session (4 points)
   - **c.** An 85–89% improvement over first client session (3 points)
   - **d.** An 80-84% improvement over first client session (2 points)
   - **e.** A 75-79% improvement over first client session (1 point)
   - **f.** Below 75% (0 Points).

B. Points for good agency citizenship (0–6 points)

1. Reports and other written work (2 points):
   - **a.** Reports are always on time and always very well done (2 points)
   - **b.** Reports are always on time and done at the expected level (1 point).
2. Goes the extra mile in helping others (1 point).
3. Is a leader in teams (1 point).
4. Attains new knowledge and teaches it to others (1 point).
5. Is involved in the community and the profession through board memberships, leadership roles, consulting, and other activities (1 point).

To give you a better idea of how this would work, Tables 10.1 and 10.2 outline how points would be given and how they equate to an actual amount of money and a designated rating of worker performance.

A Model Evaluation

End of the Year Evaluation: Sara Smith received three quarterly evaluations this year which outline her general functioning at the agency. This evaluation is a summary of the three former evaluations including any new behaviors noted in the fourth quarter of the year.

This is Ms Smith's second full year with the agency. She continues to work at the norm established by the agency. Her work with clients, while consistent, is never beyond expectations and all aspects of her client work are average. Her reports are on time and use the agency format. While basically accurate, her reports sometimes use non-technical language and Ms Smith has been told on eight occasions not to use slang or familiar language when more descriptive professional language is available. Ms Smith is always on time and has missed only 4 days during the year because of illness. The agency's policy is to pay the worker for unused sick days at 25% of their cost. Ms Smith will be paid for the 8 unused sick leave days for the year.

Ms. Smith has very good working relationships with her co-workers and is well liked by the support staff. On a number of occasions she has filled in for sick workers or stayed late to help with agency overloads. Her work is usually quite ethical but on a few occasions I have overheard her talking about clients in the lunch room. While she never identifies the client by name, it isn't difficult to know who she's talking about. In the times I've overheard her talking about clients it has never been derogatory or overly informative. Still, it's against agency policy and she has been notified that this behavior should stop. To my knowledge it has.

Ms. Smith is a very good team member and is always willing to offer suggestions to other workers. She is always on time for supervision and takes our meetings seriously. To improve the quality of her practice with clients I have sent her to a conference on the use of the strengths perspective and another on competency-based practice. I see little evidence that she is applying either approach and her ability to use the Internet to answer practice questions, as I've instructed her to do, has been minimal. In her self-evaluation for the year, Ms Smith notes no community involvement, although she's been encouraged to become more involved and has even been offered released time to join a committee working on problems of our clients.

While she is well liked by her clients as is evidenced by high scores on the client satisfaction scale (an average score of 4.5 on a 5 point scale) clients complain in the written portion of the survey that she is overly non-direct and much too passive. We have discussed this, and she agrees, but it is difficult for her to be more directive and she continues to allow clients to work things out by themselves and to be a passive participant in sessions. Nonetheless, her clients improve at an average level. I am therefore recommending a salary increase of 3 merit points for her client satisfaction (see the merit scale) as outlined in the agency's merit pay schedule for salary increases, 1 point for better client functioning, and 1 point for achieving goals set for treatment. I've given her 1 additional point for her good agency citizenship. Each point is worth $200. Ms Smith's salary increase will be $1,200.

In summary, Ms Smith is a good agency citizen who is well liked and regarded by others. She is hard working and goes the extra mile in filling in for others. Her work with clients remains average and she continues to be too passive and non-directive with clients. We will continue to work on this area of practice in the coming year.

Table 10.1 Appraisal Score, Salary Increase, and Evaluation Rating in an Example Merit Pay Scheme

Performance appraisal score	Rating	Salary increase at $200/point
18.00–20.00	Outstanding	$3,600–4,000
14.00–17.99	Significantly exceeds expectations	$2,800–3,598
10.00–13.99	Exceeds expectations	$2,000–2,798
5.00–9.99	Meets expectations	$1,000–1,998
0.00–4.99	Unsatisfactory	0

Table 10.2 Rating Scale for Evaluating Performance in the Example Merit Pay Scheme to which Table 10.1 Refers

Score	Standard
18–20	Outstanding—Performance in this category is clearly exceptional. Must be properly documented with examples applicable to the individual performance category.
14.00–17.99	Significantly exceeds expectations—Significantly exceeds performance standards established for the position. Must be properly documented with examples applicable to individual performance category.
10.00–13.99	Exceeds expectations—Exceeds performance standards established for the position. Must be properly documented with examples applicable to the individual performance category.
5.00–9.99	Meets expectations—Meets all standards of performance established for the position.
0.00–4.99	Unsatisfactory—Not acceptable. If an employee is not to be terminated for non-performance, a written plan for improvement must be developed with the supervisor. No merit raise will be granted for the performance review period in which an unsatisfactory performance rating is earned. A follow-up evaluation shall be provided as determined by management. In the case of a ninety (90)-day performance improvement plan, an evaluation session will be conducted each thirty (30) days and a final evaluation issued at the end of ninety (90) days.

A Case to Evaluate

You are supervising a young woman whom you like very much as a person. She is warm, funny, and kind but does a very poor job with clients. It's not that she doesn't like them or want to help but her helping impulses often get in the way and she relates to clients, not as a professional, but as an overly involved parent. She's taken clients home with her, she's bought them gifts when they are feeling blue, she buys them food from her own pocket and often drives them to places when they are perfectly capable of doing this by themselves. In essence, she is developing severe dependency by doing what they should be doing for themselves if they are to achieve better social functioning. The clients aren't getting better but have regressed. You have given her an unsatisfactory evaluation which means she is automatically placed on probation without a salary increase for the year which can result in the loss of her job if she doesn't improve over the next 6 months. You need to develop a plan with her which will attempt to make her a sounder and more effective professional without destroying her strong desire to help her clients.

Questions

1. Why is she acting in such an unprofessional way? Surely her training would suggest to her that she needs to be more professional in her work with clients, or does it?
2. What readings would you give her to help her better understand that by causing her clients to be dependent on her, they meet her needs rather than the other way around?
3. What activities might you do jointly to help her move toward a professional role with her clients?
4. Some people would say that what your worker is doing is really what helping is all about. How can you help her see that her clients are actually not being helped?
5. Might this type of problem suggest the need to treatment because it so closely parallels co-dependent behavior? Go to the literature and find out what treatment approaches seem to help reduce co-dependent behavior in workers.

SUMMARY

In this chapter on competency-based evaluations special attention is paid to understanding the need for objective, measurable work objectives that are at the same time realistic, relevant, and ethical. Discussion includes merit systems and ways to set them up in a human service agency. In a case presentation at the end of the chapter, you are asked to consider how you might work with a member of your team whom you supervise who, while a wonderful person with concern for others and loyalty to the agency, at the same time isn't very effective.

REFERENCES

American Board of Examiners in Clinical Social Work (2008). *A model practice act for clinical social work*. Retrieved August 23, 2012 from <http://www.abecsw.org/images/Center%20Model%20Practice%20Act%20Final%207.3.08.pdf>.

Clive, C. N. (2004). *Does merit pay really reward performance? Compensation and Benefits Forum*. Retrieved August 23, 2012 from <http://www.baylights.com/articles/0503employeemotivation.html>.

Dee, T. S., & Keys, B. J. (2004). *Dollars and sense.* The Hoover Institute. Available at <http://www.educationnext.org/20051/60.html>.

Glicken, M.D. (2008). *A competency-based approach to supervision in the human services.* Unpublished manuscript.

Kohn, A. (2003). The folly of merit pay. *Education Week*, 46–53 September.

Saleebey, D. (1996). The strengths perspective in social work practice: Extensions and cautions. *Social Work*, *41*(no. 3), 296–305.

Van Ark, B. (2002). Understanding productivity and income differentials among OECD countries: a survey. In: *The review of economic performance and social progress 2002: Towards a social understanding of productivity.* Retrieved August 23, 2012 from <http://ideas.repec.org/h/sls/repsls/v2y2002bva.html>.

Walzer, M. (1983). *Spheres of justice.* New York: Basic Books.

Witkin, S. L, & Harrison, W. D. (2001). Editorial: Whose evidence and for what purpose? *Social Work*, *46*(no. 4), 293–296.

PART *Four*

Effective Treatment for Work-Related Problems

CHAPTER 11

Treating Work-Related Problems

INTRODUCTION

This chapter discusses best evidence for treating job dissatisfaction, worker burnout, and one of the major problems resulting from job unhappiness, substance abuse. The approaches suggested in this chapter are those with best evidence of effectiveness, but problems related to substance abuse and long-term depression require thoughtful review of the literature and are difficult to resolve for many workers because of the length of the problem and because our efforts to date to find effective treatments are still at an early stage. The approaches included in this chapter are: life coaching; brief and long-term treatment for mild depression associated with early stage burnout; treating anxiety often associated with demanding work that creates overstimulation; the use of groups in treating work-related problems; and treatment approaches for substance abuse, including those informed by research findings that many early substance abusers improve with brief interventions or may never use professional treatment at all but resolve problems on their own or with self-help programs that offer support and a sense of community. Case examples are provided throughout the chapter to show how each approach is applied to a client.

LIFE COACHING FOR JOB DISSATISFACTION

Life coaching is a brief, goal-oriented way of problem solving that generally works on a specific problem with healthy people for a very limited amount of time. It is highly performance oriented and is much less concerned with the development of insight or broader application to other areas of life. Clients are generally people who have intrusive problems requiring quick solution. Work-related problems, job changes, divorce work, and relationship problems may all be issues that respond well to coaching.

The elements of life coaching that may be useful for work with job dissatisfaction are the following. (1) Life coaching is geared to here and

Treating Worker Dissatisfaction During Economic Change
DOI: http://dx.doi.org/10.1016/B978-0-12-397006-0.00011-7

now problems. It doesn't assume that a problem has its origins in the past, and it tries to find quick, logical solutions. (2) Life coaching is very practical. It uses advice, homework assignments, asking other people for information, and searching the Internet and journals for answers to problems. Life coaches often suggest that clients keep logs or write down ideas that are then shared with the coach. This technique seems efficient to many dissatisfied workers who believe that taking responsibility for change will speed up the process. (3) Life coaching encourages the use of behavioral charting to analyze a problem and to track success.[1] (4) Coaching assumes that clients are emotionally healthy and functioning well but just need some practical and supportive assistance with problem solving. Compare this to counseling and psychotherapy that assumes dysfunction, describes people in unhealthy ways, and often uses labels. (5) Coaching is very positive and optimistic. It is founded on belief that problems can be resolved in a short period of time and that people have the necessary inner resources and skills to resolve problems with just a little direction from the coach.

Case Example: Life Coaching with a Job Dissatisfied Worker

June Addison has all the signs of job dissatisfaction and came to a life coach with concerns about her job performance. Her most recent work evaluation was mediocre to poor. Given the company's current economic condition, Jane worries that she might lose her job. With a family to support and no other possibilities of similar work in her field in the community, she is very determined to improve her work performance even though she is admittedly unhappy with her job and doesn't much like the company she works for. Still, it's a good job and she doesn't want to lose it because of her attitude. The coach looked at her written performance and saw three areas that definitely needed improving. Over two sessions, Jane and the coach worked together on practical ways to improve her performance. They also set up a way of measuring whether improvement was taking place.

[1] The senior author's daughter developed a chart to determine which graduate schools she should focus on when applying to schools in public health. Two or three indicators were suggested by her father to determine which schools were most likely to provide a good experience (rankings, availability of assistantships, program focus). By the time she finished the chart, she had over 20 indicators. When she was done filling in the information under each indicator, it was clear that four or five programs stood out. She indicated that charting cut down on extraneous efforts to problem solve and that it was very time and energy efficient.

After the initial two sessions, Jane sent the coach a weekly progress report by email. Brief telephone calls augmented the reports. Several times Jane was clearly not following through on the strategies they had decided on and the coach called her in for a chat about why things didn't seem to be going better and what could be done about it. The coach and Jane also worked out a "360," a management technique used to get maximum feedback from others on Jane's work performance. With work evaluations coming every 3 months, they had less than 3 months to resolve the problem, and they did. The next evaluation placed the clients' performance in the low excellent range and her job was secure.

How did this differ from counseling? The client had initially gone for therapy when she saw her work evaluations begin to deteriorate. She was also working longer and longer hours but getting little done and feeling more and more unhappy at work and stressed. The counselor felt that Jane was experiencing a mild depression in response to being passed over for a promotion. There were also some conflicts in the family that seemed to be troubling her and could have been responsible for her poor work performance. Counseling consisted of trying to find out more about her feelings regarding the promotion and her concerns about her family. There were some very good discussions and the counselor felt that therapy was certainly helping her until a quarterly evaluation suggested that her performance had slipped even more. Concerned that counseling wasn't helping, Jane sought out the life coach on the advice of some co-workers who had used her in the past with good success. In comparing the two forms of help, Jane said,

> *"I liked both people. I thought they were very competent and caring. I think the counselor was helpful in getting me to talk about my reaction to not getting the promotion and my family problems. She was right in thinking that I was depressed. I was. I just didn't know what to do about work and in that regard, she wasn't very helpful.*
>
> *"When I went to the coach, all she talked about was work. I felt there were other things that needed dealing with but that work was the most important thing. She helped a lot. She was very nice in a no-nonsense sort of way, and she knew her stuff. In no time, I was back on track at work but felt there were other issues I needed to deal with before the same thing that happened at work started happening again. So I went back to the therapist and I'm very happy with the work we're doing together. Why didn't I stay with the coach? I don't know. My life is a lot more complicated than work. I thought I needed someone who would listen and help me figure it all out. I don't think charts and 360s work well for all life problems, but maybe they do. I'd recommend a coach for very practical problems and a counselor for more complicated problems. That's my read on it, anyway."*

TREATING WORK-RELATED BURNOUT AND DEPRESSION

Worker burnout is a form of depression in which the worker has little emotional energy to perform work-related functions. Burnout negatively affects a worker's attitude toward the organization and often creates problems in a worker's personal life. For that reason, treating burnout as a form of depression is a primary way to help workers redefine their attitudes toward work, make necessary changes in their careers, and energize them to seek new careers, jobs or, when necessary, additional specialized training.

In terms of the research on treatment effectiveness for depression, Gallagher-Thompson, Hanley-Peterson, and Thompson (1990) followed older clients of an age where layoffs and burnout are common for 2 years after completion of treatment and found that 52% of the clients receiving cognitive treatment, 58% of the clients receiving behavioral treatment, and 70% of the clients receiving brief dynamic treatment had no return of depressed symptoms 2 years after treatment. The authors report that these rates of improvement are consistent with those of a younger population of depressed clients. However, Huffman (1999) reports high rates of recurrence of depression in older workers following treatment. For subjects aged 60–69, the recurrence rate was 65%. Subjects treated with just an antidepressant and scheduled office visits to check on their progress did least well, with a 90% recurrence rate for both age groups (Huffman, 1999).

Lebowitz et al. (1997) found that certain types of psychotherapy are effective treatments for depression. For many adults, especially those who are in good physical health, combining interpersonal psychotherapy with antidepressant medication appears to provide the most benefit. The authors note that about 80% of adults with depression recovered with this kind of combined treatment and had lower recurrence rates than with psychotherapy or medication alone. The authors conclude that the more cognitively and physically healthy the client, the more likely therapy will be beneficial.

Lenze et al. (2002) studied the effectiveness of interpersonal treatment in conjunction with antidepressants with depressed clients. The authors found improved social adjustment attributable to combined interpersonal psychotherapy and maintenance medication. While improvement in social functioning could not be directly related to therapy, maintenance of the gains made in social functioning seemed directly related to therapy. The most significant gains reported by the authors were in the areas of interpersonal conflict role transitions and abnormal grief.

Zalaquett and Stens (2006) believe we have "a great body of data supporting the use of medication and/or psychosocial therapy to help the person with depression return to a happier, more fulfilling life ... and shorten the time to recovery" (p. 192). Pinquart and Sörensen (2001) suggest that using psychosocial therapy with adults is valuable because it decreases depression and promotes general psychological well-being. O'Connor (2001) reports that adults usually get better after their first episode of depression, but that the relapse rate is 50%. Clients with three episodes of depression are 90% more likely to have additional episodes. O'Connor suggests that we need to accept depression as a chronic disease and that therapists must be prepared to "give hope, to reduce shame, to be mentor, coach, cheerleader, idealized object, playmate, and nurturer. In doing so, inevitably, we must challenge many of our assumptions about the use of the self in psychotherapy" (p. 508).

Brief and Group Therapy for Burnout

Plopper (1990) believes that brief and focused approaches to the treatment of depression are preferable to intensive psychodynamic psychotherapy. Psychodynamic treatment, which aims to provide clients with both support and a personal understanding of their current difficulties, emphasizes the importance of interpreting the patient's emotional experience through the therapeutic relationship.

Roth and Fonagy (1996) report that group therapies with adults experiencing depression showed promise of reducing symptoms of depression. In one study, psychodynamic group therapy and cognitive behavioral group therapy approaches were compared and found to be equally effective in reducing levels of depression. Another study evaluated the effectiveness of self-help books with mildly to moderately depressed adults (Floyd, Scogin, McKendree-Smith, Floyd, & Rokke, 2004). Participants were randomly assigned to a cognitive bibliotherapy group, a behavioral bibliotherapy group, or a delayed treatment control group. Participants in the cognitive bibliotherapy group received a cognitive therapy self-help book, while participants in the behavioral bibliotherapy group received a behavioral therapy self-help book. Participants were told to read the books and were contacted in 4 weeks with follow-up questions to determine the impact of the books on depression. The results suggested "a clinically significant change" in depression with both cognitive and behavioral therapy self-help books. Gains continued at 6-month and 2-year follow-ups.

Table 11.1 Best Evidence of Treatment Effectiveness for Depression

Therapy	Major depression	Dysthymia	Maintenance
CBT	Probably efficacious	Potentially useful/helpful	Incomplete evidence
IPT	Incomplete evidence	Potentially useful/helpful	Useful with medication
BDT	Probably efficacious	No data	No data
RT	Potentially useful/helpful	No data	No data
Family	Incomplete evidence	Incomplete evidence	Incomplete evidence
Group	Has been researched with incomplete evidence	Incomplete evidence	Incomplete evidence

BDT, brief dynamic therapy; CBT, cognitive-behavioral therapy; IPT, interpersonal therapy; RT, reminiscence therapy.

Table 11.1 (Zalaquett and Stens, 2006, p. 197) shows our current state of research-based knowledge about treatments that work best with adults experiencing depression.

In summarizing treatment effectiveness with older clients experiencing depression, Myers and Harper (2004) report that many interventions have been found effective with older adults "... diagnosed with subclinical or clinical depression. These include reminiscence; individual behavioral, cognitive, and brief psychodynamic therapies; group psychodynamic and cognitive-behavioral therapies; and self-help bibliotherapy" (p. 210).

TREATING WORK-RELATED ANXIETY

Beck and Stanley (1997) report positive results with anxious clients using cognitive-behavioral therapy and relaxation training. Benefits for older clients experiencing anxiety appear as positive as they are with younger clients. Smith, Sherrill, and Celenda (1995) have found that adults respond well to psychotherapy for anxiety, "especially if it supports their religious beliefs and encourages life review that helps to resolve both hidden and obvious conflicts associated with specific events in the patient's life history" (p. 6). The authors recommend medications only after all options have been considered. Most anxiety problems in younger clients are treated with benzodiazepines, but these have only a "marginal efficacy for chronic anxiety and are especially bad for older adults because the body accumulates the drug and may produce excess sedation, diminished sexual desire, worsening of dementing illness, and a reduction in the general level of energy" (p. 6). The authors also warn that Prozac may actually cause anxiety as a side effect and recommend pinpointing the cause of the anxiety problem before considering the use of medications.

Although the effects of cognitive-behavioral approaches seem positive, Lang and Stein (2001) recommend that treatment of anxiety should be tailored to the individual needs and cognitive abilities of the client. Anxious clients may find relaxation approaches inappropriate or childish. Systematic desensitization may be seen as unrelated to their situation or to the origins of their anxiety, and they may view changes in the way they are told to perceive life events as dangerous to their survival since long-held beliefs and behaviors have often served them well in the past. Being asked to view a situation with clarity and rationality may suggest to the client that workers believe they are lying about an event. Clients may discount psychological explanations for their anxiety and prefer to think that it has a physical origin. All of these cautionary suggestions should be taken into account when working with anxious clients or one runs the risk of having psychological treatments dismissed completely.

A suggestion to encourage better acceptance of any intervention is to give clients reading materials to help them understand the origins of their anxiety and the approach most likely to help relieve their symptoms. Testimonials from other clients might also be helpful, or suggestions made by other professionals they trust could help the client accept treatment. Keep in mind that anxious clients are like all of us. They may be suffering, but they also fear that accepting new ways of approaching life may actually increase their level of anxiety. However, as Lang and Stein (2001) report, there are harmful side effects to the long-term use of many anti-anxiety medications. While some of the cognitive-behavioral approaches used in the treatment of anxiety may not always fit a client's frame of reference, it's wise to let them know about medical treatments and the potential for harm as one way to acknowledge that medications have risks that should be considered, just as there are associated risks in doing nothing.

DIAGNOSING AND TREATING SUBSTANCE ABUSE

The DSM-IV (American Psychiatric Association, 1994) uses the following diagnostic markers to determine whether substance use is abusive—a dysfunctional use of substances causing impairment or distress within a 12-month period as determined by one of the following: (1) frequent use of substances that interfere with functioning and the fulfillment of responsibilities at home, work, school, etc; (2) use of substances that impair functioning in dangerous situations such as driving or use of machines; (3) use of substances that may lead to arrest for unlawful behaviors; (4) substance use that seriously interferes with relations, marriage, child rearing, and other interpersonal responsibilities (p. 182). Substance abuse may lead to slurred speech, lack of coordination, unsteady gait, memory loss, fatigue and depression, feelings of euphoria and lack of social inhibitions (p. 197).

Short Tests

Several tests may be helpful in determining whether substances are used to an extent that may be causing serious problems functioning on the job. They are as follows.

Miller (2001) reports that two simple questions asked of substance abusers have an 80% chance of diagnosing substance abuse: "In the past year, have you ever drunk or used drugs more than you meant to?" and, "Have you felt you wanted or needed to cut down on your drinking or drug abuse in the past year?" Miller reports that this simple approach has been found to be an effective diagnostic tool in three controlled studies using random samples and laboratory tests for alcohol and drugs in the bloodstream following interviews.

Stewart and Richards (2000) suggest that four questions from the CAGE questionnaire are predictive of alcohol abuse. CAGE is an anachronism for Cut, Annoyed, Guilty, and Eye-opener (see the questions below). Since many people deny their alcoholism, asking questions in an open, direct and non-judgmental way may elicit the best results. The four questions are:

1. **Cut:** Have you ever felt you should cut down on your drinking?
2. **Annoyed:** Have people annoyed you by criticizing your drinking?
3. **Guilty:** Have you ever felt guilty about your drinking?
4. **Eye-opener:** Have you ever had a drink first thing in the morning (Eye-opener) to steady your nerves or get rid of a hangover? (Bisson, Nadeau, and Demers, 1999, p. 717)

Stewart and Richards (2000) write, "A patient who answers yes to two or more of these questions probably abuses alcohol; a patient who answers yes to one question should be screened further" (p. 56).

Short-Term Treatment of Substance Abuse

Herman (2000) believes that individual psychotherapy can be helpful to substance abusers and suggests five situations where therapy would be indicated: (1) as an appropriate introduction to treatment; (2) as a way of helping mildly or moderately dependent drug abusers; (3) when there are clear signs of emotional problems such as severe depression, since these problems will interfere with the substance abuse treatment; (4) when clients progressing in 12-step programs begin to experience emerging feelings of guilt, shame, and grief; (5) when a client's disturbed interpersonal functioning continues after a long period of sustained abstinence. Therapy might help prevent a relapse.

One of the most frequently discussed treatment approaches to addiction in the literature is brief counseling. Bien, Miller, and Tonigan (1993) reviewed 32 studies of brief interventions with alcohol abusers and found that, on average, brief counseling reduced alcohol use by 30%. In an evaluation of a larger report by Consumers Reports on the effectiveness of psychotherapy, Seligman (1995) notes that, "Alcoholics Anonymous (AA) did especially well, ... significantly bettering mental health professionals [in the treatment of alcohol and drug related problems]" (p. 10).

Bien et al. (1993) found that two or three 10–15 minute counseling sessions are often as effective as more extensive interventions with older alcohol abusers. The sessions include motivation-for-change strategies, education, assessment of the severity of the problem, direct feedback, contracting and goal setting, behavioral modification techniques, and the use of written materials such as self-help manuals. Completion rates using brief interventions are better for elder-specific alcohol programs than for mixed-age programs (Atkinson, 1995), and late-onset alcoholics are also more likely to complete treatment and have somewhat better outcomes using brief interventions (Liberto & Oslin, 1995).

Miller and Sanchez (1994) summarize the key components of brief intervention using the acronym FRAMES: feedback, responsibility, advice, menu of strategies, empathy, and self-efficacy.

1. **Feedback:** Includes the patient's risk for alcohol problems, his or her reasons for drinking, the role of alcohol in the patient's life, and the consequences of drinking.
2. **Responsibility:** Includes strategies to help patients understand the need to remain healthy, independent, and financially secure. This is particularly important when working with older clients and clients with health problems and disabilities.

3. **Advice:** Includes direct feedback and suggestions to clients to help them cope with their drinking problems and other life situations that may contribute to alcohol abuse.
4. **Menu:** Includes a list of strategies to reduce drinking and to cope with such high-risk situations as loneliness, boredom, family problems, and lack of social opportunities.
5. **Empathy:** Bien et al. (1993) strongly emphasize the need for a warm, empathetic and understanding style of treatment. Miller and Roilnick (1991) found that an empathetic counseling style produced a 77% reduction in patient drinking as compared with a 55% reduction when a confrontational approach was used.
6. **Self-efficacy:** This includes strategies to help clients rely on their inner resources to make a change in their drinking behavior. Inner resources may include positive points of view about themselves, helping others, staying busy, and good problem-solving and coping skills.

Babor and Higgins-Biddle (2000) discuss the use of brief interventions with people involved in "risky drinking" who are not as yet classified as alcohol dependent. Brief interventions are usually limited to 3–5 sessions of counseling and education. The intent of brief interventions is to prevent the onset of more serious alcohol-related problems. According to Babor and Higgins-Biddle, "Most programs are instructional and motivational, designed to address the specific behavior of drinking with information, feedback, health education, skill-building, and practical advice, rather than with psychotherapy or other specialized treatment techniques" (p. 676).

Higgins-Biddle, Babor, Mullahy, Daniels, and Mcree (1997) analyzed 14 random studies of brief interventions, which included a total of more than 20,000 risky drinkers. They report a net reduction in drinking of 21% for males and 8% for females. To improve the effectiveness of short-term interventions, Babor and Higgins-Biddle (2000) encourage the use of early identification of problem drinking, life-health monitoring by health and mental health professionals, and risk counseling that includes screening and brief intervention to inform and motivate potential alcohol abusers of the risk of serious alcohol dependence and to help change their alcohol use. This approach requires a high degree of cooperation among health and education personnel, who are often loathe to identify very young people as having "at risk" alcohol problems because they fear that doing so will exacerbate the problem through public identification and often believe that more moderate drinking will take place as the child matures.

Fleming and Manwell (1998) report that people with alcohol-related problems often receive counseling from primary care physicians or nursing staff in five or fewer standard office visits. The counseling consists of rational information about the negative impact of alcohol use as well as practical advice regarding ways of reducing alcohol dependence and the availability of community resources. Gentilello, Donovan, Dunn, and Rivara (1995) report that 25–40% of the trauma patients seen in emergency rooms may be alcohol dependent. The authors found that a single motivational interview, at or near the time of discharge, reduced drinking levels and readmission for trauma during 6 months of follow-up. Monti et al. (1999) conducted a similar study with 18- to 19-year-olds admitted to an emergency room with alcohol-related injuries. After 6 months, all participants had decreased their alcohol consumption; however, "the group receiving brief intervention had a significantly lower incidence of drinking and driving, traffic violations, alcohol-related injuries, and alcohol-related problems" (Monti et al., 1999, p. 3).

Lu and McGuire (2002) studied the effectiveness of outpatient treatment with substance-abusing clients and came to the following conclusions. (1) The more severe the drug use problem before treatment was initiated, the less likely clients were to discontinue drug use during treatment when compared with other users. (2) Clients reporting no substance abuse 3 months before admission were more likely to maintain abstinence than those who reported abstinence only in the past 1 month. (3) Heroin users were very unlikely to sustain abstinence during treatment, while marijuana users were less likely to sustain abstinence during treatment than were alcohol users. (4) Clients with a "psychiatric problem" were more likely to use drugs during treatment than clients without psychiatric problems. (5) Clients with legal problems related to their substance abuse had reduced chances of improving during the treatment. (6) Clients who had multiple prior treatments for substance abuse were less likely to remain abstinent during and after treatment. (7) More-educated clients were more likely to sustain abstinence after treatment. (8) Clients treated in urban agencies were less likely to maintain abstinence than those treated in rural agencies.

Natural Recovery

Granfield and Cloud (1996) estimate that as many as 90% of all problem drinkers never enter treatment and that many suspend problematic use of alcohol without any form of treatment. Sobell, Sobell, Toneatto, and Leo (1993) report that 82% of the alcoholics they studied who terminated their addiction did so by using natural recovery methods that excluded the use of a professional. In another example of the use of natural recovery techniques, Granfield and Cloud (1996) indicate that most ex-smokers discontinued their tobacco use without treatment. while many addicted substance abusers "mature-out" of a variety of addictions, including heavy drinking and narcotics use. Biernacki (1986) reports that addicts who naturally stop their addictions use a range of strategies that include breaking off relationships with drug users, removing themselves from drug-using environments, building new structures in their lives, and using friends and family to provide support for discontinuing their substance abuse.

Granfield and Cloud (1996) studied middle-class alcoholics who used natural recovery alone without professional help or self-help groups. Many of the participants in their study felt that the "ideological" base of many self-help programs was inconsistent with their own philosophies of life. For example, many felt that some self-help groups for substance abusers were overly religious, while other self-help groups believed in alcoholism as disease which suggested a lifetime struggle. The subjects in the study also felt that some self-help groups encouraged dependence on the group and that associating with other alcoholics would probably make recovery more difficult. In summarizing their findings, Granfield and Cloud (p. 51) report that:

> *Many [research subjects] expressed strong opposition to the suggestion that they were powerless over their addictions. Such an ideology, they explained, not only was counterproductive but was also extremely demeaning. These respondents saw themselves as efficacious people who often prided themselves on their past accomplishments. They viewed themselves as being individualists and strong-willed. One respondent, for instance, explained that "such programs encourage powerlessness" and that she would rather "trust her own instincts than the instincts of others."*

Humphreys (1998) studied the effectiveness of self-help groups with substance abusers by comparing two groups: one receiving inpatient care for substance abuse, and the other attending self-help groups for substance abuse. At the conclusion of the study, the average participant assigned to a self-help group (AA) had used $8,840 in alcohol-related health care resources as compared with $10,040 for the inpatient treatment participants. In a follow-up study, Humphreys (1998) compared outpatient services utilized by two separate groups for the treatment of substance abuse. The clients in the self-help group had decreased alcohol consumption by 70% over 3 years and consumed 45% less health care services (about $1,800 less per person) than the clients receiving professional substance abuse treatment.

Case Study: A Young Worker Deals with Substance Abuse

Albert White is a 26-year-old associate at a law firm in Chicago. Albert had an excellent record as a law student at a prestigious law school in the midwest but his current work has been anything but stellar. He is perpetually late, blaming it on traffic and car problems. A number of his colleagues have seen him in bars after work and late into the night; he has asked many of them to join him. Although his work is generally adequate, the firm's general manager has begun to think that Albert is a liability to the firm and a potential embarrassment should his drinking affect his work at some point. There has been talk of releasing him from his job, an action that would have a highly negative impact on his future job prospects.

After an evening of heavy drinking, he was taken to the emergency room when his car spun out of control and hit an embankment. Three passengers in the car were slightly injured. Albert and his friends had been binge drinking. All four friends were highly intoxicated and had walked a block and a half from a party they were attending to their car wearing tee-shirts in zero degree weather. Albert sustained minor injuries. After he became sober enough in the emergency room to recognize the seriousness of the accident and that his blood alcohol level was in excess of 0.25%, three times the allowed drinking and driving level of 0.08%, he became antagonistic and withdrawn.

A social worker and nurse met with Albert three times over the course of a 2-day stay in the hospital. They gave out information about the health impact of drinking and did a screening test to determine Albert's level of abusive drinking. They concluded that Albert was at very high risk of becoming a substance abuser because his drinking impaired his judgment, affected his work and was thought to be responsible for high blood sugar readings consistent with early onset diabetes and moderately high blood pressure. A psychosocial history taken by the social worker revealed that Albert had begun experimenting with alcohol at age 10 and was frequently using it at home and with friends from age 13 and on. He was drinking several bottles of hard liquor a week. As a result of the accident and subsequent blood level readings, Albert's driver's license was revoked by the court and, on the basis of the report made by the emergency room personnel, Albert was sent for mandatory alcohol counseling.

Albert is now in treatment and is a reluctant client. He discounts his drinking problem, claiming that he drinks no more than his friends. Were it not for the accident, he argues, he would not be in counseling since he was not having any serious problems in his life. That isn't altogether true, however, given an evaluation by his work supervisor indicating, just the day before the accident, that Albert was in serious jeopardy of being terminated at work.

After months of treatment where Albert would often sit in silence and stare at the therapist, he has begun to talk about his feelings. He feels strong when he drinks, he told the therapist, and loves the peaceful feeling that comes over him as he gets drunk. He romanticizes his drinking and can hardly wait to have his first drink of the day. Sometimes he drinks when he wakes up and often drinks rather than eat. He is aware that this cycle of drinking to feel better about himself can only lead to serious life problems, but doesn't think he is capable of stopping.

Albert's therapist asked him to do an Internet search to find the best approach to help Albert with his drinking problem. It seemed like a silly request to Albert since the therapist was supposed to be the expert, but Albert was intrigued and did as he was asked. When he met next with the therapist, Albert had printed out a number of articles suggesting ways of coping with young adult alcoholism that seemed reasonable to him and to the therapist. From the work of Kuperman et al. (2001), they agreed that Albert had a number of problems that should be dealt with, including problems at work, with friends, and with his alcohol abuse. They decided that a cognitive-behavioral approach would work best, with homework assignments and cognitive restructuring as an additional aspect of the treatment. Albert was intrigued with an article he found on the strengths approach and showed the therapist an article by Moxley and Olivia (2001) that they both found quite useful. Another article by Humphreys (1998) convinced them that a self-help group for young adult abusers might also be helpful.

Albert has been in treatment for over a year. He is applying himself at work. His drinking has modified itself somewhat. Although he still drinks too much at times, he won't drive when he is drinking or engage in risky behavior. He feels much less angry and has developed new friendships with peers who don't drink or use drugs. The changes seem very substantial, but it's too early to know if the alcoholism is likely to become problematic when he deals with additional life stressors. Albert is unsure and says that, "Yes, it's all helping me but my head isn't always on straight and sometimes I do dumb stuff. I'm more aware of it now, but I still do it. My new friends are real friends, not drinking buddies. I don't know. I looked at some studies on the Internet and it looks like I have a pretty good chance of becoming an alcoholic. I like to drink. It makes me feel strong. I'm in a profession where there's a lot of heavy drinking and sometimes you do it with superiors and clients to fit in and for advancement but, yes, I know I'm better. I just hope it keeps up."

Albert's therapist said, "Albert has a good handle on himself. I wouldn't argue with anything he said. He has lots of potential but he also has enough problems to make me unwilling to predict the future. What I will say is that he works hard, is cooperative, and seems to be trying to work on some longstanding issues about his perception of himself. I think that addictions are transitory and you never know when his desire to drink will overwhelm his desire to stay sober. The self-help group he's in keeps close tabs on his drinking, and his new friends are helpful. I'd caution anyone who works with substance abusers not to expect too much from treatment. I do want to applaud the professionals he worked with in the hospital. Even though the treatment was brief, it made a lasting impact on Albert to hear that he was considered an alcoholic, and it did bring him into treatment. That's exactly what you hope for with serious alcoholics who are in denial."

SUMMARY

In this chapter on treatment, three types of work-related problems frequently seen in Employee Assistance Programs and by other mental health professionals working with job unhappiness and anxiety, burnout, and substance abuse are discussed. Evidence-based practice (EBP) and substance abuse research findings are reported that suggest the effectiveness of certain types of treatment, particularly very brief treatment with high-risk abusers. Promising research on natural recovery and self-help groups suggests that treatment effectiveness may be consistently positive with these two approaches. Research issues are discussed that make the development of best evidence on the efficacy of all forms of treatment of substance abuse questionable, and the suggestion is made that before we can develop best evidence, more effective studies must take place that include adequate research designs and controls. A case study is provided that demonstrates the use of EBP with substance-abusing clients.

REFERENCES

American Psychiatric Association (1994). *Diagnostic and statistical manual of mental disorders* (4th ed.). Washington, DC: APA.

Atkinson, R. (1995). Treatment programs for aging alcoholics. In T. Beresford, & E. Gomberg (Eds.), *Alcohol and aging* (pp. 186–210). New York: Oxford University Press.

Babor, T. F., & Higgins-Biddle, J. C. (2000). Alcohol screening and brief intervention: Dissemination strategies for medical practice and public health. *Addiction, 95*(Issue 5), 677–687.

Beck, J. G., & Stanley, M. A. (1997). Anxiety disorders in the elderly: The emerging role of behavior therapy. *Behavior Therapy, 28*, 83–100.

Bien, T. J., Miller, W. R., & Tonigan, J. S. (1993). Brief interventions for alcohol problems: A review. *Addictions, 88*(3), 315–335.

Biernacki, P. (1986). *Pathways from heroin addiction: Recover without treatment.* Philadelphia: Temple University Press.

Bisson, J., Nadeau, L., & Demers, A. (1999). The validity of the CAGE scale to screen heavy drinking and drinking problems in a general population. *Addiction, 94*, 715–723.

Fleming, M., & Manwell, L. B. (1998). Brief intervention in primary care settings: A primary treatment method for at-risk, problem, and dependent drinkers. *Alcohol Research and Health, 23*(2), 128–137.

Floyd, M., Scogin, F., McKendree-Smith, M. L., Floyd, D., & Rokke, P. L. (2004). Cognitive therapy for depression: A comparison of individual psychotherapy and bibliotherapy for depressed older adults. *Behavior Modification, 28*, 297–318.

Gallagher-Thompson, D., Hanley-Peterson, P., & Thompson, L. W. (1990). Maintenance of gains versus relapse following brief psychotherapy for depression. *Journal of Consulting and Clinical Psychology, 58*, 371–374.

Gentilello, L. M., Donovan, D. M., Dunn, C. W., & Rivara, F. P. (1995). Alcohol interventions in trauma centers: Current practice and future directions. *JAMA, 274*(13), 1043–1048.

Granfield, R., & Cloud, W. (1996, Winter). The elephant that no one sees: Natural recovery among middle-class addicts. *Journal of Drug Issues, 26*, 45–61.

Herman, M. (2000). Psychotherapy with substance abusers: Integration of psychodynamic and cognitive-behavioral approaches. *American Journal of Psychotherapy, 54*(4), 574–579.

Higgins-Biddle, J. C., Babor, T. F., Mullahy, J., Daniels, J., & Mcree, B. (1997). Alcohol screening and brief interventions: Where research meets practice. *Connecticut Medicine, 61*, 565–575.

Huffman, G. B. (1999). Preventing recurrence of depression in the elderly. *American Family Physician, 59*(9), 2589–2591.

Humphreys, K. (1998). Can addiction-related self-help/mutual aid groups lower demand for professional substance abuse treatment? *Social Policy, 29*(2), 13–17.

Kuperman, S., Schlosser, S. S., Kramer, J. R., Bucholz, K., Hesselbrock, V., Reich, T., et al. (2001). Developmental sequence from disruptive behavior diagnosis to adolescent alcohol dependence. *The American Journal of Psychiatry, 158*, 2022–2026.

Lang, A. J., & Stein, M. B. (2001). Anxiety disorders. *Geriatrics, 56*(5), 24–30.

Lebowitz, B. D., Pearson, J. D., Schneider, L. S., Reynolds, C. F., III, Alexopoulos, G. S., Bruce, M. L., et al. (1997). Diagnosis and treatment of depression in late life.

Consensus statement update. *Journal of the American Medical Association, 278*(14), 1186–1190.

Lenze, E. J., Dew, M. A., Mazumdar, S., Begley, A. E., Cornes, C., Miller, M. D., et al. (2002). Combined pharmacotherapy and psychotherapy as maintenance treatment for late-life depression: Effects on social adjustment. *American Journal of Psychiatry, 159*(3), 466–468.

Liberto, J. G., & Oslin, D. W. (1995). Early versus late onset of alcoholism in the elderly. *International Journal of Addiction, 30*, 1799–1818 [number 13–14].

Lu, M., & McGuire, T. G. (2002). The productivity of outpatient treatment for substance abuse. *Journal of Human Resources, 37*(2), 309–335.

Miller, K. E. (2001). Can two questions screen for alcohol and substance abuse? *American Family Physician, 64*, 1247.

Miller, W. R., & Roilnick, S. (1991). *Motivational interviewing: Preparing people for change.* New York: Guilford Press.

Miller, W. R., & Sanchez, V. C. (1994). Motivating young adults for treatment and lifestyle change. In G. S. Howard, & P. E. Nathan (Eds.), *Alcohol use and misuse by young adults* (pp. 55–81). Notre Dame, IN: Univ. of Notre Dame Press.

Monti, P. M., Colby, S. M., Barnett, N. P., Spirito, A., Rohsenow, D. J., Myers, M., et al. (1999). Brief intervention for harm reduction with alcohol-positive older adolescents in a hospital emergency department. *Journal of Consulting and Clinical Psychology, 67*(6), 989–994.

Moxley, D. P., & Olivia, G. (2001). Strengths-based recovery practice in chemical dependency: A transperson perspective. *Families in Society, 82*, 251–262.

Myers, J. E., & Harper, M. C. (2004). Evidence-based effective practices with older adults. *Journal of Counseling & Development, 82*, 207–218.

O'Connor, R. (2001). Active treatment of depression. *American Journal of Psychotherapy, 55* (4), 507–530.

Pinquart, M., & Sörensen, S. (2001). How effective are psychotherapeutic and other psychosocial interventions with older adults? A meta-analysis. *Journal of Mental Health & Aging*, 7, 207–243.

Plopper, M. (1990). Evaluation and treatment of depression. In B. Kemp, K. Brummel-Smith, & J. W. Ramsdell (Eds.), *Geriatric rehabilitation* (pp. 253–264). Boston: College-Hill.

Roth, A. D., & Fonagy, E. (1996). *What works with whom? A critical review of psychotherapy research.* New York: Guilford Press.

Seligman, M. E. P. (1995). The effectiveness of psychotherapy: The consumers report study. *American Psychologist, 50*(12), 965–974.

Smith, S. S., Sherrill, K. A., & Celenda, C. C. (1995). Anxious elders deserve careful diagnosing and the most appropriate interventions. *Brown University Long-Term Care Letter*, 7(10), 5–7.

Sobell, L., Sobell, M., Toneatto, T., & Leo, G. (1993). What triggers the resolution of alcohol problems without treatment? *Alcoholism: Clinical and Experimental Research, 17* (2), 217–224.

Stewart, K. B., & Richards, A. B. (2000). Recognizing and managing your patient's alcohol abuse. *Nursing, 30*(Issue 2), 56–60.

Zalaquett, C. P., & Stens, A. N. (Spring 2006). Psychosocial treatments for major depression and dysthymia in older adults: A review of the research literature. *Journal of Counseling & Development, 84*, 192–201.

FURTHER READING

Apgar, K. R. (2003). Solutions to workplace substance abuse: Prevention and treatment strategies. *Issue Brief*, *2*(1), 1–16. Retrieved May 6, 2012 from <http://www.businessgrouphealth.org/pdfs/substance_brief.pdf>.

Heathfield, S. M. (n.d.) *360 Degree feedback: The good, the bad, and the ugly.* About.com website. Retrieved May 6, 2012 from <http://humanresources.about.com/od/360feedback/a/360feedback.htm>.

National Committee on Employer-Sponsored Behavioral Health Services. (n.d.). *An employers guide to behavioral health services: A roadmap for evaluating, designing and implementing behavioral health services. Center for Prevention and Health Services.* Retrieved May 6, 2012 from <http://www.businessgrouphealth.org/pdfs/fullreport_behavioralHealthservices.pdf>.

Trachtenberg, A. I., & Fleming, M. F. (n.d.). *Diagnosis and treatment of substance abuse in family practice. National Institute on Drug Abuse.* Available at: <http://archives.drugabuse.gov/diagnosis-treatment/diagnosis.html>.

CHAPTER 12

A Quality of Life Approach to Understanding and Measuring Workplace Problems

INTRODUCTION

A major aim of this chapter is to describe how quality of life (QoL) measures can be responsive to displaced workers' perceptions of their feelings and attitudes during the recent economic downturn. There is a recently renewed interest in QoL issues in both the academic and popular literature. The World Health Organization Quality of Life Group (WHOQOL Group, 1995) defines quality of life in terms of "an individual's perception of their position in life in the context of the culture and value systems in which they live and in relation to their goals, expectations, standards and concerns." The field of medicine has demonstrated that the problems of illness cannot be fully described merely by measures of disease and body systems. Psychosocial factors that include restricted mobility and other functional impairments, difficulty fulfilling personal and family responsibilities, financial burdens, and reduced cognition must also be considered.

Beyond the direct tangible impact of illness, the medical field has examined some of the negative effects that illnesses and treatments have on life satisfaction and subjective well-being. Although QoL assessments were almost unknown 15 years ago, they have become an integral measure of assessment and outcome in medical research. It has been reported that over a thousand articles on QoL are added to the literature each year (Muldoon, Barger, and Flory, 1998). For example, Eriksson et al. (2010) reported that lifestyle assessments and interventions delivered along with primary care that included increased physical activity and improved diet can help reduce both specific diseases and generic risk factors in order to help improve overall QoL.

It would seem reasonable, given the importance of including QoL methods in medical treatment, that other disciplines would consider its potential value for advancing care in mental health, life satisfaction, and personal happiness as well. It appears that few helping professionals in

Treating Worker Dissatisfaction During Economic Change
DOI: http://dx.doi.org/10.1016/B978-0-12-397006-0.00012-9

fields other than medicine are very familiar with the value of QoL as an assessment tool and intervention potential in practice. This chapter contends that QoL research findings that have emerged from evidence-based, positive psychology could better apprise mental health workers, social workers, counselors, and other human services professionals of its value to their work. Other helping disciplines might improve client care by applying principles of QoL along with their regular assessment and treatment methods. A number of client problems that are complex and hard to measure could possibly be treated more effectively and with greater insight into individual client's felt needs.

DEFINITION AND BACKGROUND OF QUALITY OF LIFE

Quality of life has emerged as a multidimensional concept, and there have been increased efforts to better understand it. An important purpose of QoL is how it helps describe connections between various dimensions of a person's life from their own point of view. Individual QoL has been broadly defined by some writers as the degree of excellence in life relative to a particular expressed or implied standard of comparison that most people in a particular society would agree upon (Veenhoven, 1984). Another way of explaining QoL is its potential to provide people with improved opportunities to have a decent level of living. This requires including the individual perceptions of people in order to help mediate the negative effects of difficult challenges to their lives. QoL is not only defined as the quantity or degree of a desired aspect of life but also as a measure that includes both satisfaction and happiness in an individual's life. For example, it has been found that longevity of life may be very desirable for one person but may not be perceived by another person as being fulfilling or even important. Some descriptions of QoL have included excellence of personal growth and mastery, economic stability, psychological well-being, and meaningful work, as being more important to some people than mere subsistence or longevity (Seed & Lloyd, 1997).

Other debates regarding what should be considered as a "working" definition of quality of life have expanded greatly and can be perceived from a variety of perspectives. One perspective that has evolved is described as Integrative Quality of Life Theory (IQOL). The idea of IQOL is that quality of life can be viewed as an integrative value system by which an individual can perceive their goals, hopes, standards, needs, and beliefs as interacting and changing, based upon a range of methods, disciplines, and indicators (Ventegodt, Merrick, & Andersen, 2003).

There has been some general agreement about what constitutes "a good quality of life." A good quality of life is related to achieving a positive attitude about what is important in life that is closely linked to the culture and society of which one is a part. Chambers and Kong (1996) described this view of a good-quality life as seen through a filter of cultural conditioning in which people include happiness and fulfillment of needs in a specific social context. This idea draws upon a multicultural model that is consistent with definitions of health and health promotion provided by the World Health Organization Group (WHOG) Profile and the World Health Organization Quality of Life (WHOQOL) definition (WHOQOL Group, 1995). The WHOG Profile emphasizes a good quality of life as embodying individual physical health, psychological well-being, and spiritual functioning in connection with the environment. One of the most important ideas to emerge was alignment with the individual's view of achieving the important possibilities of their life.

King and Napa (1998) and others found that cultural differences in beliefs have often complicated the understanding of how QoL is to be defined. The issue is further conflicted when QoL measures have been initially developed in a particular culture and later translated for people who have a different cultural background. For example, a Western or individualistic perception of happiness in the United States will differ for people who come to live there from a familial or group-oriented society. Although this issue is too extensive for elaboration in this chapter, many of the basic tenets for assessing QoL from a cultural context can be found in the work developed in the Schedule for the Evaluation of Individual Quality of Life (SEIQL; O'Boyle, Browne, Hickey, McGee, & Joyce, 1993).

Two constructs that have emerged as central to understanding and defining QoL are subjective well-being and life satisfaction. These related constructs were developed in the field of Positive Psychology and have had various interpretations and interrelated meanings (Diener, 1984; Strack et al., 1991). The earlier emphasis was on subjective quality of life, which has been described as the perceived satisfaction each individual has about their life as they make personal evaluations through their feelings and emotions. When an individual is content with life and feels happy, this reflects their subjective quality of life. Objective quality of life is how a person's life is perceived in relation to the outside world. Objective quality of life has also been described as a person's ability to adapt to the values and standards of the culture of which they are a part. An example might be the particular rankings of social status in a given culture or the status symbols that one covets in order to be considered a respected member of that culture.

EVIDENCE-BASED QUALITY OF LIFE CONCEPTS AND MEASURES

Quality of life measures may be generic while assessing QoL across different populations or different issues, or they can focus on specific issues or problems. Neither approach independently or directly influences life satisfaction or subjective well-being (SWB) or happiness, because they depend on how they are cognitively perceived and individually evaluated (American Psychiatric Association, 2000; Diener & Larsen, 1993; Michalos, 1991).

A search of the Institute for Scientific Information (ISI) database from 1982 to 2005 revealed over 55,000 academic citations utilizing the term "quality of life" spanning a wide range of academic disciplines. Quality of life has also been included in broader areas of discourse concerning economic prosperity and sustainability. It has been generally assumed that more income and consumption are the primary reasons for a better quality of life. The notion of a primary or major emphasis on financial well-being has been challenged by several authors, notably Sen (1985) and Nussbaum (1995). It has also been challenged in a fair amount of the psychological research (e.g., Diener & Lucas, 1999; Easterlin, 2003).

QoL research has focused more often on objective measures of QoL that are quantifiable indicators, such as economic and health indices obtained from the United Nations Human Development Index (UN Development Programme, 2012). For example, objective measures frequently include factors of economic production, literacy rates, and life expectancy. These measures can usually be gathered without directly surveying or interviewing the individuals being assessed. Objective indicators of QoL have generally been used independently or in combination to form summary indexes such as the UN Human Development Index (Sen, 1985; UNDP, 2012). It is acknowledged that these measurements only provide a brief assessment of how certain physical and social QoL needs are met. They often represent a narrow and sometimes biased viewpoint. Although useful, this does not always allow an opportunity to incorporate many measures that contribute to QoL that are sensitive and relevant. These indicators would include perceived need, happiness, life satisfaction, and psychological well-being. It has been found that many surveys and interview measures only represent the findings that were identified from the point of view of the researcher.

Rather than assume an understanding of the importance of various life domains, subjective measures can tap into the perceived importance of the domain to the individual respondent (Diener & Suh, 1999). It is universally acknowledged that subjective QoL indicators are valid when they measure what they were intended to measure about what people perceive to be important to their happiness and well-being. It was also found that there are a number of limitations to using objective and subjective approaches separately. It has been generally acknowledged that the approach to QoL that connects objective and subjective approaches is the most meaningful.

Quality of life methods are beneficial because of the inclusion of individual personal feelings that are not accounted for in a great deal of the literature. QoL concepts incorporate personal feelings in both individualized and standardized measurements for the assessment of physical, mental, and social well-being. Carr, Higginson, and Robinson (2003) reported that there are literally hundreds of QoL measures specifically designed to address health-related issues. It has been explained that the reason for a preponderance of specific health-related QoL measures is that they are more likely to be valid and reliable on account of their focus on a problem or issue. Generic measures such as the Nottingham Health Profile (Hunt, McEwen, & McKenna, 1985) are used to assess more broad and general QoL issues across a range of different populations.

The following are some examples of specific and generic QoL standardized instruments.

- Generic measures:
  - General Health Questionnaire (Goldberg, 1972);
  - Goteborg Quality of Life Instrument (Tibblin, Tibblin, Peciva, Kullmna, & Svardsudd, 1990);
  - Life as a Whole Index (Andrews & Withey, 1976);
  - Life Satisfaction Index (Neugarten, Havighurst, & Tobin, 1961);
  - (Multifaceted) Life Satisfaction Scale (Harner & Neal, 1993);
  - Quality of Life Inventory (Frisch, Cornell, Villanueva, & Retzlaff, 1992);
  - Satisfaction With Life Scale (Diener, Emmons, Larsen, & Griffen, 1985).

- Specific measures:
  - Health Measurement Questionnaire (Kind & Gudex, 1994);
  - Quality of Life in Depression Scale (Hunt & McKenna, 1992);
  - Quality of Life Index for Mental Health (Sainfort, Becker, & Diamond, 1996);
  - Quality of Life Scale (Heinrichs, Hanlon, & Carpenter, 1984);
  - Schedule for the Evaluation of Individual Quality of Life (O'Boyle, 1994).

Diener and Suh (1999) were instrumental in the development of the Quality of Life Model and the Integrative Quality of Life Model.

Quality of Life Model (QoL)

This model conceptualizes QoL as the extent to which objective human needs are fulfilled in relation to personal or group perceptions of subjective well-being and life satisfaction.

- Subjective well-being or happiness is assessed by individual or group responses to questions about happiness or life satisfaction. Life satisfaction is an empirically valid construct that has been defined as a subjective measure that an individual can identify when their needs or desires are being successfully fulfilled (Frisch, 2006). The positive aspects of happiness come from feeling that their standards for achieving life satisfactions have been met. As stated by Frisch (2006), "the perceived gap between what we have and what we want to have in valued areas of life determines our level of life satisfaction or dissatisfaction." The relation between specific human needs and perceived life satisfaction involves both factors being affected by mental capacity, cultural context, information, education, temperament, etc. This includes:
  - The extent to which desires are matched by experience;
  - The domains that individuals consider as important in their lives;
  - Distinct but related factors which are sometimes viewed as separate domains in QoL measures;
  - Both cognitive and affective measures obtained by weighting the sum of all separate domains that equate to overall Quality of Life.

Integrative Model of QoL

Quality of life is also represented as the interaction of human needs and the subjective perception of their fulfillment, mediated by the opportunities available to meet needs. Diener and Suh (1999) noted that the models listed above were derived primarily from an integration of other research regarding basic human needs that includes:

- Maslow's (1954) hierarchy of needs;
- Sirgy and Samli's (1995) Need Hierarchy Measure of Life Satisfaction;
- Greenley, Greenberg, and Brown's (1997) Quality of Life Questionnaire;
- Frisch's (1998, 2006; Frisch et al., 1992) Quality of Life Inventory.

Frisch (2006) provides an extensive discussion of this issue, which is the main perspective of this chapter. This perspective of QoL was described as Quality of Life Therapy (QOLT):

- a multidimensional construct based upon multiple individual needs that reflect community, national, and global levels.
- Each need is assumed to contribute in a different degree to each other and to overall QoL.
- It relates to the subject of this chapter in that involuntary job displacement can create a change in the QoL work domain and impact other related categories and factors, or "domains," of a worker's life.

WORKPLACE QUALITY OF LIFE AND THE ECONOMIC DOWNTURN

This section will address various implications of the recent economic downturn, involuntary job displacement, and how worker quality of life may be affected by these issues. Brand, Becca, and Burgard (2008) and other writers have written about how involuntary job displacement such as layoffs and plant closings independently affect mental and physical health as well as financial well-being. Fewer studies have investigated the overall effects on QoL when workers are suddenly displaced as a result of a severe economic downturn. For example, a number of studies looked at the onset of depression and other mental health conditions among workers who were nearing retirement (e.g., Brand, Levy, & Gallo, 2008). They found significantly less depression among imminent retirees than among workers who experienced unanticipated involuntary job displacement.

Other areas of inquiry have investigated the greater impact of economic downturns on job-displaced workers who experience disparities due to racial and ethnic categories, gender, age, types of industry, etc. (Smeeding, 2010). Other writers recognized the economic downturn's negative effect on issues such as family divorce and fertility rates and the use of leisure time. Research into economic downturns and subsequent job displacement could benefit from a better perspective of diversity and job-displaced workers by selecting appropriate QoL measures.

Despite a long history of challenges to its validity and reliability, Quality of Life theory has developed a number of empirically grounded multidimensional, assessment and intervention tools. Many of these measures can provide a better understanding of the needs and concerns of displaced workers. Frisch (2006) developed a number of studies and models that demonstrated the value of using QoL independent and objective measures in alliance with other methods. In spite of a number of challenges, QoL methods have demonstrated the value of recognizing the expressed feelings of laid-off workers and what's important to them. This chapter presents QoL methods as a means to understanding the broader social and personal well-being indicators of job-displaced workers. This chapter is related to how the recent economic downturn and job displacement impacts a wide range of social domains as well as financial and psychological quality of life domains.

Consistent with the QoL approach, McKee-Ryan, Song, Wanberg, and Kinicki (2005) identified specific measures that include increased levels of distress and depression, as a consequence of involuntary job loss. The study extended beyond individual workers to include families and community domains and indicators. Vinokur, Price, and Caplan (1996), Westman, Etzion, and Horovitz (2004), and others found that most people respond to job displacement in the context of relationships with significant others who are often regarded as among the most important QoL concerns (Frisch, 2006).

As a result of the economic downturn and work loss, it may be useful to understand some of the interrelated circumstances that displaced workers can experience within the overall quality of their lives. QoL is a concept that has the potential to identify a wide range of complex implications related to both abrupt and long-term involuntary job displacement. Previous economic research has shown how poor mental and physical health can negatively impact a worker's employment success and the quality of their work life. This chapter is concerned with how involuntary job displacement indirectly impacts mental and physical health domains as well as other work-related QoL factors.

David Grusky et al. (2011) noted that, during 2008 and 2009, the United States suffered one of the largest drops in labor force employment since the Great Depression. The massive number of jobs that were suddenly lost during this recent economic downturn has had an effect on displaced worker's quality of life that is not well understood. This raises the question of what happens to workers' and their families' quality of life that goes beyond financial difficulties. The overall consequences of job loss are becoming more important due to the unpredictability of the longer-term prospects for economic recovery.

Other studies, including work by Grusky (2011) and colleagues, have addressed various dimensions of the economic downturn, but far less is known about its broader QoL consequences. For example, unemployment statistics are cited almost daily in the media, but very little is reported about how displaced workers' self-esteem, goals, and values are affected by the economic downturn.

Bohen & Viveros-Long (1981) wrote about how the quality of work life (QWL) was related to the overall well-being of displaced Federal government employees and their families. It described how, along with financial compensation, the work environment also contributed positively to workers' intellectual, physical, and social well-being. A report by the Gallup-Healthways Well-Being Index (WBI) (Gallup Well-Being, 2012) also describes how the 2009 economic downturn affected the well-being of millions of Americans after losing their jobs. Many displaced workers observed that the loss of workplace benefits was almost as distressing as leaving the workforce. The WBI is composed of a combination of six attributes of life: Life Evaluation, Emotional Health, Basic Access, Physical Health, Work Environment, and Healthy Behavior. The WBI measure had been fairly stable during the previous year. It went from a high of 67.0 to a low of 63.3, and by the end of the year had declined overall by 8.2%.

The WBI saw the greatest decline in the Life Evaluation attribute of QoL domains. The index indicated that the greatest long-term concern was in the decrease in Healthy Behaviors. Another finding in the study was evidence of declining trends in attributes described as Thriving, Struggling, or Suffering. The data suggested that people are experiencing the economic downturn in more personal ways than previously realized. Changes in these well-being measures were found to be associated with how people have become increasingly concerned about their overall mental, social, and physical health, along with their negative financial outlook for the future.

As a multidisciplinary concept, QoL may gain increased attention during the recent economic downturn as a generic measure. It may also represent appropriate indicators of multidisciplinary and integrative quality of life (IQOL). This includes interrelated and interdependent life satisfaction and subjective well-being measures of displaced workers' perspectives of home, work, and community. QoL can also help explain how loss of work can contribute to feelings of "sadness, depression, anxiety or anger" (Lucas et al., 2004).

Case Study: Diminished Quality of Life and Job Loss

This case offers a typical example of the many ways in which a person may experience job displacement and a diminution of quality of life, in respect of their unique individual circumstances, during the recent economic downturn. This older, well-educated, and experienced professional woman expresses her present dilemma in 2012 as a result of the downturn.

> *"A few days before my 71st birthday in 2009 I was advised that my services were no longer required at the financial institution where I had been employed for the past 33 years! I had received exceeds-expectation ratings from the beginning of my employment, and therefore my dismissal as a part of the downsizing being implemented by my company as a part of the economic downturn of the economy was unexpected. I was an Assistant Vice President of the company and my immediate supervisor had informed me that his direct line superior had indicated that my job was secure.*
>
> *Because of the nature of the organization I was informed that I should 'take my purse and leave the building immediately.' I should make an appointment to return at a later date to pick up any other personal items still remaining, at which time a security officer of the bank would escort me out. In retrospect, I was in shock because I remained calm throughout and my immediate supervisor appeared more upset than I was at this outcome. It was not until the following Saturday when I returned for my personal items and was sitting in my car surrounded by the accumulation of personal effects from a 33-year job that it finally hit me.*
>
> *It had not been my intention to retire at this time, although I was 71 years of age. I was in excellent health, energetic and considered more than competent to perform the expectations of my job. Now at the age of 71 years I was thrown into a job market comprised of young people just out of college looking for employment, other younger individuals who also were now out of work as well as the other senior citizens in the same situation that confronted me in an economy in serious decline.*
>
> *When I considered the cause for this situation I realized that the company had probably looked at the salary that I had achieved over a 33-year span and the benefits that they paid for me as well as my having passed the normal age of retirement and decided that they could hire someone for less without comparable benefits and make a significant cut in their bottom line. My loyalty to the company, acquired knowledge and experience in the positions I had held were not a part of that equation.*

Furthermore, the profit-sharing package that I had expected to have as a significant part of retirement, although not nearly enough to sustain me along with Social Security, had been decimated by the stock market hit that year and my little 'nest egg' had been seriously reduced. However, I was in better shape than many of the other seniors I encountered and was able to pay off much of my outstanding debt and could see that. While collecting unemployment, I could possibly find something else to do to supplement my diminished income.

So the quest began. The first job I found was commission-only and soon proved to be less fruitful than hoped. Through that employment I acquired a more satisfactory situation with a base income plus commission. But soon, once again the economic market kicked in and that employer determined that they could no longer pay the base and would only be able to pay commission. Back to square one.

My subsequent attempts to find suitable employment proved less than fruitful. Living on a Social Security income without even the possibility of collecting unemployment because none of the jobs held had been salaried where the employers paid into the unemployment system has proved interesting. Because of periodic jobs where I have been paid on a cash basis and because I had been able to reduce my expenses by paying off all of my debt, I am able to live from Social Security check to Social Security check and handle my current expenses. The reality of the situation is that, while the cost of living has gone up, the increases provided by Social Security have not matched. At some point I am fully aware that I may have to give up my car, downsize my living space, and hope that my health remains good.

Fortunately, I am an optimistic individual who finds the obstacles I may be facing interesting and a challenge rather than the end of the world I once knew in better financial days."

This example suggests that many subjective aspects of this person's life are being affected as a result of the involuntary job loss. It was clear that this person was not only enduring financial hardships but a number of other QoL issues as well. After several years without finding employment this person has been able to develop some positive ways of coping with the situation. Other job-displaced individuals may experience a great deal more dissatisfaction and lack of success in various areas of their lives and less capacity to cope.

Work loss factors might include the following:

- Loss of self-esteem due to failure to obtain satisfactory standards of success in employment;
- Feelings of guilt as a result of the inability to achieve key personal goals;
- Not engaging in favorite pastimes as often because of perceived financial constraints;

- Disengagement from helping activities because of a perceived lack of time or motivation;
- Lacking the motivation to engage in learning activities because of a lack of career goals;
- Feeling alienated from friends, relatives, and children because of perceived inadequacy and interpersonal conflicts.

Because unemployment is a shared life event that affects people differently in various life domains, it is important to recognize the value in better understanding how individuals, families, and numerous other systems might be affected during the economic downturn. Unemployment situations can be plagued by a variety of complex reactions that are unique to specific individuals and generic with respect to other QoL domains (Westman et al., 2004).

DISPLACED WORKERS AND SUBJECTIVE WELL-BEING OR HAPPINESS

Relative to the recent economic downturn, both life satisfaction and subjective well-being or feelings of happiness have gained increased attention in the psychological and social sciences. Rollero and Tartaglia (2009) investigated factors that addressed life satisfaction during the economic downturn. Diener et al. (2006) and others cite subjective well-being or happiness as an important concept that explains how people evaluate important personal aspects of their lives. Individuals respond to the objective circumstances of their economic adversity such as financial insecurity and unemployment in a variety of predictable and objective ways. This might include how one will pay the rent or the car note and their children's school tuition. Diener et al. (2006) and others explain that life satisfaction is manifested in the cognitive appraisal that one makes of the economic circumstances within the context of all of the other aspects of one's life.

Subjective well-being or happiness is not just being cheerful and content but comprises an intense personal experience of feeling in one's life. The intensity of the experience is a dimension that does not separate happiness from other aspects of the quality of life. For example, in the event of job loss, subjective well-being or happiness is related to complex non-rational dimensions such as love, close ties with the community, etc., but not necessarily with money, state of health, and other objective factors.

Elizur and Shye (1990) stated that subjective well-being or happiness has often been differentiated from the broader concept of a quality working life. Happiness can be viewed as a complex process that is related to specific domains of QoL that are directly affected by the loss of a working life. The relationship of the loss of a quality working life to the happiness aspect of QoL remains relatively unexplored and unexplained. A review of the literature reveals relatively little on this subject, and this issue may lead to not using appropriate QoL measures or indicators. A consideration of the value of a quality working life provides a greater context for understanding other subjective well-being issues related to displacement from the workplace such as loss of self-esteem and family stress.

Hackman and Oldham (1975) and other authors proposed components of quality of working life measures which included a range of positive factors that would no longer contribute to a worker's overall quality of life were he or she to be displaced. Warr, Cook, and Wall (1979) describe some of the subjective well-being aspects of quality of working life that might be lost to displaced workers:

- A positive and secure work environment;
- An intrinsic job motivation;
- Positive goals and values;
- Enhanced self-esteem;
- Opportunity for creativity;
- Enabling of helping;
- Feeling of happiness and contentment;
- Supportive relationships.

Lawler (1982) found that quality of working life is conceptually similar to the subjective well-being or happiness of workers but differs from job satisfaction, which primarily relates to the workplace domain. Quality of working life has been viewed as incorporating a range of needs that not only include work-based factors such as job satisfaction, pay and relationships with supervisors and workplace colleagues, but also includes feelings concerning relationships between work and non-work life domains (Danna & Griffin, 1999).

Diener and Seligman (2004) reported that unemployment and job insecurity are related to "depression, fear, anxiety, insomnia and somatic symptoms." It was found that individuals who are affected by economic adversity rely upon psychological support as well as other subjective factors. As a result of the current economic downturn job-displaced workers are more than likely to experience challenges to issues such as parenting roles, love relationships, social lives, and achieving personal goals.

QUALITY OF LIFE THERAPY

Michael Frisch (2006) developed the "CASIO" model as part of Quality of Life Therapy (QOLT), which is a linear, additive model of life satisfaction where QoL intervention may lead to an improvement in other domains of life. This model is applicable to work-related issues since it is generic and can be used as a non-clinical measure. Frisch defined non-clinical as applying to individuals or groups without mental health problems defined as a disorder in the DSM-IV-TR manual of disorders (American Psychiatric Association, 2000). Quality of Life Therapy rests on an assumption that an individual's overall life satisfaction consists largely of the sum of specific satisfactions, in particular "domains" or areas of life that are valued as important by the individual. Diener (1984) and Clark, Beck, and Alford (1999) set forth an underlying concept that is addressed in this chapter as a combined cognitive-affective or life satisfaction model which is synonymous with personal happiness. There is general support for this concept based upon a number of studies by researchers who were instrumental in developing the QOLT/CASIO model (Campbell Converse, & Rodgers, 1976; Diener & Diener, 1995; Evans, 1994; Frisch, 2006; Michalos, 1991). Frisch offers an example of this approach that states "a working mother might be more content than a homemaker because satisfactions in one domain (e.g., work, family life and children) may minimize the effects of dissatisfaction in other areas of life."

Frisch (2006) described some basic elements of Quality of Life Therapy with the CASIO construct, which outlines the individual life satisfaction and subjective well-being model as follows:

- C: Objective characteristics and living *conditions*;
- A: Perceived or subjective characteristics or *attitudes*;
- S: Evaluation based on personal standards of fulfillment and overall *satisfaction*;
- I: Satisfaction weighted by *importance* or value;
- O: *Overall* satisfaction in valued areas of life.

This model essentially describes how individual satisfaction with a particular area of life is composed of the five components that are listed above.

These QoL measures may determine that a worker's subjective satisfaction with work could be related to the work itself, such as relationships with co-workers, management, the work environment, and job security. As a result of work loss an individual might perceive that the "objective characteristics" of work life have been destructive to their overall QoL. Workers may need to be encouraged to make objective efforts to alter or adjust other areas of their lives as a result of the work loss. Quality of Life Therapy may be used to assess a person's subjective perception or attitude as a result of losing work. This may also influence their QoL in unpredicted life domains. QOLT can assist in helping a person understand how they cognitively interpret work loss circumstances once they are perceived. This could include deciding what individual choices and values are given to one's overall QoL.

There are numerous standardized QoL instruments that have empirically demonstrated strengths for particular purposes and tasks. Some instruments are used for clinical assessment purposes and others for screening and monitoring activities. The scale and inventory described above was initially derived from the Satisfaction with Life Scale, a cognitive-therapy-based model developed by Diener, Emmons, Larson and Griffen (1985) primarily to measure the judgmental component of subjective well-being. This instrument was determined to be a good multidimensional item scale with very good relationship between measures and reliability. The Frisch (1992) Quality of Life Inventory (QOLI) which borrowed from this concept was selected as a generic model and is applicable to the assessment of displaced workers. It also possesses fair to good internal consistency and reliability. The QOLI has been found to have good convergent validity with the Diener Satisfaction with Life Scale and various other Quality of Life Index scores. The Frisch QOLT conceptual model is consistent with the approach of the World Health Organization (WHO, 2006). Combining elements of QOLT with the WHO's and other approaches emphasizes considerations that can be related to job-displaced workers' cultural, psychological, and spiritual functioning.

ISSUES RELATED TO QUALITY OF LIFE OUTCOMES

Carr, Scott, Thompson, and Silman (1996) suggested that QoL measures can assist in depicting both the personal and social context of job displacement outcomes. QoL outcome measures can be used in screening for work-loss-related problems, prioritizing problems, monitoring change, and identifying clients' personal feelings and preferences. QoL outcomes that are related to the economic downturn are often portrayed as short-term events, but a substantial body of literature that was described earlier, shows that the economic downturn is a potentially long-term experience. The consequences of sudden unemployment and long-term economic inactivity can have serious and unpredictable QoL consequences for displaced workers and families. For example, job loss and falling incomes can force a family to delay or forgo education and training for themselves or college for their children. Many families may neglect health screening and dental care. In such cases, an economic recession can lead to what has been described as "scarring." Scarring has been explained as long-lasting damage not only to an individuals' economic situation, but social, physical, and emotional scarring can occur as well.

The *New York Times* editorial page reported in March, 2012 that the job market started to show a slow trend of improvement but it is predicted that the US economy would require at least 5 years to regain its previous status. This projection suggests that economic opportunities as well as broader QoL outcome prospects for many job-displaced workers will probably be permanently marred. Unemployment and income losses can:

- Reduce educational achievement;
- Threaten early childhood nutrition;
- Reduce families' abilities to provide a supportive learning environment;
- Prevent adequate health care;
- Eliminate summer activities;
- Reduce stable housing;
- Cause the delay or abandonment of educational or college plans.

The article further reported that there was substantial evidence that potential hardships resulting from the economic downturn will be passed across generations. The economic hardships experienced by job-displaced families will mean more than just enduring economic hurdles. It should be recognized that there are effects upon social and emotional domains that go far beyond the financial consequences of the economic downturn. The lessons of the Great Depression have taught that a severe, sudden, and long-term loss of work will result in reshaping the overall economic and social fabric of society. Many QoL outcome issues will not be realized until long after the economic damage has occurred.

For example, various aspects of the economic downturn are interconnected and can impact future educational outcomes for children in a variety of ways. A substantial body of literature recognizes that quality early childhood education is primarily driven by parental options and adequate funding (Heckman & Masterov, 2007). Economic outcomes such as work loss can reduce family resources that impact the quality of education outcomes for their children. Evidence has also shown that job displacement factors impact other areas such as early childhood nutrition, which can impact cognitive development. Other studies have shown that improved nutrition factors can lead to greater grade attainment, reading comprehension, and cognitive abilities. The health and nutrition problems that can have a long-term effect on the the lives of children during an economic downturn suggests the need for using QoL measures related to work loss (Vincent & Higginson, 2003).

Although there has been increasing support for using Quality of Life measures as explicated by Frisch (2006), Seed and Lloyd (1997), and others in Chapter 13 of this book, it is generally agreed that QoL outcome measures can have some bias due to their many interrelated subjective and objective dimensions. Bowling (2003) and others cautioned that, due to many mediating variables other than specific and individualized QoL outcome measures, it can be a complex process to understand. Stephens and Schaller (2009) noted increasing evidence that laid-off workers are prone to suffer QoL outcome declines in health that may prove difficult to fully understand or measure. There may also be a need to more fully explain how sudden work loss influences outcomes that are associated with stress-related health problems. Diener and Suh (1999) provide supportive evidence that QoL measurements are a valid means to determine what people feel are important to their subjective well-being and life satisfaction. Diener and Seligman (2004) noted that economic adversity and unemployment can have a detrimental effect on people's lives. QoL indicators provide measures and strategies to address issues related to unemployment, such as depression and emotional and physical health. Due to some of the limitations of QoL measures, this approach can be most effectively used in conjunction with other disciplines, to better address job loss outcomes and develop strategies to deal with them.

SUMMARY

Quality of Life (QoL) is a dynamic concept that is determined by a range of interacting objective and subjective measures. The degree to which an individual's desires and ambitions are met often depends upon their perception of the position they hold in the context of their culture. In relation to job-displaced workers the concept of QoL is an appropriate method to measure an individual's goals and personal concerns. Both generic and specific appraisals can be made with QoL of an individual's circumstances and attitudes measured against an ideal standard. QoL is also determined by the extent to which a person's feelings, hopes, and desires are matched by their achievement. There are a variety of interacting objective and subjective dimensions of an individual's QoL, measured by sixteen domains and other areas (QOLI) that constitute their overall quality of life. Quality of life has been further explained by Diener and Seligman (2004) as a tool to support treatment outcomes of cognitive therapy and ongoing therapeutic treatment as required. Quality of Life assessment and intervention has also been found to be beneficial in working with non-clinical populations such as unemployed workers (Clark, Beck, & Alford, 1999).

Quality of Life Inventory (QOLI) measures provide a useful means of assessing the feelings, goals, and the value of work for displaced workers in the context of the recent economic downturn. Assessments of the economic downturn have primarily focused upon unemployment and financial considerations. A number of findings have shown how the financial impact of the economic downturn has disrupted and sometimes devastated the quality of people's lives. The subjective well-being of displaced workers is affected in various dimensions, including health, children, family, social belonging, and leisure activities. Fewer stories have been written about the consequences of work loss on individuals' overall quality of life. A greater understanding is needed of how to measure the feelings, goals and circumstances of people who have experienced loss of work.

Quality of Life Therapy (QOLT) as an assessment and intervention method can provide a way of including an individual's personal feelings within a social context that is important to them. Quality of Life Therapy can provide a useful multidisciplinary approach to assess a wide range of individual domains that constitute a person's quality of life. It can be potentially useful in addressing issues related to the economic downturn and worker job displacement. Quality of Life Inventory measures can be applied as both generic and specific measures depending on whether the purpose is for assessment, treatment, or evaluation of a job-displaced worker's quality of life.

REFERENCES

American Psychiatric Association (2000). *Diagnostic and statistical manual of mental disorders* (4th ed.). Washington, DC: APA.

Andrews, F. M., & Withey, S. B. (1976). *Social indicators of well-being: Americans' perceptions of life quality.* New York: Plenum.

Bohen, H. H., & Viveros-Long, A. (1981). *Balancing jobs and family life: Do flexible work schedules help?* Philadelphia: Temple University Press.
Brand, J. E., Becca, R., & Burgard., S. A. (2008). Job displacement and social participation over the life course: Findings for a cohort of joiners. *Social Forces, 87(1)*, 211–242.
Brand, J. E., Levy, B. R., & Gallo, W. T. (2008). Effects of layoffs and plant closings on subsequent depression among older workers. *Research on Aging, 30*, 701–721.
Cambell, A., Converse, P., & Rodgers, W. (1976). *The quality of American life.* New York: Russell Sage Foundation.
Carr, A. J., Scott., D. L., Thompson., P. W., & Silman, A. (1996). Quality of life measures. *British Journal of Rheumatology, 35*, 275–281.
Carr, A. J., Higginson, I. J., & Robinson, P. G. (2003). *Quality of life.* London: BMJ Books.
Chambers, J. W., & Kong, B. W. (1996). *Assessing quality of life: Construction and validation of a scale.* Cobb & Henry: Hampton, VA.
Clark, D. A., Beck, A. T., & Alford, B. A. (1999). *Scientific foundations of cognitive theory and therapy of depression.* New York: John Wiley & Sons.
Danna, K., & Griffin, R. W. (1999). Health and well-being in the workplace: A review and synthesis of the literature. *Journal of Management, 25*, 357–384.
Diener, E. (1984). Subjective well-being. *Psychological Bulletin, 95*, 542–575.
Diener, E., Emmons, R. A., Larson, R., & Griffen, S. (1985). The satisfaction with life scale. *Journal of Personality Assessment, 49*, 71–75.
Diener, E., & Larsen, R. J. (1993). The experience of emotional well-being. In M. Lewis, & J. M. Haviland (Eds.), *Handbook of emotions* (pp. 405–415). New York: Guilford Press.
Diener, E., & Diener, M. (1995). Cross-cultural correlates of life satisfaction and self-esteem. *Journal of Personality and Social Psychology, 68*, 653–663.
Diener, E., & Lucas, R. (1999). Personality and subjective well-being. In D. Kahneman, E. Diener., & N. Schwarz (Eds.), *Well-being: The foundations of hedonic psychology* (pp. 213–229). New York: Russell Sage Foundation.
Diener, E., & Suh, E. (1999). National differences in subjective wellbeing. In: D. Kahneman, E. Diener, & N. Schwarz (Eds.), *Well-being: The foundations of hedonic psychology* (pp. 434–452). New York: Russell Sage Foundation.
Diener, E., & Seligman, M. E. P. (2004). Beyond money: Toward an economy of well-being. *Psychological Science in the Public Interest, 5*(1), 1–31.
Diener, E., Lucas, R. E., & Scollon, C. N. (2006). Beyond the hedonic treadmill: Revising the adaptation theory of well-being. *American Psychologist, 61*, 305–314.
Easterlin, R. A. (2003). Explaining happiness. *Proceedings of the National Academy of Sciences, 100*(19), 11176–11183.
Elizur, D., & Shye, S. (1990). Quality of work life and its relation to quality of life. *Applied Psychology, 39*, 275–291.
Eriksson, M. K., Hagberg, L., Lindholm, L., Malmgren-Olsson, E. B., Osterlind, J., & Eliasson, M. (2010). Quality of life and cost-effectiveness of a 3-year trial of lifestyle intervention in primary health care. *Archives of Internal Medicine, 170*, 1470–1479.
Evans, D. R. (1994). Enhancing the quality of life in the population at large. *Social Indicators Research, 33*, 47–88.
Frisch, M. B. (1992). Use of the Quality of Life Inventory in problem assessment and treatment planning for cognitive therapy of depression. In A. Freeman, & F. M. Dattilio (Eds.), *Comprehensive casebook of cognitive therapy* (pp. 27–52). New York: Plenum.
Frisch, M. B. (1998). Quality of life therapy and assessment in health care. *Clinical Psychology: Science & Practice, 5*, 19–40.

Frisch, M. B. (2006). *Finding happiness with quality of life therapy: a positive psychology approach*. Woodway, TX: Quality of Life Press.

Frisch, M. B., Cornell, J., Villanueva, M., & Retzlaff, P. J. (1992). Clinical validation of the quality of life inventory: A measure of life satisfaction for use in treatment planning and outcome assessment. *Psychological Assessment*, *4*, 92–101.

Gallup Well-Being (2012). *Gallup-Healthways Well-Being Index*. Available at <http://www.gallup.com/poll/123215/gallup-healthways-index.aspx>.

Goldberg, D. (1972). *Detecting psychiatric illness by questionnaire*. Oxford: Oxford University Press.

Greenley, J. R., Greenberg, J. S., & Brown, R. (1997). Measuring quality of life: A new and practical survey instrument. *Social Work*, *42*, 244–254.

Grusky, D. B., Western, B., & Wimer, C. (2011). *The great recession*. New York: Russell Sage Foundation.

Hackman, J. R., & Oldham, G. R. (1975). Development of the job diagnostic survey. *Journal of Applied Psychology*, *60*, 159–170.

Harner, C. J., & Neal, L. W. (1993). *The life satisfaction scale*. Columbus, OH: International Diagnostics Systems.

Heckman, J. J., & Masterov, D. V. (2007). The productivity argument for investing in young children. *Applied Economic Perspectives and Policy*, *29*(3), 446–493.

Heinrichs, D. W., Hanlon, T. E., & Carpenter, W. T. (1984). The quality of life scale: An instrument for rating the schizophrenic deficit syndrome. *Schizophrenia Bulletin*, *10*, 388–398.

Hunt, S. M., & McKenna, S. P. (1992). The QLDS: A scale for the measurement of quality of life in depression. *Health Policy*, *22*, 307–319.

Hunt, S. M., McEwen, J., & McKenna, S. P. (1985). Measuring health status: a new tool for clinicians and epidemiologists. *Journal of the Royal College of General Practitioners*, *35* (273), 185–188.

Kind, P., & Gudex, C. M. (1994). Measuring health status in the community: A comparison of methods. *Journal of Epidemiology and Community Health*, *48*, 86–91.

King, L. A., & Napa, C. K. (1998). What makes a life good? *American Psychologist*, *75*, 156–165.

Lawler, E. E. (1982). Strategies for improving the quality of work life. *American Psychologist*, *37*, 486–493.

Lucas, R. E., Clark, A. E., Georgellis, Y., & Diener, E. (2004). Unemployment alters the set point for life satisfaction. *Psychological Science*, *15*, 8–13.

Maslow, A. (1954). *Motivation and personality*. New York: Harper.

McKee-Ryan, F., Song, Z., Wanberg, C. R., & Kinicki, A. J. (2005). Psychological and physical well-being during unemployment: A meta-analytic study. *Journal of Applied Psychology*, *90*, 53–76.

Michalos, A. C. (1991). *Global report on student well-being, Life satisfaction and happiness* (*Vol. 1*). .New York: Springer-Verlag.

Muldoon, M. F., Barger, S. D., & Flory, J. D. (1998). What are quality of life measurements measuring? *British Medical Journal*, *316*, 542.

Neugarten, B. L., Havighurst, R., & Tobin, S. (1961). The measurement of life satisfaction. *Journal of Gerontology*, *16*, 134–143.

Nussbaum, M. (1995). Human capabilities, female human beings. In M. Nussbaum, & J. Glover (Eds.), *Women, culture and development* (pp. 61–104). Oxford: Clarendon Press.

O'Boyle, G. A. (1994). The Schedule for Evaluation of Individual Quality of Life (SEIQoL). *International Journal of Mental Health*, *23*, 3–23.

O'Boyle, C. A., McGee, H. M., Hickey, A., Joyce, C. R. B., Browne, J., O'Malley, K., & Hiltbrunner, B. (1993). *The Schedule for the Evaluation of Individual Quality of Life (SEIQoL). Administration manual.* Dublin: Royal College of Surgeons in Ireland.

Rollero, C, & Tartaglia, S. (2009). Preserving life satisfaction during the economic crisis: Which factors can help? *Psicologia Politica, 39*, 75–87.

Sainfort, F., Becker, M., & Diamond, R. (1996). Judgments of quality of life of individuals with severe mental disorders: Patient self-report versus provider perspectives. *American Journal of Psychiatry, 153*, 497–501.

Seed, P., & Lloyd, G. (1997). *Quality of life.* London: Jessica Kingsley.

Sen, A. K. (1985). *Commodities and capabilities.* Oxford: Elsevier Science.

Sirgy, M. L., & Samli, A. (1995). Developing a life satisfaction measure based on need hierarchy theory. In M. J. Sirgy, & A. Samli (Eds.), *New dimensions of marketing and quality of life.* Westport, CT: Greenwood Press.

Smeeding, T. (2010). Prolonged recession creates a new, possibly permanent poor. *Economic Opportunity Report, 45*(4), 25.

Strack, F., Argyle, M., & Schwarz, N. (Eds.), (1991). *Subjective well-being. An interdisciplinary perspective.* Oxford: Pergamon Press.

Tibblin, G., Tibblin, B., Peciva, S., Kullman, S., & Svardsudd, K. (1990). The Goteborg Quality of Life Instrument – An assessment of well-being and symptoms among men born 1913 and 1923. *Scandinavian Journal of Primary Health Care, 8*(*Suppl 1*), 33–38.

United Nations Development Programme (2012). *Human Development Index (HDI).* Available at <http://hdr.undp.org/en/statistics/hdi/>.

Veenhoven, R. (1984). *Conditions of happiness.* Boston: Reidel.

Ventegodt, S., Merrick, J., & Andersen, N. J. (2003). Quality of Life Theory I. The IQOL theory: An integrative theory of the global quality of life concept. *The Scientific World Journal, 3*, 1030–1040.

Vinokur, A. D., Price, R. H., & Caplan, R. D. (1996). Hard times and hurtful partners: How financial strain affects depression and relationship satisfaction of unemployed persons and their spouses. *Journal of Personality and Social Psychology, 71*, 166–179.

Warr, P., Cook, J., & Wall, T. (1979). Scales for the measurement of some work attitudes and aspects of psychological well-being. *Journal of Occupational Psychology, 52*, 129–148.

Westman, M., Etzion, D., & Horovitz, S. (2004). The toll of unemployment does not stop with the unemployed. *Human Relations, 57*, 823–844.

WHOQOL Group (1995). The World Health Organization Quality of Life assessment (WHOQOL): position paper from the World Health Organization. *Social Science & Medicine, 41*, 1403–1409.

World Health Organization (2006). *Constitution of the World Health Organization.* Available at <http://www.who.int/governance/eb/who_constitution_en.pdf>.

FURTHER READING

Brand, J. E. (2008). Job displacement and social participation over the life course: Findings for a cohort of joiners. *Social Forces, 87*, 211–242. Retrieved 20 February, 2012 from <http://sf.oxfordjournals.org/content/87/1/211.short>.

Diener, E. (1997). Measuring quality of life: Economic, social, and subjective indicators. *Social Indicators Research, 40*, 189–216 Retrieved 26 February, 2012 from <http://www.springerlink.com/content/p1j7507112p6u744/>.

Hanisch, K. A. (1999). Job loss and unemployment research from 1994 to 1998: A review and recommendations for research and intervention. *Journal of Vocational Behavior, 55*, 188–220. Retrieved 16 February, 2012 from <http://www.sciencedirect.com/science/article/pii/S0001879199917220>.

Irons, J. (2009). Economic scarring: The long-term impacts of the recession. *Economic Policy Institute website.* Retrieved 10 March, 2012 from <http://www.epi.org/publication/bp243/>.

Von Wachter, T. (2010). *Testimony before the Joint Economic Committee of U.S. Congress on Long-term Unemployment: Causes, consequences and solutions.* newsweek.com website. Retrieved 30 January, 2012 from <http:/ndn.newsweek.com/media/94/JEC_testimony-4_29_10.pdf>.

CHAPTER 13

Quality of Life Treatment and Workplace Problems

DEVELOPING APPLIED QUALITY OF LIFE THERAPY (QOLT)

Literally hundreds of studies have been carried out for the primary purpose of addressing individual health and disease-specific quality of life (QoL) issues (Bowling, 2001). Regardless of the purpose for which it is used, QoL has been seen as a way of explaining an individual's personal life expectations and goals. QoL can be best determined by how an individual's hopes and desires are matched by what they are actually experiencing. Individuals also view their QoL from the perspective of their personal value system, culture, goals, and standards. People measure their present circumstances in relation to a standard that they perceive as most ideal. An individual places the highest QoL value on the extent to which certain desires, ambitions, goals, and beliefs are most satisfying to them (Frisch, 2006).

QoL has been defined earlier as the degree of excellence in living relative to some expressed or implied standard that exists in a particular society (Veenhoven, 1984). Frisch (2006) and others found that most often QoL can be personally determined by any aspect of life. For example, work can be excellent, satisfying, enjoyable, necessary, or distasteful to an individual. From this perspective, the quality of an individual's work life can go beyond mere economic or financial well-being. The goal of an ideal quality of life is related to the subjective well-being or happiness aspects of life that are particularly enjoyable and worthwhile might be found that, beyond a satisfying work life, there might be an enjoyable family life, excellent health, or the full development of one's talents and self-expression.

Verdugo, Schaluck, Keith, and Stancliff (2005) reported that the QoL construct has changed since its origin as a general organizing concept. It has been more recently seen from an assessment and intervention perspective. QoL has become more useful as a framework for assessing quality of life outcomes and a social construct that guides quality of life improvement

Treating Worker Dissatisfaction During Economic Change
DOI: http://dx.doi.org/10.1016/B978-0-12-397006-0.00013-0

strategies. Quality of life methods provide a basis for enhancing the effectiveness of other strategies. This enhancement role places additional emphasis on the need for more valid QoL assessment and intervention measures.

QoL and Quality of Life Therapy (QOLT) represents the conceptual and practical framework used throughout this chapter (Frisch, 2006). This approach help explain many of the relationships between the QoL approach and involuntary job displacement during the recent economic downturn. For example, QoL measures have the potential of expressing a worker's personal feelings and values such as health, self-esteem, happiness and other factors as being a more prominent concern related to the workplace. QOLT constitutes a way for individuals to evaluate their overall satisfaction with life within and beyond the workplace (Eid & Larson, 2008; Frisch, 2006).

Diener and Larsen (1993) and Frisch (2006) indicated how QoL theory can help explain the relationship between:

- Subjective well-being (SWB) or happiness, which is related to the degree to which a person's emotional and cognitive evaluations of their most important needs, goals, and wishes have been fulfilled;
- Life satisfaction, which is viewed as the subjective evaluation or perceived gap between what a person has and what they desire to have in valued areas of life.

Quality of Life is expressed as the combination of these two components.

This chapter expands upon the definition of a working alliance. The Frisch (2006) definition of QoL articulated the working alliance as the agreement between helping professionals and clients on the goals and tasks of treatment and the presence of a strong bond between helping professionals and clients. A stronger working alliance was associated with positive appraisals of subjective quality of life (Bordin, 1983). Outcome research has indicated that clients' perceptions of working alliances are major predictors of the success of various types of interventions, such as psychotherapy and case management services. The professional therapist or case manager needs various strategies to establish and maintain working alliances with patients and their supportive networks.

Beck, Rush, Shaw, and Emery (1979), Frisch (1992), Lewinsohn, Redner, and Seeley (1991), and others saw QoL factors as contributing causes or the consequences of various psychological or physical life challenges. In order to provide for more comprehensive assessments or interventions, QoL integrative approaches between a client's supportive networks should be considered as co-equal or in collaboration with others' efforts aimed at addressing social, psychological, financial, and other problems related to workplace challenges.

Based upon the work of Diener and Larsen (1993), later supported by Frisch (2006), an integrated QoL approach can be particularly beneficial in addressing problems related to the recent economic downturn as follows.

- As a result of the economic downturn, work life and the workplace is changing rapidly and putting increased pressure on businesses and human service organizations to conduct joint assessments and interventions.
- Comprehensive approaches should be emphasized that address clients' workplace problems and functioning in all domains of life.
- The need for QoL constructs and procedures that allow for integration across disciplines in order to increase treatment efficacy and flexibility should be recognized.
- The feelings and needs of new and diverse clientele, including displaced workers, using both traditional and creative interventions should be included.
- The interdisciplinary research on QoL and subjective well-being that may further the clinical enterprise in psychology, medicine, and gerontology should be applied.
- An understanding of human behavior in general, and clinical disorders such as depression in particular should be increased.
- A theoretical framework that facilitates clinical and conceptual integration should be further developed.
- Clinical assessment to a new, relevant, and practical realm of human functioning should be extended.
- The development and use of brief QoL work-related interventions should be encouraged.

Integrated Quality of Life Therapy (IQOLT) helps to support the perspective that improved work-related outcomes can be achieved with an integrated and multidisciplinary helping approach (Frisch, 1992). A major concern that is frequently noted in the QoL literature is the need for a more valid and methodologically reliable basis for supporting QoL theory. Concerns have been raised regarding QoL in general and its contribution as a valid assessment and treatment outcome measure (Frisch et al., 2005). This chapter is guided by several useful models and constructs which have been found to be valid, reliable, comprehensive, and integrative treatment approaches, including:

- World Health Organization Quality of Life (WHOQOL) Group (1998);
- Schedule of the Evaluation of Individual Quality of Life (SEIQOL) (Broadhead et al., 1998);
- Quality of Life Inventory (QOLI) (Frisch, 1994a,b);
- Quality of Life Therapy (QOLT) (Frisch, 2006).

The model developed by Frisch (2006) that is primarily used in this chapter, Quality of Life Therapy (QOLT), was selected as an integrative and multidimensional construct. This model focuses on generic interactive objective and subjective measures that are very relevant for addressing work-related issues. The QOLT model is related to an individual's satisfaction with work circumstances, personal attitudes, and standards. It is also recognized that defining, measuring, and scaling these concepts will need further articulation and refinement. In spite of some limitations, the QOLT model presents an opportunity to enhance assessment and treatment, for individuals, families, and communities at risk for job displacement and workplace-related problems.

As an example, for years a faith-based social services agency has served literally thousands of people in a primarily low- to middle-class downtown area in Phoenix, Arizona. Before and during the recent economic downturn, it became readily apparent that the financial crisis that resulted in drastic job displacement was the tip of the proverbial iceberg. In many cases unemployment was not always initially presented as the primary problem, but it invariably became a prominent issue. People came to the agency by way of various emergencies, circumstances, and conditions.

A diverse group of individuals came to the agency needing help for reasons that included substance abuse, re-entry from penal institutions, and work loss. QOLT screening assessments were used to help assess and determine the type of intervention that was deemed most appropriate for this group of clients. QOLT provided guidance and screening for potential DSM disorders and support during job displacement. The QOLT core techniques that were used for assessment and interventions placed an emphasis on those areas of specific concern to the individual. For example, the QOLT assessment may have found that spiritual values were of greater interest to a recently displaced worker with a minimal interest in immediate paid employment. In this case, all areas would be considered, but spiritual goals and values would be emphasized and work interventions would be de-emphasized for this individual for a period of time.

Although QOLT was able to emphasize specific areas of interest depending upon the clients' concerns and needs, it was recommended that the overall areas or domains be assessed. It was found that concerns of relevance were often found in areas that clients thought initially to be irrelevant to their situation. For example, the work domain for many displaced workers contained various areas of concern, such as discrimination claims, interpersonal conflicts with co-workers, or disputes with bosses. Other issues involved several workers' feelings about unfulfilling work and excessive work demands. Overall, the QOLT Inventory revealed that client life satisfaction was enhanced across unanticipated domains through QOLT interventions.

The QOLT model provides a rationale for allowing clients to consider any areas of life that they personally value. QOLT may also be helpful in cases where several related problems beyond job loss for an individual may exist, such as a chronically unhappy marriage, chronic illness, or an unsatisfactory work situation. Lewinsohn et al. (1991) and Frisch (2006) found that QoL measures have been found to help identify those at risk for serious unanticipated mental health-related problems such as depression, so that it may also be used as a referral or preventive measure (Frisch, 2006).

In related studies, Baruffol, Gisle, and Corten (1995) found that low life satisfaction contributes to the prediction of clinical depression. The results of those studies were supported and extended in more recent studies and practice. Findings have demonstrated that the Frisch QOL Inventory (1994a,b), which measures low life satisfaction, significantly predicted the onset of depression. Other studies found that low life satisfaction is a major risk factor for several other forms of psychological disturbance.

These findings suggest that individuals at risk for losing or who have lost employment should be routinely screened with QOLT assessments for low life satisfaction. This may help identify those at risk for more severe mental disorders to be more objectively evaluated. The characteristics of different types of work have also been found to contribute to varying degrees of satisfaction. For example, a person's degree of satisfaction with work may involve the type of work, pay, relationships with co-workers and managers, the work environment, work loss and job security. A person's subjective perception of work or a workplace may include their self-esteem, creativity, and goals, which could also influence their satisfaction within the overall aspects of work (Frisch, 1994a,b, 2006).

A central premise of QOL theory is that life satisfaction in highly valued areas of life has a greater influence on evaluations of overall life satisfaction than does that in areas of lesser importance. For example, a person who is satisfied with both work and recreational pursuits but values work more highly will have their overall judgments of life satisfaction influenced more by work than by recreational satisfaction. Lazarus (1991) and Pavot and Diener (1993) noted that changing the value or importance attributed to specific areas of life can dramatically affect overall life satisfaction. For example, involuntary loss of work that was previously highly valued may reduce the value of work to a marginal place in a person's life, whereby a person might then focus on being a better spouse or parent.

Campbell, Converse, and Rodgers (1976) discovered in their study that all of the measures of the work domain on QoL were positively inter-correlated. This was found to be especially true for workers with the highest levels of satisfaction with their job. This group of workers also expressed the highest levels of satisfaction with non-work domains such as family life and friendships. Satisfaction with the job and non-work domains was also high among all other workers in the study.

The QoL measures described by Higginson and Carr (2001) as having the potential to assist routine clinical practice that can be related to the workplace are as follows:

- prioritizing problems of displaced workers;
- active communication with at-risk and displaced workers;
- screening workers for potential problems;
- identifying workers' QoL preferences;
- monitoring change or response to treatment of workers.

VALIDITY AND RELIABILITY OF QOLT MEASURES

In the past there have been few assessment and intervention studies directly aimed at increasing an individual's QoL, outside of specific medical or psychological areas that were empirically evaluated (Evans, 1994). In general, QoL interventions were often considered to be impractical and invalid measures. This was especially true when attempts were made to directly administer QoL interventions independently to functional, non-clinical subjects, with no apparent QoL deficits or risk factors. It is most likely that employing QOLT became more useful for health providers and other helping professionals while treating a specific physical illness/disability or a psychological disturbance.

QOLT (Frisch, 1998a,b) was initially used while studying a sample of clients selected for both low QoL and in conjunction with various psychological disturbances and clinical depression. The findings revealed that QOLT had a clinically significant effect upon the sample treatment group. This study demonstrated that the treatment group's statistical means were well within one standard deviation of the mean for samples at post-test and follow-up. It was determined by a National Institute of Mental Health (NIMH) panel of experts (Newman, Ciarlo, & Carpenter, 1999) that the Frisch Quality of Life Inventory (QOLI) met the eleven essential criteria for a useful assessment instrument. The evaluation of the QOLI resulted in its being rated as very good to excellent according to the following criteria:

- Psychometric strength in clinical and non-clinical settings;
- Clinically significant and practical;
- Understood by non-professional audiences;
- Compatible with diverse theories and clinical practices;
- A low measure of cost relative to its uses;
- Useful in assessing treatment progress as well as outcomes;
- Relevant to a broad target group;
- Predictive, convergent, discriminant, and treatment validity;
- Test-retest and internal consistency reliability;
- Based upon a nationwide normative study.

The QOLI (Frisch, 1994a,b) provides a valid score that indicates a person's overall satisfaction with life, based on how well their needs, goals, and wishes are being met in important areas of their life. It was noted by Frisch that the data from this QoLT Inventory should also be used in conjunction with professional judgment based upon other pertinent information concerning the individual client.

The general application of Quality of Life Therapy (QOLT; Frisch, 2006) to work-related issues can be outlined as follows.

- The Quality of Life Inventory (QOLI; Frisch, 1992, 1994a,b) provides a measure of positive life satisfaction based on QoL theory. The QOLI can be designed to comprehensively screen for problems and strengths related to job-displaced individuals. QOLI scores can also be used to plan treatment, monitor progress, and evaluate the symptoms of potentially depressed individuals. Frisch (1994b) describes the procedure as follows.
- The QOLI consists of 16 items. The items are selected to include all domains of life, including work, that have been empirically associated with overall QoL.
- Respondents rate how important each of the 16 domains including work is related to their overall happiness and satisfaction.

- The importance and satisfaction ratings for each item are multiplied to form weighted satisfaction ratings ranging from −6 to +6.
- A weighted life satisfaction profile is then computed by averaging all weighted satisfaction ratings with non-zero importance ratings. This score reflects a person's satisfaction in only those areas of life that he or she considers important.
- The total raw score is converted to a T-score and percentile-score which reflect a person's overall quality of life measure.
- Respondents also indicate, on a supplementary section of the QOLI answer sheet, what problems interfere with their satisfaction in each area.

The 16 areas of quality of life that can be calculated to accurately account for the positive or negative degree of overall life satisfaction are listed in Box 13.1.

CULTURALLY RELEVANT QOLT ASSESSMENT AND INTERVENTION MEASURES

Quality of life measures usually originate in one cultural setting and can be translated when used in another social context. Unless the cultural

Box 13.1 Areas of QoL in the Quality of Life Inventory

Health: being physically fit, without illness, pain or disability
Self-esteem: liking and respecting oneself
Goals and values: attitude of life, beliefs about what matters most
Money or earnings: what is owned, secure future, money security
Work: type of job, career, duties, employed, unemployed
Recreation or play: use of free time, relaxation, self-improvement
Learning: gaining new skills or information
Creativity: using imagination to discover new ways of doing things
Helping: social service and civic action, helping others in need
Love relationship: a person in a close romantic relationship with you
Friendships: people you know and care about with like interest
Relationships with children: how you get along with family children
Relationships with relatives: how you get along with relatives
Home: place where you live and how you feel about it
Neighborhood: area near your home and how you feel about it
Community: whole city or town and how you feel about all aspects of it.

Source: Frisch (1994a,b).

equivalence of the measure is taken into consideration, the validity of the measures may not be met. Measures that have consistently met the conditions of cultural relevance are those of the WHO (World Health Organization Quality of Life Group, 1998). Grassi and Riba (2012) and others explain how competent interventions require culturally relevant assessment instruments and inventories for effective delivery in a multicultural workplace.

Previous studies have demonstrated the importance of measures that accurately reflect distinctive cultural differences. Culturally grounded assessment models are needed that emphasize a special awareness of the client's culture. The WHOQOL Group (1998) has viewed QoL measures as having the capacity of assessing various groups across cultures. The Group provides an opportunity to conduct research in a number of diverse workplaces and the results can then be compared between the different workplaces. By using a cultural perspective, more than standardized questions can be used to identify a client's life satisfaction and subjective well-being that is related to the workplace.

Culturally relevant QOLT assessment and treatment incorporates the client's racial and ethnic perspective. In order to better assess the benefits of an intervention in employment-related quality of life, it is important to provide culturally appropriate evidence from the worker's perspective. For example, quality of life may be perceived differently by the general culture and other cultures. This may reflect different experiences and life-style perspectives of a displaced worker's physical, emotional, and subjective well-being.

In order to help address the issue of cultural relevance for reasons outlined above, QOLT measures are primarily generic measures and have been found to be appropriate constructs when related to workplace issues. Many QoL measures are useful when addressing specific medical issues but are not relevant when addressing generic QoL measures. An advantage of QOLT is its potential to be used in partnership as part of a supportive network of human services providers. Culturally relevant measures have wide applicability, which allows for comparisons of assessments and treatments related to diverse settings such as the workplace. The major downside of combining some generic measures is the lack of validity and reliability.

QOLT (Frisch, 1998a,b) offers suitable area-specific treatment strategies for the 16 areas of life that may constitute an individual's overall QOL. In addition to area-specific strategies, QOLT offers general treatment strategies referred to by the acronym CASIO, and its techniques are applicable to any area of life. The format of QOLT questions, measures, and administration are suitable for most workplace settings and cultures. The general model of QOLT or CASIO is used for overall problem solving that supports the findings related to the QOLI described earlier. Specifically, the four components of life satisfaction depicted below are combined with a fifth that is concerned with increasing overall satisfaction by increasing life satisfaction in other areas of life that are not of immediate concern (Frisch, 1994a,b).

The CASIO model for increasing happiness and fulfillment considers change in five paths:

- The objective *Circumstances* of an area
- The *Attitude* or perception/interpretation of an area
- The *Standards* of fulfillment for an area
- The *Importance* placed on an area for one's overall happiness
- *Other* areas not of immediate concern that can be applied to any particular area of dissatisfaction to enhance clients' quality of life.

Box 13.2 Outlines strategies for improving QoL according to the CASIO approach.

INTEGRATED QOLT METHOD AND THE ECONOMIC DOWNTURN

During the recent economic downturn the high unemployment and related social disruption is disheartening. Besides economic policies that are needed to help stimulate the economy, government officials and policymakers hesitate to enact social policies that can better assist people in coping with work loss challenges. There is a vital need for society, organizations and businesses to also help buffer the mental and social impact that accompanied the economic downturn. It is also important to recognize that the serious social cost of the economic downturn will most likely be much longer lasting than originally anticipated.

The benefits of integrated IQOL methods related to an individual's quality of life are well documented (Diener & Seligman, 2004). During the recent economic downturn, some businesses may be resistant to providing the type of work environment that can be seen as supportive toward employees. The workplace can potentially provide for problem solving through cooperative and innovative workplace approaches. Insuring successful IQOL opportunities across diverse cultures in the

Box 13.2 The Five CASIO Strategies for Increasing Your Quality of Life

Instructions. Pick an area of your life that you are unhappy with and are willing to work on. Make a plan to improve your happiness with this part of your life based on the five strategies below. You can also use these strategies to make a plan to deal with other problems or difficult situations in your life.

What Is Happiness? Happiness, or quality of life, can be defined as the extent to which your most important needs, goals, and wishes have been fulfilled. For any area of life that you are unsatisfied with and that is important to you, there are five strategies you can use to boost your satisfaction and thereby increase your overall happiness.

1. *Change Your Circumstances.* The first strategy involves changing your circumstances to improve a particular area of your life. You could change your circumstances by changing things like your relationships, where you live, where you work, or what you do for fun. For example, if you are unhappy with your marriage, you may seek couples counseling to improve your relationship with your partner.
2. *Change Your Attitude.* The second way to improve your happiness in a particular area of life is to change your attitude about the situation, to correct any distortions or negativity in your thinking. Changing your attitude involves taking a new look at any part of your life by asking two key questions: (a) "What is really happening here?" and (b) "What does it mean to me?" Many times our view of a situation or what we think the situation means for our self-worth, our well-being, and our future is not based on the facts; that is, our view is distorted. For example, you may believe that your boss is unhappy with your work because he or she seems to be ignoring you, when in fact your boss is preoccupied with a personal problem.
3. *Change Your Goals and Standards.* The third strategy for boosting your satisfaction in an area of life such as work or love is to change your goals and standards for that area. The key idea here is to set realistic goals and to experiment with raising and lowering your standards of fulfillment for particular areas of life that you are unhappy with. To do this you have to answer questions like "What do I really want in this part of life? How much is enough? What realistic goals and standards can I set for success in this particular part of my life?" Often it helps to lower your standards somewhat so that you can gain some fulfillment in an area of life that you are worrying about.
4. *Change Your Priorities.* The fourth strategy for improving life satisfaction or happiness is to change your priorities or consider changing what you think is important in your life. This strategy involves reevaluating your

priorities and emphasizing those areas that are most important to you and that are most under your control, that is, areas that you can do something about. For example, if you have an unbeatable health problem, you may deemphasize the importance of health in your life and instead focus on relationships or your work. These may be two areas that you can change to make yourself happier.

5. *Boost Your Satisfaction in Other Areas Not Considered Before.* The fifth and final strategy for improving your quality of life is to boost your satisfaction in other areas that you haven't considered before. You can boost or increase your overall quality of life by increasing your satisfaction with other areas of life that are not of immediate concern. This is especially helpful when you are working on an area that is very difficult and slow to change, such as a love relationship. While a particular area of concern, like love, may be moving slowly toward improvement, you can boost your overall quality of life by focusing on other areas of life that you care about, such as recreation and friendships, even though these areas are not your "number one" concern at the moment.

Summary. To apply these five strategies to your situation, all you need to do is (a) identify the areas of life that you are unhappy with and want to change, and (b) creatively brainstorm about ways to apply one or more of these five strategies with the goal of improving your satisfaction. As the above strategies suggest, you can improve your satisfaction in any area of life by actually improving the objective circumstances or by changing your attitudes, goals, standards, and priorities. Finally, because your overall quality of life is made up of your happiness with all of the particular parts of life that you care about, you can increase your overall quality of life by doing what you can to boost your satisfaction in any area that you care about, even ones that are not of pressing concern right now.

Source: Questionnaire handout from the Quality of Life Therapy: Therapist Manual (Frisch, 1998b).

workplace is a very complex task. It requires that supportive workplace networks employ flexible and multidisciplinary approaches.

Tzafrir & Mano-Negrin (2006) reported that downsizing has been a very pervasive organizational issue. During the recent economic downturn many organizations have done little to prepare their employees for a mass layoff. A main focus of this study is to examine how workplace QOLT methods and alliances during a period of downsizing can enhance the QoL of employees. This includes both those who are dismissed and others who remain in an organization. Several findings indicate that QOLT methods can have a twofold effect. For example, staff from a community-based social service agency (FIBCO Family Services Inc.) interviewed workers who were displaced as a result of company downsizing. Many of the displaced workers had participated in joint pre-dismissal interviews with companies and job placement agencies. Workers who had participated in these interviews were found to express a more positive adjustment to their dismissal than displaced workers who had not participated in such efforts. Individuals who did participate in the QOLT assessments and interventions were found to increase their morale and reduce some of the negative outcomes that can occur as a result of downsizing.

Community mental health programs have identified problem areas that could benefit from QOLT. Many communities have been increasingly affected by rising social problems resulting from the economic downturn. There has also been a noticeable increase in the occurrence of violence and mental health issues in the workplace. As a response to this issue, some programs have expanded support for social service referrals to include marriage and family counseling, child and elder care services. legal advice, financial planning, and debt counseling (Walker, 2009).

These programs have also seen fit to expand service referrals that should offer a challenge to researchers, service providers, and government programs to develop new approaches including QOLT as a way to address involuntary work loss. Job displacement during this recent economic downturn should be viewed as a long-term social issue. This will require comprehensive and collaborative societal support that must also address diminishing employment labor contracts and disappearing pension benefits. It will require sustained and increased human resources to address real and perceived increases in future job instability and related QoL concerns.

Case Study: Using QOLT and Work Loss Experiences

The QOLT assessment and CASIO intervention was used as a tool in assisting the following client. The process demonstrates the unique feelings, hopes, goals, values, and levels of life satisfaction that can be felt by an individual. This client came to an inner- city, faith-based social services agency initially requesting employment assistance after being laid off from work. During the QOLT initial interview process it was clear that this individual had very important personal priorities beyond their recent work loss. After administering the CASIO intervention technique and QOLT Weighted Satisfaction Profile, the measures revealed the following.

- Very strong dissatisfaction in the areas of (1) Health, (2) Love.
- The Profile indicated low satisfaction in the areas of (1) Money, (2) Work, (3) Home, (4) Relatives.
- The Profile revealed average satisfaction in the areas of (1) Self-esteem, (2) Play, (3) Children, (4) Friends.
- The areas of the Profile in the highest satisfaction range were (1) Goals & Values, (2) Learning, (3) Creativity, (4) Helping.

All of the areas improved slightly after several administrations, with the exception of love, health, and relatives. The client's final overall quality of life classification score was in the average range and did not suggest that they were at risk for depression. During the course of the QOLT process the client became noticeably more interested in learning, trusting others, less anxious, becoming more financially independent from significant others, became more confident in finding a career, and became more inclined to perform helping activities. By supporting the client in boosting satisfaction in other areas of life such as spirituality, there were improvements in other areas including work.

The client provided the following narrative about their experiences during this period:

> *"I had a very different experience than most with the economy. I learned that the workforce is not very favorable for individuals or families that may be experiencing any type of trauma, such as illness. You either go to work at the appointed times or you don't have a job and have to suffer the consequences of it. My husband became very ill and was hospitalized for close to one year. My kids and I still had to live, pay rent and utilities and buy food but with my attention and time needed at the hospital, I was unable to find a position that would work around my personal life. It was then that I learned the key in dealing with any of life's situation, faith in God.*
>
> *I had always been able to find work quickly and easily. I have over 10 years of experience in financial aid processing for students and with education being so popular, there was no shortage of positions. I would send resume after resume and went on some interviews but was not hired. I didn't realize at the time that if I had taken a position, that my husband's illness would most likely cause me to lose it anyway. So, I did the only thing I knew how to do, I just trusted in my faith to get me through.*
>
> *Before my husband got sick, the townhouse that we were renting went into foreclosure. The owner did not inform us. We were going to be making our first payment on our own since I cancelled my Section 8 Housing Assistance after I got married. My husband went into the hospital and that month and the next went by. At the beginning of the third month, I got a notice from the bank that they had bought the property and I would have 30 days to move. To make a long story short, I received money from the bank to move, since I had not been informed by the owner. Then I attempted to rent another house, gave the woman the money to move in and was notified by her when I came with my truck to move in, that she*

could not rent the house. By the way, she didn't return all of my money on that day and was unable to be reached after that. So, I wound up in my friend's shelter for about 6 months but she allowed me to stay totally free, which was a blessing because remember, I am not working.

Around the beginning of 2010, I did get a temporary assignment with the US Census Bureau and was able to rent a four-bedroom house in S. Phoenix. My children had been living with their dad for the past 6–8 months so I was ready to have us all together again. The Census assignment ended much sooner than expected so I was evicted. The landlord was very nice though and agreed not to issue a judgment against me as long as I moved and left the house in good condition. From there, I took a job as a cab driver and was able to get an apartment in East Mesa, which I was evicted from within 2 months.

Here's the good part. I was really trusting God to provide my rent for that place; I didn't want my daughter to have to go through another eviction. Well, the constable came at 8am to lock me out and that same day at 5pm, I received a call from an agency where I had applied for a housing program. They told me that I would be a great candidate for a program that would pay a portion of my rent for one year. I moved in with a girlfriend temporarily until all of my paperwork was completed, and in December 2010, I moved into my own place. Starting in February, they started paying all of my rent and did so until September 2011. They still paid a large portion of my rent in October, November, and December 2011.

Through this experience, I learned to really trust that my life was in the hands of another. We may have plans but His plans supersede anything that we may want to do. And He is able to provide what we need during the time that He is preparing us. So, my advice for dealing with a bad economy or any other crisis, TRUST GOD!!!"

During the next 6 months the client was provided with several administrations of the QOLT Inventory and CASIO treatment interventions. The client's overall QOL Inventory moved closer to a higher satisfaction classification. There was also a clear shift toward a happier, creative, and more confident affect. After a year had passed, the client sent this note thanking the agency for its support and presented the following statement:

"My experience inspired me to create a women's ministry, whose mission is to educate and encourage women to embrace their true identity, to make women aware of the potential life changing consequences of compromising in relationships, and to release women affected by illness and other issues from their shame and restore them to their wealthy place in a spiritual life."

WORK LOSS CIRCUMSTANCES AND QOLT ASSESSMENT

Overall economic adversity has been found to have a negative impact on the well-being and life satisfaction of people (Deckker & Shaufeli, 1995), since work occupies a central place in people's lives. Subjective well-being or happiness and life satisfaction are not only affected by unemployment but there is a lasting effect after individuals regain employment (Aytac & Rankin, 2009). As noted earlier in this chapter a central premise of QoL theory (Lazarus, 1991; Pavot & Diener, 1993) is that changing the value or importance attributed to specific areas of life can dramatically affect overall life satisfaction. For example, involuntary loss of work that was previously highly valued may be compensated for by reducing the value of work to a marginal place in a person's life. A displaced worker might then focus on being a better spouse, parent, enhancing self-esteem, improving health, developing friendships, bettering the neighborhood, or boosting other life domains.

Work Loss Circumstances and Children

McLoyd (1989) found that one of the most significant circumstances related to an economic downturn was the effect that it has on how displaced workers get along with their children. Research on the impact of paternal job loss on children shows that some direct effects have been found, but most effects are indirect. Loss of work due to the economic downturn will often result in changes in a particular parent's behavior and disposition. Loss of work may cause changes in a parent's lifestyle or career and how that affects their children's self-esteem. It will also determine how a parent spends most of their time. Loss of work can result in missing creative challenges that employment brought, resulting in a lack of positive engagement with children. Lack of money earned on a job might alienate children from friends and neighbors. Parents who become unemployed may not engage in favorite hobbies or pastimes with their children. Loss of income may require children to relocate to new schools and establish relationships with people with whom they are unfamiliar. Displaced workers' families will experience a variety of factors that influence the downgrading of their QoL.

Circumstances related to the effect of parent's involuntary work loss can be quite serious. McLoyd (1989) found that some parents may respond to economic loss with increased irritability and pessimism and become less supportive, more punitive and arbitrary in their interactions with the child. This behavior increases the risk for socio-emotional problems, deviant behavior, and reduced aspirations in children. Children may model the unemployed parent's negative temperament and relationship with other family members following the economic loss. A parent's job loss may influence a child's social development indirectly through events such as divorce related to job loss.

Work Loss Circumstances and Self-Esteem

Self-esteem has been defined as the degree to which a person likes and respects themselves measured against their perceived strengths, weaknesses, and ability to cope with life challenges. Frisch (1994b) noted that a person tends to experience low self-esteem when they see failure in themselves based upon their own standards in many valued QoL areas of life, including work. Loss of meaningful work means a number of things to a person, including how they define themselves. This includes how they perceive the quality of how they spend most of their time. Meaningful work includes the feeling of a sense of pride about their duties associated with the job. The money that is earned and the people with whom one works is a major standard against which a person measures their self-esteem.

An individual may feel very inadequate in losing or failing to find a job. Loss of work represents a challenge to liking and respecting oneself in light of perceived work-loss-related successes and failures, and ability to obtain employment. Other key areas of life such as school, parenting, and love relationships can be linked to this perceived failure experience (Diener & Seligman, 2004). Vaillant (2002) found that the loss of work can disrupt a displaced worker's life in other ways. This includes a lessening of overall mental, physical, and emotional health.

Work Loss Circumstances and Health

Linn, Sandifer, and Stein (1985) assessed the effects of involuntary unemployment on the mental and physical health of middle-aged men who became unemployed. The unemployed men reported more physician visits, symptoms of somatization, depression, and anxiety than those who continued to work.

Frisch (1994a,b) and others defined good health essentially as being physically fit without pain, ailments, or disability as a domain of QoL. Loss of work may cause a person to suffer from a loss in happiness due to an increase in poor fitness and health habits, chronic illness or disability, heart disease, poor mental health, or alcohol and drug abuse. It should be noted that many displaced workers are able to successfully adapt to their illness or disabilities related to job loss. They can find other avenues of happiness and well-being and take steps to improve in other domains.

Diener and Seligman (2004) in a related study indicated that a number of studies confirmed that happiness may help people adjust to health problems. By assessing the well-being of individuals with mental disorders it was found that happiness also alleviates regular physical health problems such as immunity to colds and viruses that may emerge. Mental disorders resulting from the economic downturn have caused widespread suffering, and their impact is growing. Several QoL studies have found that suffering due to work-loss-related mental disorders can be lessened by QOLT treatment. In order to offer more comprehensive treatment to a greater number of displaced workers who may be prone to physical health problems and mental disorders, QOLT can be a viable option.

Work Loss Circumstances and Friends

Friends are non-relatives whom you know well and care about and who have interests and opinions similar to your own. Friends also have fun together, discuss personal problems and help each other when needed. Since people spend a great deal of time at work, relationships with friends on the job often take on a great deal of significance. When a displaced worker loses close friends on the job he or she may feel alienated from one or more of them. The displaced worker may have neglected other friendships and have difficulty in knowing how to reestablish those friendships. If the person has no close friends outside of the job, he or she may yearn for the work-related friendships and feel unable to develop new or previous friendships. The displaced worker may find it difficult to share personal problems or may experience mistrust that gets in the way of making new friends which can affect their QoL.

Work Loss Circumstances and the Neighborhood

QOLT defines the neighborhood as the area around the house or apartment where one resides. The perception one has about the neighborhood depends upon a number of characteristics: e.g., how nice it looks, the amount of problems in the area, and how well you like the people. Displaced workers may find they can no longer afford to live in a neighborhood which will affect their QoL. If required to move, they may be unable to improve or maintain general maintenance of the new neighborhood. The physical setting of the new neighborhood may be perceived as unsafe, unattractive, or unfriendly. Supportive, positive social relationships are necessary for well-being. There are data suggesting that well-being leads to good social relationships. In addition, evidence indicates that people suffer when they are displaced from groups or have poor relationships in new groups. The fact that positive neighborhood relationships are important to the well-being of displaced workers, there are many implications for the QoL in other life domains.

Work Loss Circumstances and Overall QoL

Displaced workers will need to reconsider the priorities in their lives and emphasize what is most important and controllable. For instance, as a result of job loss, displaced workers should carefully consider the issues related to relocating to a new neighborhood. They will also need to recognize that losing a job may sever long-term friendships and therefore be detrimental to their well-being.

Displaced workers who deal with work loss circumstances with positive life satisfaction will have a better overall QoL and subjective well-being. They can be more helpful to other people at home and in other areas of their life domains and have better social relationships than people with a low sense of well-being. For example, they are more likely to get married, stay married, and have rewarding marriages. Finally, a positive QoL is related to health and longevity, although the pathways linking these domains are not fully understood. Happiness or well-being is not only valuable because it feels good, but also has overall beneficial consequences.

CONCEPTUAL DOMAINS USED IN QOLT ASSESSMENT AND INTERVENTION

Subjective well-being or happiness has been defined as QoL in a number of ways. It has been generally agreed that it is defined with regard to how people evaluate the emotional reactions and cognitive judgments of their lives. This can include a sense of peace, personal fulfillment, and life satisfaction. Subjective well-being encompasses moods and emotions and how well an individual evaluates their satisfaction with general and specific areas of their lives. When they are integrated, subjective well-being and life satisfaction constitute one's quality of life (Diener & Larsen, 1993; Frisch et al., 1992).

Grant, Salcedo, Hynan, and Frisch (1995) reported that QoL refers to the extent that people experience positive thoughts and feelings.

A person's emotions are seen as adaptive in that they provide continuous feedback on their progress toward personal goals. This provides for the perception that important needs, goals, and wishes have been met, achieved, or fulfilled. Unpleasant feedback or negative affect signals a lack of fulfillment in valued areas of life. A person's subjective perception of domain will also influence their satisfaction with the area. QoL assessment and intervention procedures can be expected to boost an individual's QoL and may also reduce the symptoms of disorders that are not directly related to a specific area of concern such as loss of work.

FUTURE TRENDS FOR THE USE OF QOLT

The purpose of this section is to examine how employers in the future can ease the job loss situation for employees. It has been found that job counseling and training programs can be vehicles shifting human resources to where they are needed in the labor market. On the organizational level, they can enhance human resource utilization, decrease perception of psychological contract breach, and minimize internal strains and organizational conflict. On the individual level, QOLT appears to be an efficient and useful way of dealing with dismissed or remaining workers. Consequently, many of the organizational, psychological, family, and social difficulties brought on by job dismissals during an economic crisis may be avoided or minimized.

Integrated QoL service delivery systems should be considered coequal with and conducted concurrently with other symptom-oriented assessments and intervention methods. QOLT should be evaluated in terms of its potential for effective assessment and treatment. The goal of workplace interventions should be to maintain or enhance QoL in addition to addressing the effects of involuntary job displacement. Routine QOLT assessment and intervention alliances with psychology and medicine can be expected to improve displaced workers QoL. QOLT interventions can directly reduce life dissatisfactions in areas such as self-esteem and goals and values related to job displacement. This can occur even when such interventions are not directly related to work domains (Frisch, 1994b).

Integrated service delivery systems that include greater alliances between QOLT, medicine, psychology, and other disciplines have been recommended. These types of partnerships are already being successfully employed in medical, comprehensive social service, and mental health settings. In the future, health care diagnosis and treatment may routinely involve QOLT assessments. This is highly possible if researchers continue to find that such assessments can identify displaced workers who are at high risk for future disorders. Preventative treatment of those identified on the basis of QOLT assessments as high risk could ultimately prove to be extremely cost-effective.

There is a pressing need to develop a better way to address the social cost of involuntary job displacement. QOLT is a tool to help address the impact of the social costs related to unemployment. The recent economic downturn should be viewed as an opportunity to deal with a potentially long-term social problem. A comprehensive and collaborative effort will be required to utilize sustained and increased human resources needed to address chronic job displacement.

SUMMARY

During this recent serious economic downturn there are a number of ways to understand its effect on job-displaced workers' subjective well-being (SWB) and life satisfaction. Taken together, these constructs constitute an individual's QoL. SWB or happiness has been defined as what people make of their lives and the circumstances in which they live. The cognitive component of SWB has been defined as life satisfaction. Marital problems and various other issues can also be related to the financial crisis. Diener and Seligman (2004) also found that there are a number of QoL effects connected to factors other than income loss.

Quality of life has been found to be a lot more than economic or financial well-being. It also emphasizes the value people place on non-material factors such as social relationships, personal contentment, or the relationship to one's work life. If meaningful work can be a source of psychological and physical well-being, it follows that the loss of employment can be detrimental to psychological and physical well-being during unemployment. Coping resources refers to the personal social and financial aids a person can utilize to offset the negative effects of unemployment. Personal resources refer to the internal constructs that include self-esteem and self-efficacy.

Quality of Life Therapy (QOLT) is presented as an appropriate and useful method of addressing some of the consequences of the recent economic downturn on the lives of working people. The domains or areas of life and settings that are impacted are appropriate and important for the application of QOLT. While addressing the issues that affect job-displaced workers, QOLT is a coping resource that boosts personal, social, and emotional attributes that a person can utilize to offset the negative financial impact of involuntary unemployment.

REFERENCES

American Psychiatric Association (2000). *Diagnostic and statistical manual of mental disorders* (4th ed., (*DSM-IV*)). Washington, DC: APA.

Aytac, I. A., & Rankin, B. H. (2009). Economic crisis and marital problems in Turkey: testing the family stress model. *Journal of Marriage and Family, 71*, 756–767.

Baruffol, E., Gisle, L., & Corten, P. (1995). Life satisfaction as a mediator between distressing events and neurotic impairment in a general population. *Acta Psychiatrica Scandinavica, 92*, 56–62.

Beck, A. T, Rush, A. J., Shaw, B. F., & Emery, G. (1979). *Cognitive therapy of depression.* New York: Guilford.

Bordin, E. S. (1983). Supervision in counseling: contemporary models of supervision, a working alliance based model of supervision. *Counseling Psychologist, 11*, 35–42.

Bowling, A. (2001). *Measuring disease. A review of disease specific measurement scales* (2nd ed.). Buckingham: Open University Press.

Broadhead, J. K., Robinson, J. W., & Atkinson, M. J. (1998). A new quality-of-life measure for oncology: The SEIQoL. *Journal of Psychosocial Oncology, 16*, 21–35.

Campbell, A., Converse, P. E., & Rogers, W. L. (1976). *The quality of American life.* New York: Russell Sage.

Decker, S. W. A., & Schaufeli, W. B. (1995). The effect of job insecurity on psychological health and withdrawal: A longitudinal study. *Australian Psychologist, 30*, 57–63.

Diener, E., & Larsen, R. J. (1993). The experience of emotional well-being. In M. Lewis, & J. M Haviland (Eds.), *Handbook of emotions* (pp. 405–415). New York: Guilford Press.

Diener, E., & Seligman, M. E. P. (2004). Beyond money: toward an economy of well being. *Psychological Science in the Public Interest, 5*(No. 1), 1–31.

Eid, M., & Larson, R. J. (2008). *The science of subjective well-being.* New York: Guilford.

Evans, D. R. (1994). Enhancing the quality of life in the population at large. *Social Indicators Research, 33*, 47–88.

Frisch, M. B. (1992). Use of the quality of life inventory in problem assessment and treatment planning for cognitive therapy of depression. In A. Freeman, & F. M. Dattilio (Eds.), *Comprehensive casebook of cognitive therapy* (pp. 27–52). New York: Plenum.

Frisch, M. B. (1994a). *Quality of Life Inventory (QOLI).* Minneapolis, MN: National Computer Systems.

Frisch, M. B. (1994b). *Manual and treatment guide for the quality of life inventory (QOLI)* Minneapolis, MN: National Computer Systems.

Frisch, M. B. (1998a). *Quality of life therapy: patient manual.* Waco, TX: Author.

Frisch, M. B. (1998b). *Quality of life therapy: therapist manual.* Waco, TX: Author.

Frisch, M. B. (2006). *Quality of life therapy, applying a life satisfaction approach to positive psychology and cognitive therapy.* Hoboken NJ: John Wiley & Sons.

Frisch, M. B., Clark, M. P., Rouse, S. V., Rudd, M. D., Paweleck, J. K., Greenstone, A., et al. (2005). Predictive and treatment validity of life satisfaction and the quality of life inventory. *Assessment, 12*, 66–78.

Grant, G., Salcedo, V., Hynan, L. S., & Frisch, M. B. (1995). Effectiveness of quality of life therapy. *Psychological Reports, 76*, 1203–1208.

Grassi, L., & Riba, M. (2012). *Pscho-oncology: an international perspective*. Hoboken, NJ: John Wiley & Sons.
Higginson, I. J., & Carr, A. J. (2001). Measuring quality of life: using quality of life measures in the clinical setting. *British Medical Journal, 322*, 1297–1300.
Lazarus, R. S. (1991). *Emotion and adaptation*. New York: Oxford University Press.
Lewinsohn, P., Redner, J., & Seeley, J. (1991). The relationship between life satisfaction and psychosocial variables: new perspectives. In F. Strack, M. Argyle, & N. Schwartz (Eds.), *Subjective well-being* (pp. 141–169). New York: Plenum Press.
Linn, M. W., Sandifer, R., & Stein, S. (1985). Effects of unemployment on mental and physical health. *American Journal of Public Health, 75*, 502–507.
McLoyd, V. C. (1989). Socialization and development in a changing economy: The effects of paternal job and income loss on children. *American Psychologist, 44*, 293–302.
Newman, F. L., Ciarlo, J. A., & Carpenter, D. (1999). Guidelines for selecting psychological instruments for treatment planning and outcome assessment. In M. E. Maruish (Ed.), *The use of psychological testing for treatment planning and outcome assessment* (2nd ed., pp. 153–170). Mahwah, NJ: Erlbaum.
Pavot, W., & Diener, E. (1993). Review of the Satisfaction With Life scale. *Psychological Assessment., 5*, 164–172.
Tzafrir, S. S., & Mano-Negrin, R. (2006). Downsizing and the impact of job counseling and retraining on effective employee responses. *Career Development International, 11*, 125–144.
Vaillant, G. E. (2002). *Ageing well: surprising guideposts to a happier life from the landmark Harvard study of adult development*. Carlton North, Victoria: Scribe.
Veenhoven, R. (1984). *Conditions of happiness*. Boston: Reidel.
Verdugo, M. A., Schaluck, R. L., Keith, K. D., & Stancliff, R. J. (2005). Quality of life audits and its measurements, important principles and guidelines. *Journal of Intellectual Disability Research., 49*, 707–717.
Walker, D. (2009). *Nonprofit organization workplace fairness promotes and educates on work place issues. Business and Finance*. Available at <http://www.examiner.com/article/non-profit-organization-workplace-fairness-promotes-and-educates-on-workplace-issues>.
World Health Organization Quality of Life Group (1998). Group development of the world health organization WHOQOL-BREF quality of life assessment. *Psychological Medicine, 28*, 551–558.

FURTHER READING

Angstman, S., Schuldberg, D., Harris, K. J., Cochran, B., & Peterson, P. (2009). Use of the quality of life inventory for measuring quality of life changes in an inpatient psychiatric population. *Psychological Reports, 104*, 1007–1014. Retrieved 20 April, 2012 from <http://www.amsciepub.com/doi/abs/10.2466/pr0.104.3.1007-1014?journalCode=pr0>.
Corless, I. B., Nicholas, P. K., & Nokes, K. M. (2001). Issues in cross-cultural quality-of-life research. *Journal of Nursing Scholarship, 33*, 15–20.
Diener, E. (2000). Subjective well-being: The science of happiness and a proposal for a national index. *American Psychologist, 55*, 34–43.
Jordan, T. E. (2011). A La Recherche Du quality of life. *Social Indicators Research, 100*, 149–154.
Samuel, P. S., Rillotta, F., & Brown, I. (2011). The development of family quality of life concepts and measures. *Journal of Intellectual Disability Research, 56*, 1–16.

CHAPTER 14

Some Final Words

In this book on job satisfaction, burnout, work-related problems, and quality of life issues, we've tried to provide informed data regarding the rates of worker unhappiness and the growing problem of worker burnout and other difficulties during the economic downturn. This chapter offers some recommendations and solutions.

As we point out in Chapter 1, even though the economy has done badly since 2007, resulting in high unemployment and underemployment, job satisfaction has steadily decreased when logic would suggest that having a job at all should increase worker satisfaction. Part of the explanation is that employers are asking workers to do more and more with less, and refusing to provide proper rewards. Mirhaydari (2012) presents this case when he writes, "Companies appear to be hiring more less-skilled and less-motivated workers at low pay levels to get the same amount of work done" (p. 1). These workers feel little loyalty to the employer, only work as hard as they need to, and, when faced with the loss of a job because of performance or the fact that they're burned out, sometimes leave the workplace for good.

The draining of worker energy by companies who overwork employees and offer few incentives to work harder, diminishing the work ethic and the desire to seek work elsewhere, has resulted in the workplace of the future facing a crisis of increasing significance for the country. More to the point the current thinking seems to be that the economy is coming out of a recession and that, in time, things will be back to normal. We don't agree.

Instead, we see high unemployment as far into the future as one can predict and a loss of skilled jobs because American workers and employers aren't preparing themselves for the new workplace. Nor do we think that employers are looking beyond the bottom line at ways to train and keep workers who are motivated and show promise. For all too many educated and motivated workers, the workplace has become a place of drudgery where work is unvarying and repetitive and low-skilled tasks are more the norm than the exception. We think fundamental changes in the workplace coupled with a dramatic improvement in the American work ethic

Treating Worker Dissatisfaction During Economic Change
DOI: http://dx.doi.org/10.1016/B978-0-12-397006-0.00014-2

are required to resolve the problem of an unproductive workforce and long-term high unemployment. Those suggested changes are as follows.

1. The free market system works remarkably well for well educated, highly motivated workers with strong work ethics and the ability to be self-directed, but it works badly for many others. To keep people employed, we think government and business together will need to prime the pump for a long time to come by training workers, creating new jobs, and retaining jobs for the less well trained and able among us. Business doesn't get a pass while sitting on trillions of dollars that could help train and hire more workers to improve the economy. Businesses too often see outsourcing jobs to foreign countries as a solution.
2. Organizations will need to continue to train workers and provide the opportunity to gain new skills. Where families and the educational system have failed, employers will need to step in. With increasing numbers of people leaving the job market for good, organizations will have to devise ways of keeping workers or face a likely labor shortage. That is, a labor shortage of people who are motivated to work.
3. The idea that you can hire people for little and work them to the point of exhaustion is repugnant and has no place in the American workplace. It is a notion that ultimately results in people leaving jobs, with no one to take their place. The attack on unions and the belief that the economy will prosper if we pay low wages are myths that result in the high levels of work unhappiness and burnout that we've reported throughout the book. No one looking at the data could possibly believe that the country will prosper if we mistreat workers.
4. The American education system needs a proper shakeup. As educators, we can attest to the fact that students are not being held to high standards and that grade inflation and social passes are robbing the country of its competiveness. No American should be content to see the current system continue to produce poorly trained workers who have a sense that they are entitled to high grades just for showing up or that the most memorable thing about college was the football team, as more than a few alumni studies have shown.
5. You don't make a problem go away merely by wishing the country to go back to better times in the past, as if doing so will negate the realities of the present. The reality is that emerging economies are producing jobs and workers who are hungry to achieve the American dream of a high-paying job, a happy personal and family life,

community status and opportunity. When other countries act on the American dream and we don't, it's inevitable that new economies will outwork and outperform us and that the grand dream we have of an exceptional America will fade away.

6. Personal responsibility is not something one can legislate for; the common dialogue needs to reinforce notions of hard work, social engagement, and self-direction. Without those worker attributes, you can't build a strong labor market, regardless of how well workers are treated. We have a great deal of work ahead of us to change the dialogue from entitlement to hard work and self-direction, but the time has come for us to recognize that we're producing generations of people who, if we were less kind, would be called slackers. Since we are kind, we believe that American families need to stop treating children as eternal adolescents and welcome them to the world as many of us were welcomed: with the recognition that if we don't develop the skills to make it in this world, no one will do it for us.
7. The society's regard for men is somewhat equivalent to the way women were and, in many cases, continue to be treated. Men aren't doing well, and as they become less and less important to the workplace, the decline we see in men seeking new skills and their retreat from higher education will continue to have a troubling impact on American society. Just as we recognized the needs of women through educational opportunities and affirmative action, we need to do the same for men, particularly minority men who fare very badly in today's America.

The idea that people can and will do the same job for most of their working lifetime is a complete misunderstanding of how people function. We urge employers to offer every opportunity for people to frequently change their work functions and to move up the ladder as fast and as far as their skills allow. In this fast-paced world, boredom often sets in quickly, and managers should understand that changing assignments from time to time is the best way to reduce burnout.

1. We think that the competency-based management model we offer in Chapter 8 will go a long way toward strengthening a workplace that continues to use the carrot and the stick in its treatment of workers. We also believe that employee assistance programs (EAPs) focused on employees' needs are necessary, when burnout, job unhappiness, and problems in a worker's personal life intrude. Providing mental health benefits for workers recognizes that, just as the body wears out

physically, it can also wear out emotionally. Investing in the positive mental health of workers can only have the best of outcomes for the bottom line of any organization.

2. To those who think unions have too much power and that the deck is stacked against employers, we see nothing of the kind. To the contrary we think that workers who are secure and have advocates to help them in time of need are happier and healthier, and we remind the reader of the time in America when labor practices were so inhumane that they gave rise to unions. From what we've seen, workers are currently too afraid to complain about working conditions for fear of job loss. Because workers need support in the best of economic times as well as the worst, in our view, unions and other advocates protect workers from harmful labor practices and are necessary for a safe and effective workplace.

JOB DISPLACEMENT AND WORKING ALLIANCES

Quality of life researchers (Frisch, 2006) have indicated that working alliances can be a major predictor of success for various types of interventions, such as psychotherapy and case management services. The professional therapist or case manager in order to employ successful strategies must establish and maintain working alliances with clients and their supportive networks. Chapters 12 and 13 of this book described a Quality of Life Therapy (QOLT) approach, which promotes the use of working alliances between mental health and other human services providers. The QOLT approach employs methods that demonstrate the value of working alliances and coordinated arrangements for assisting displaced workers and families. Working alliances can also be used to help validate the effectiveness of services, addressing changes in needs, and revising plans in collaboration with displaced workers and their family networks.

Livingston and Cohn (2010) clearly described how the financial implications of the recent economic downturn influenced the decline in birth rates for families in the United States. As noted earlier, this book deals with a number of concerns that go well beyond the financial impact of the recent economic downturn. A major focus of this book is the social and psychological impact that the economic downturn has had on displaced workers and families. Many workers will also experience the problems associated with long-term job displacement, which have been referred to as "scarring."

One purpose of this chapter is to summarize some of the insights related to the value of collaborations and working alliances. Joint working agreements can help address the complex circumstances of displaced workers and families. The economic downturn has impacted the lives of many people who were previously unaffected by involuntary work loss. A large number of these people were unprepared for the lost investments, home foreclosures, and bankruptcies. Many workers and families are finding it increasingly difficult to meet their obligations and successfully make the necessary adjustments in their lives without unemployment benefits and other forms of assistance.

As a consequence of the recent economic downturn, people have experienced new types of personal difficulties. Therefore, they are increasingly turning to community social service agencies, government services, and faith-based programs for help. Community service organizations and many other agencies are also under great financial stress and finding it difficult to meet the increasingly complex needs of people. Their ability to respond is also hampered by a history of limited collaboration and integration among service providers. The long-term projections for the economic downturn will continue to challenge the capacity of agencies to independently provide adequate support and services to address the needs of displaced workers and families.

The question of organizational collaboration as an effective tool to enhance program effectiveness and efficiency has been debated for a long while. Woodland and Hutton (2012) examined collaboration as a widely utilized strategy for facilitating organizational innovation and performance and the development and effects of interagency collaboration. In their report, the authors present the Collaboration Evaluation and Improvement Framework (CEIF) used to increase capacity to engage in efficient and effective collaborative practices. Use of the CEIF to operationalize and assess the construct of collaboration can help enable the evaluator to ascertain how collaborative efforts correlate with indicators of organizational impact and outcomes (Janz, Soi, & Russell, 2009).

Fleury and Mercier (2002) described how organizing services in an integrated network, as a model for transforming healthcare systems, is often presented as a potential remedy for service fragmentation and should enhance system efficiency. In the mental health sector, integration of services is often a part of a diversified response to the multiple needs of clients. This is particularly important when assisting people with serious mental health disorders. The authors describe how the notion of integrated service networks came to serve as a model for transforming the mental health system in Québec, and this provides a frame of reference for this chapter. This approach addresses some of the challenges and issues raised in the mental health sector and more generally as a context for improving other human service systems.

Foster-Fishman, Berkowitz, Lounsbury, Jacobson, and Allen (2001) presented the results of a comprehensive qualitative analysis of 80 articles, chapters, and practitioners' guides that focused on collaboration and coalition functioning. The purpose of this review was to describe how an integrative and collaborative approach captured the core competencies and processes needed within collaborative bodies to facilitate their success. The resulting framework for building collaborative capacity described four critical levels of collaborative capacity: member capacity, relational capacity, organizational capacity, and programmatic capacity. Each level described the effective strategies for building each type of capacity. The overall implication of this analysis was that core competencies and programmatic capacity were supported on each of the collaborative levels.

During the economic downturn, working alliances between social services programs, medical providers, and other professionals can be important for the provision of more effective services for the most vulnerable members of the workforce. Hudson, Hardy, Henwood, and Wistow (1999) describe recommendations and findings concerning the increasing need for working alliances and collaboration between health and social services providers. They also suggest how some obstacles might be overcome in order to improve the integration of services for displaced workers.

Johnson, Wistow, Schulz, and Hardy (2003) noted that many human service providers had been unable to adequately provide many preventative services, because of an increase in crisis management requests. During the recent economic downturn, community service agencies such as FIBCO Family Services (2012) in Phoenix, Arizona have also reported an increase in the urgent needs of vulnerable people. Not only has there been an increase in crisis situations, but FIBCO and many other agencies have reported that problems have also become much more complex. There has been an increase in the needs of people who are new to receiving services such as emergency shelter and food banks. Increased financial burdens are also associated with greater mental health issues, addictions, domestic abuse, and suicide. Other related concerns include children who are no longer receiving childcare and youth who are unable to participate in summer camps or other recreational activities.

As the increased need for services and supportive care continues to become more critical, agencies such as FIBCO have found it necessary to share their resources and develop effective working alliances. Service providers will be required to support more people with the same amount of staff, less financial resources, and the need to reallocate existing resources. Agencies will need to reassess their capacity to share staff duties and seek additional volunteer support. As organizations begin to see greater demands on their staff and volunteers, burnout will become more common among front-line workers. Many workers will experience related trauma as they witness increased suffering and multiple impacts of the recession. Resources that are required to recruit and train volunteers will also shrink and become less available under these conditions (Social Planning Network of Ontario, 2010).

The increased need for supportive working alliances as a result of the economic downturn and subsequent unemployment will require extended investments by companies and government in collaborative efforts. People in need who require multiple services may have to wait for longer periods before the necessary assistance is available. As a result, many people will not receive timely services and will obtain assistance only by chance. Others will only see their health and overall quality of life become increasingly more fragile as the economic downturn persists. The following is a summary of supportive and collaborative approaches recommended by Hossfeld (2008) during a downturn in the economy.

- During the economic downturn community service agencies will need to identify and develop supportive alliances that can effectively shore up their capacity to sustain effective services. Due to the increased need for financial support, agencies need to develop strategies for long-term support in order to fortify the existing non-profit community and government service programs.
- Increased funding will be necessary to support job-related collaborative strategies that expand programs for job-displaced workers and families, including youth, seniors, women, and people with disabilities. Supportive services need to be expanded in areas that include child care, affordable housing, and food security initiatives.
- Special efforts are necessary to improve collaboration and increase access to social assistance programs in order to reduce stressful mental and physical health circumstances faced by displaced workers and families.

Hossfeld (2008) recommends support for individual community service delivery systems that normally provide crisis management and services independently. Although it is seen as desirable, inter-agency collaboration often remains elusive and difficult to achieve. Supportive alliances have been recognized as being effective and efficient in providing services, but have not been specifically applied to displaced workers. Wolff (2001) reported that building successful community coalitions is a highly complex process and identified nine elements that are critical to successful coalitions:

1. coalition readiness
2. intentionality
3. structure and organizational capacity
4. taking action
5. membership
6. leadership
7. dollars and resources
8. relationships
9. technical assistance.

The following example describes a successful faith-based collaborative working alliance that demonstrates the recommendations cited above.

The Faith Opportunity Zone (FOZ) (data.ed.gov, 2012) is a non-profit, faith-based community partnership initiated by FIBCO Family Services in Phoenix, Arizona. This alliance connected three of the largest and predominantly African American churches located in the heart of south-central Phoenix. The formation of this consortium represented a new level of community development and capacity building for south Phoenix by bringing these three churches together and leveraging their resources and contacts. First Intuitional Baptist Church Organization (FIBC), Tanner Community Development Corporation (TCDC), and Pilgrim Rest Baptist Church (PRBC) have individually and collectively served the south Phoenix and the greater Phoenix metropolitan area for almost 320 years.

The FOZ mission states, "The Faith Opportunity Zone (FOZ), a faith-based alliance, serves African American and African immigrant children, their families, and communities by providing a cradle-to-college pathway through partnerships, technology, rigorous academics, social responsibility, and faith." The FOZ vision states, "The Faith Opportunity Zone (FOZ) is a strong community where positive life options are limited only by personal choice."

The three organizations that comprise FOZ have also taken leadership roles in state- and community-wide coalitions that provide programs and services throughout Maricopa County and the State of Arizona. FOZ works to empower communities through community capacity building and helping people become more self-sustaining by focusing on the strengths of community through a human asset-based philosophy. It is especially notable during the recent economic downturn that FOZ demonstrated the value of capacity building through some of the following supportive and collaborative approaches.

FOZ represented a unique opportunity for addressing the needs of the community during the recent economic downturn. The FOZ member organizations each have a strong record of serving the target population of high-risk and vulnerable families. Through the combined efforts and unique strengths of all consortium members, FOZ has a significant impact on the health, well-being, and culture of families with children and adults, moving them from financial crisis or instability to greater functioning and/or self-sufficiency. FOZ seeks to accomplish this by increasing parent education and advocacy, job readiness training, academic attainment, social service support, and career development. Each member organization of the consortium offers its unique resources and expertise in the following three areas:

1. Parent education and advocacy training, provided through
   - **a.** A research-based home visitation program, Parents as Teachers, and
   - **b.** A parent advocacy research- and evidence-based Strengthening Multi-ethnic Families approach;
2. Academic enrichment using evidence-based programs and best practices, including
   - **a.** Reading programs recommended by the Children's Defense Fund Freedom School, and
   - **b.** Big Math for Little Kids, recommended and sponsored by ASU-Polytechnic;
3. Social services and workforce readiness, including
   - **a.** Connecting families with social service support systems,
   - **b.** Preparing individuals and families for gainful employment,
   - **c.** Maintaining a formal alliance with the Maricopa Workforce Connection.

The FOZ consortium leverages the collective strength of the three major partners to invest in the well-being of children and families in the community. After 320 years of replicating individual efforts, FOZ has realized the lack of leverage in that process and understands that strength lies within the collaboration. The economic downturn and job displacement has highlighted the importance of this initiative. FOZ no longer only looks for support outside of its member network, but looks more often within the FOZ member organizations for sustainable support services and change. FOZ includes a broad range of workforce opportunities to better address the challenges of its constituents and members.

The FOZ alliance supports the following workforce services and career benefits during the depressed economy:

- Access to high-quality family-centered programs to meet individual and family needs that lead to successful employment outcomes;
- Wrap-around workforce services in a single location;
- Individualized job preparation;
- Movement from instability to job readiness;
- Mentoring to minority high school students and prospective college students;
- Training for career development;
- Providing support for families during personal and financial crises;
- Connecting families to needed employment resources.

During the current economic downturn the scope of the work of FOZ lends itself to collaboration with additional community members and organizations. Arizona State University (Mary Lou Fulton School of Education) and the Arizona State University, Southwest Interdisciplinary Research Center (SIRC) serve as the research and evaluation partner providing technical assistance, writing reports, and overseeing the research and evaluation process.

IMPACT OF WORKER JOB DISPLACEMENT AND SOCIAL SUPPORT

Job layoffs not only have a big impact on workers' own lives but also cause worry about the financial and emotional support of their families. By providing and receiving adequate social support, the displaced workers' overall well-being is enhanced. This also prevents deterioration in physical/mental functioning further down the road. Social support can also reinforce the displaced workers' ability to make necessary adjustments to their lives (Mallinckrodt & Bennett, 1992).

In Quality of Life Therapy (QOLT), discussed in Chapters 12 and 13 of this book, social support for others is seen as one of the core principles of life satisfaction and happiness. It has been noted before that, when people are emotionally impacted by disruptive events such as the economic downturn, it is important that they receive work-based and non-work-based social support from friends, family, and colleagues. Lim and Sng (2006) and Zhao, Lim, and Teo (2012) indicated that there are moderating effects of work-based support on job insecurity and other work- and career-related outcomes, including:

- job dissatisfaction;
- proactive job search;
- noncompliant job behaviors;
- non-work-based support;
- life dissatisfaction.

It has been suggested that support derived from others at the workplace can contribute significantly in buffering individuals against job dissatisfaction and noncompliant job behaviors. Equally important is support provided by family and friends that may buffer individuals against negative outcomes such as life dissatisfaction associated with job insecurity. Diener and Seligman (2004) and Lyubomirsky, King, and Diener (2005) imply that helping and social support can provide purpose and focus for people going through major life crises and transitions. It was also noted that social support is an important factor in predicting the physical health and overall well-being for many people, ranging from childhood through older adults. Initial social support, when people know that they are valued by others, is a determining factor in successfully overcoming life stress. This can be an important psychological factor in helping people cope with the negative aspects of job loss. Social support not only helps improve a job-displaced worker's well-being, it is a major factor in preventing negative symptoms such as depression and anxiety.

Isaacs (2011) wrote that children throughout the United States continue to be negatively impacted by the ongoing effects of the economic downturn. Children in some states are being impacted by the recession in ways that are not always obvious. Some economic data ignore children, while other information is long delayed. Espey, Harper, and Jones (2010) reported that when social support is provided for children and other dependants of job-displaced workers, their health and social development is enhanced. The recent economic downturn has demonstrated negative effects caused by inadequate attention to support for children and the risks to their education, health, and overall well-being. There have been limited measures to address the impact of the recent economic downturn on children, even when data indicating negative consequences are available. Businesses and organizations would do well to recognize the value of support for vulnerable families and how it can buffer the effects of economic downturns. It has been recognized, however, that social support as a concept does require further empirical evidence, to clearly realize its value for enhancing the well-being and social benefits for children, (Espey, Harper, & Jones, 2010).

Social support of children and other family members is crucial to their positive well-being and social and personal development. The economic crisis has demonstrated the need for greater social support. The slow economic recovery provides less opportunity for the positive development of children, who will require even greater social support.

Besides the need for financial assistance, adolescents often have special developmental issues that require considerable family and social support. Adolescents who receive inadequate support from parents will likely have a greater chance of experiencing depression and other mental health and emotional problems. This is further compounded when adolescents become confused if they don't receive the financial support and positive reinforcement from their parents and family members that they expect (Stice, Ragan, & Randall, 2004). Root (2006) found that, during the period in which adolescents are still developing, they are more prone to experiencing anxiety and depression. These are two main psychological disorders common among many adolescents, and may be exacerbated as a result of the economic downturn and job loss.

Beside family support, peer support is also an important factor for the well-being of adolescents, who value and rely a great deal upon their friends. Peer support can be considered as an alternative method for receiving social support when adolescents are given inadequate attention from their parents. Peer support is not as reliable as family support since it can more easily be withdrawn or replaced among friends. Adolescents who become emotionally distraught or depressed can find that social support from peers is often less available. Social support is even more essential for an adolescent's well-being and ability to cope during difficult economic times (Stice et al., 2004).

Social support is also an important factor in predicting the health and well-being of entire families, ranging from childhood through older adulthood. The absence of social support reveals some difficulties among job-displaced individuals and families. In many cases, it can predict the deterioration of certain aspects of physical and mental health among vulnerable family members. Clark (2003) noted that when people receive early and sustained social support it is a positive factor in their successfully preventing or overcoming stress at a later period. When individuals and family members know that they are valued by other people, it is an important psychological predictor in helping them to cope with negative aspects of their lives. During periods of serious economic difficulties, social support can be a major factor in helping to address existing problems and prevent symptoms of depression and other difficulties from developing.

Researchers over several decades have determined that certain kinds of social support can influence the outcome of specific types of physical and mental health issues. Cutrona, Russell, and Rose (1986) described six criteria that have been used to measure the level of social support available for a specific person or situation. These criteria could also be applicable to involuntarily job-displaced workers and members of their families. They are outlined as follows:

1. The amount of attachment provided from a loved one or spouse;
2. The level of social integration of the individual, usually with a group of friends;
3. The assurance of worth from others—positive reinforcement that could inspire and boost self-esteem;
4. The reliable support that is provided by others, which means that the individual knows they can depend on receiving support from friends and/or family members whenever it is needed;
5. The guidance and assurances of support given to the individual from a high-ranking figure or person such as a teacher, employer, or parent;
6. The opportunity for nurturance, meaning the person would receive some social enhancement by having children of their own and providing a nurturing experience.

Many displaced workers and their families have been impacted by very unfamiliar work-related life changes. Some are introduced to various government and business policies and programs that have been created to assist displaced workers to adapt to job loss. Jobless benefits are often limited or unavailable for terminated workers and families who need or desire immediate or long-term help. Social support may help fill some of the gaps for displaced workers such as single-parent families or families where most of the family members have become jobless. Social support, both workplace- and non-workplace-based, is a major untapped resource for helping displaced workers and families.

AFFIRMING THE BENEFITS OF A DIVERSE WORKPLACE

Workplace diversity was described in Chapter 5 of this book as acknowledging the value, acceptance, and contributions of all people. It was further explained as understanding that each person is unique and important, while recognizing their individual differences. Workplace diversity can also provide a variety of positive benefits that can be brought to an individual, organization, or business setting. As demonstrated during the current economic downturn, an organization's success and competitiveness will increasingly depend upon its ability to embrace the benefits gained from the diverse backgrounds and experience of its workers. By not affirming diversity, an organization's ability to obtain the best creative talent from its workforce is clearly limited. Employers who promote equality of opportunity among their workforce can draw upon a much wider pool of the culture in the workforce. In the rapidly changing social and economic environment, diversity must be fostered or supported if an organization or business is to remain truly competitive (Fine, 1996).

For most businesses, surviving the economic downturn has meant using drastic cutbacks in every possible area, from plant renovation to personnel or health costs. For a number of businesses and organizations the elimination of many employee benefits and programs was deemed as absolutely necessary. In order to plan for the future survival of a business and the economic severity of the times, it has often felt essential that costs be cut down to a basic operational level. The idea of maintaining diversity programs in the workplace has been challenged, but it has proven to be a good investment in the overall stability and financial returns to many businesses (Society for Human Resource Management, 2010).

Diversity programs that were found to be an asset to a company and workforce during better economic times can continue to have a positive benefit during an economic downturn. The dynamic of a diverse work environment has historically been a catalyst for greater creativity and can help maintain employee loyalty during a recession. Businesses that are committed to employing and showing commitment to a diverse workforce are creating positive labor relations. A diverse workforce provides a unique distribution of talent from a wide range of the population. Individual characteristics, experiences, and the backgrounds of each employee make for a more flexible and innovative workforce. Harvey and Allard (2012) noted that the recession has posed problems and challenges that extend far outside the realm of normal business, and a team of diverse problem solvers is critical to business competiveness. Diversity in the work place offers businesses a competitive advantage on both a local and global level.

The recession has changed business at many levels and also resulted in a greater number of older workers seeking employment and forced many of them to work past retirement age. Companies that strive for diversity in age as well as culture and ethnicity have an advantage when it comes to meeting the challenges of new market opportunities and changing demographics. By maintaining a good reputation concerning age diversity and offering older workers opportunities during difficult times, those companies will be held in higher regard by both employees and consumers. Despite some concerns about the value of diversity and discrimination in the workplace, Wentling, and Palma-Rivas (1998) discussed the place of diversity in the future workplace, arguing that various demographic trends indicate that it will be increasingly important to recognize the talents of older workers and people with differences.

The following summary lists some findings of the poll by the Society for Human Resource Management (SHRM) (2010), indicating key benefits to organizations and workers by having diversity in the workforce.

(I) Diversity can be beneficial to both the organization and workers by bringing substantial benefits such as:

- Better decision making;
- Improved problem solving;
- More creativity and innovation;
- Enhanced product development;
- Successful marketing to different types of customers;
- Ability to compete in global markets and link the variety of talents within the organization;
- Allowing those employees with these talents to feel needed and to have a sense of belonging;
- Increases a worker's commitment to a company;
- Allowing each worker to contribute in a unique way.

It has been well established by a number of surveys and the US Department of Commerce (DeNavas-Walt, Proctor, & Smith, 2011) that African Americans, Hispanics, and other minorities do less well economically than white Americans in good or bad times. These differences have persisted over time and will continue until there is a better way of addressing the lack of inclusion of marginalized people in the workplace. Policies that can address these disparities require an investment in direct job creation that deals with long-neglected needs in order to help the most vulnerable populations. Additional government financial assistance is needed during the economic downturn to encourage states, localities, and businesses to invest in a more diverse workforce. Due to the continuing economic downturn and increasing global economic interconnectedness, diversity is becoming an even more essential factor in the workplace.

(II) The SHRM (2010) report describes workplace diversity as "an inclusive corporate culture that strives to respect variations in employee personality, work style, age, ethnicity, gender, religion, socio-economics, education and other dimensions in the workplace." The SHRM study provides encouraging information about the current state of diversity in the workplace. The study reported increases in the:

- Percentage of companies that provide training on diversity issues;
- Number of organizations that have a diverse board of directors;
- Percentage of organizations reporting that their diversity practices were effective in achieving their organization's desired outcomes.

Recently, there has been only a slight decrease in the percentage of organizations with practices that address workplace diversity, and this is likely related to the recent economic downturn. However the SHRM (2010) report provides some highlights that describe the correlation between workplace diversity, enhanced organizational performance, and benefits to workers.

(III) The following list describes how diversity among employees improves organizational effectiveness, efficiency and client relations.

- Decreases recruiting costs and training costs.
- Leads to higher worker retention, fewer complaints and litigation.
- Improves the organization's ability to move into emerging markets.
- Promotes a better understanding of the marketplace.
- Increases creativity and innovation.
- Produces more effective problem-solving.
- Enhances the effectiveness of corporate leadership.
- Promotes more-effective global relationships.

Substantial costs exist for firms that do a poor job of integrating their diverse workforce.

Carter, Simkins, and Simpson (2003) reported that supporting diversity in the workplace improves a company's opportunities to develop strategic partnerships with clients and suppliers between generations. According to Scott Page (2007), workplace teams that are made up of people from different generations and cultures tend to form high performance teams. Diverse groups across generations are found to be capable of generating innovative ideas and executing more creative approaches than teams that are homogenous. Mask (2007) noted in a survey that the respondents indicated that managing multi-generational work teams can pose some challenges but most of the evidence supports the benefits of multi-generational workplace diversity.

According to a study by Yap, Holmes, Hannan, and Cukier (2010), executives and other professionals perceive diversity training in their organizations to be very beneficial. They reported that employee career satisfaction and organizational commitment scores are higher than for those working in organizations where diversity training is minimal or nonexistent. Even though some diversity programs have been put on hold during the economic downturn, the SHRM (2010) report found that organizations are still making significant investments in diversity training and that this is showing a positive return for those organizations.

The SHRM (2010) report describes three major workplace diversity practices that organizations indicated they were using:

- Recruiting strategies designed to help increase diversity within the organization;
- Diversity-related community outreach (e.g., links between organization and educational institutions);
- Alignment of diversity with business goals and objectives.

(IV) Diversity will increase significantly in the coming years, and organizations will benefit by taking immediate action now and by spending resources on managing diversity in the workplace, as follows.

- Increased future adaptability for workplace diversity:
  - Organizations employing a diverse workforce can supply a greater variety of solutions to future problems in service, sourcing, and allocation of resources;
  - Employees from diverse backgrounds bring individual talents and experiences in suggesting ideas that promote flexibility in adapting to future fluctuating markets and customer demands.
- Broader service range of workplace diversity: A diverse collection of skills and experiences (e.g., languages, cultural understanding) allows a company to address a variety of viewpoints in order to provide services to customers on a global basis.
- Variety of diversity viewpoints:
  - A diverse workforce that feels comfortable communicating varying points of view provides a larger pool of ideas and experiences;

  - The organization can draw from that pool to meet business strategy needs and the needs of customers more effectively.
- More effective execution with workplace diversity:
  - Companies that encourage diversity in the workplace inspire all of their employees to perform to their highest ability;
  - Company-wide strategies can be executed, resulting in higher productivity, profit, and return on investment.

Implementation of diversity-in-the-workplace policies can be a major challenge to diversity advocates. Organizations must build and implement a specialized strategy to overcome some of the challenges of diversity for their particular organization. These challenges include the following.

- Communication:
  - Perceptual, cultural and language barriers need to be overcome for diversity programs to succeed;
  - Ineffective communication of key objectives results in confusion, lack of teamwork, and low morale.
- Resistance to change:
  - There are always employees who will refuse to accept the fact that the social and cultural makeup of their workplace is changing;
  - The "we've always done it this way" mentality silences new ideas and inhibits progress.

Successful management of diversity in the workplace should take account of the following.

- Diversity training alone is not sufficient for an organization's diversity management plan.
- A strategy must be created and implemented to create a culture of diversity that permeates every department and function of the organization.

(V) Recommended diversity steps that have proven successful in world-class organizations are the following.

- Assessment of diversity in the workplace:
  - Top companies make assessing and evaluating their diversity process an integral part of their management system;
  - A customizable employee satisfaction survey can accomplish this assessment for a company efficiently and conveniently;
  - Such a survey can help a management team determine which challenges and obstacles to diversity are present in a workplace and which policies need to be added or eliminated;
  - Reassessment can then determine the success of diversity in the workplace plan implementation.

- Development of a diversity-in-the-workplace plan:
  - Choosing a survey provider that provides comprehensive reporting is a key decision;
  - That report will be the beginning structure of your diversity-in-the-workplace plan; the plan must be comprehensive, attainable and measurable;
  - An organization must decide what changes need to be made and a timeline for that change to be attained.
- Implementation of the diversity-in-the-workplace plan:
  - The organization's executive and managerial team leaders must make a personal commitment to incorporate diversity policies into every aspect of the organization's function and purpose;
  - Attitudes toward diversity originate at the top and filter downward;
  - Management cooperation and participation is required to create a culture conducive to the success of your organization's plan.

As the economy becomes increasingly global and the workforce becomes increasingly diverse, organizational success and competitiveness will depend on ability and experience in effectively managing diversity in the workplace. The following quote by Greenberg (2012) summarizes the importance of diversity management that is committed, knowledgeable, and reflected throughout an organization.

> *"This competency explores whether an organization promotes understanding and support for interaction among diverse population groups while respecting individuals' personal values and ideas. It focuses on perceived equality in the work environment. Research shows that by fostering a climate in which equity and mutual respect are intrinsic, an organization can create a success-oriented, cooperative, caring work environment that draws intellectual strength and produces innovative solutions from the synergy of its people. All businesses can benefit from a diverse body of talent bringing fresh ideas, perspectives, and views to the workplace. However, a diverse workforce means that the managers within your organization must be capable of capitalizing on the mixture of genders, cultural backgrounds, ages, and lifestyles present in your staff to respond to business opportunities more rapidly and creatively. Including this competency in your survey can provide insight into whether your organization is encouraging and leveraging a diverse workplace, as well as maximizing the potential of the people, backgrounds, and ideas of your present staff."*

The economic downturn has changed business at every level and challenged many of the stereotypes that were once associated with businesses, workers, and customers. The Equality and Human Rights Commission Inquiry Into Race Discrimination in the Construction Industry Action

Plan (EHRC, 2009) stated that good employment and training guidelines used in the recruitment and management of employees should be fair and offer equal opportunity. In this respect the "Medici Effect" (Mask, 2007) is a metaphor for deliberately bringing diverse cultures together. The purpose of this idea is to create more productivity through the intersection of different ideas, experiences, backgrounds, and beliefs. This is only possible when intercultural differences are clearly understood and intercultural communication is effectively taking place. Mask (2007) and others state that the purpose of intercultural and diversity seminars and programs is to:

- Break down cultural barriers;
- Help people accept and understand the value of diversity;
- Help people better understand their own cultural heritage;
- Help people view issues from different perspectives and different cultures;
- Encourage people to venture beyond familiar networks and develop better relationships;
- Generate high levels of understanding and acceptance of differences;
- Improve communication;
- Formulate new ideas.

Cox and Blake (1991) and Robinson and Dechant (1997) described how business management establishes a relationship between board diversity and how that contributes financial value to a business. Robinson and Dechant (1997) summarize how board diversity affects a firm's long-term and short-term financial value, saying that it:

- Helps provide a better understanding of the marketplace when demographic projections indicate that a company's potential customers are more diverse and increases the supplier's ability to penetrate those markets;
- Increases creativity and innovation—attitudes and beliefs tend to vary with demographic variables such as age, race, and gender;
- Contributes to more-effective problem-solving—the varieties of perspectives that emerge allow decision makers to evaluate more alternatives and more carefully explore the consequences of these alternatives;
- Enhances the effectiveness of corporate leadership by taking a broader view of problem solving—having diversity at the top of an organization provides for a better understanding of the complexities of the environment and allows for better decision making;
- Promotes more-effective global relationships in an international environment. Ethno-cultural diversity allows for corporate leaders to be more sensitive to non-American culture.

THE SIGNIFICANCE OF SOCIAL AND ECONOMIC "SCARRING"

This book has often described how economic downturns are portrayed as short-term events. However, a substantial body of economic literature shows how high unemployment, falling incomes, and reduced economic activity can have lasting negative consequences. In addition to the short-term economic problems that unemployment causes for people, there are serious long-term debilitating social effects (Irons, 2009; von Wachter, Song, & Manchester, 2009). Clark, Georgellis, and Sanfey (2001) and a number of other writers describe the negative long-term consequences of unemployment as "scarring effects." Those scarring effects are the result of such factors as the deterioration of job skills and forgone work experience. Scarring can also result in a potential employer's belief that long-term unemployed workers will have lost some of their productivity. The longer a person is unemployed the more severe the scarring effects are presumed to become and remain.

Katz (2010) wrote that the human costs of economic downturns are much more far reaching than temporary loss of income. This includes the long-term scarring effects of lost lifetime earnings, human capital, worker discouragement, adverse health outcomes, and loss of social cohesion. Sullivan and von Wachter (2009) and Holzer (2010) stated that some negative effects of long-term job loss are associated with higher risks of heart attacks and other stress-related illnesses. These writers noted that high unemployment, falling incomes, and reduced economic activity can also have a number of family-related consequences. For example, job loss and falling incomes can force families to delay or forego a college education for their children. Children may also experience a decline in schooling achievement (Stevens & Schaller, 2012). Palme and Sandgren (2008) found a significant relationship between a parent's reduced economic circumstances during their offspring's childhood and reduction in lifespan of the child.

Long-term job loss not only reduces a worker's probability of being quickly rehired but also leaves permanent emotional scarring on many individuals. The Department of Commerce (Census Bureau) Current Population Study (2010) found that workers are financially scarred by lost income and job benefits during periods of joblessness, and further scarred by reduced income when they find new employment. Arulampalam (2001) found that a period of initial unemployment carries an average wage penalty of about 6% upon returning to work. Three years after a second period of unemployment, workers were earning 14% less when returning to work. Irons (2009) reported the following summary of the potential consequences or scarring related to long-term economic downturns.

- Educational achievement: Unemployment and income losses can reduce educational achievement by threatening early childhood nutrition in the following manner:
  - The lowering of a family's ability to provide a supportive learning environment (including adequate health care, summer activities, and stable housing);
  - Forcing a delay or abandonment of college plans.
- Opportunity:
  - Recession-induced job and income losses can have lasting consequences on future opportunities for individuals and families;
  - The increase in poverty that will occur as a result of the recession will have lasting consequences for children;
  - A recession should not be thought of as a one-time event that stresses individuals' and families' investments for only a couple of years;
  - Economic downturns will impact the future investment prospects of all family members, and will have consequences for years to come.

Holzer (2010) stated that:

> *"High rates of child poverty exist in the United States even in the best of times, and this poverty tends to limit the health, education, and earnings of adults who grew up poor throughout their lives. This creates costs not only for the individuals themselves and their families, but for the U.S. economy as a whole. The current recession will raise child poverty rates substantially and for many years to come, thus exacerbating these problems. Even short spells of poverty or parental unemployment can scar children and youth for many years. Policies that tend to limit child poverty in the next few years by strengthening the safety net, raising employment, or improving the skills of disadvantaged children and youth might thus have a high social payoff over time."*

This chapter has focused on the long-term "scarring" effects of a parents' unemployment on children. Not only does unemployment affect children during their childhood, but children who face parental unemployment have been shown to grow into adults with decreased earnings. According to Taylor et al. (2011), African Americans and other minorities have lost disproportionally more wealth during the economic downturn, due to the real estate and foreclosure crisis. Because of the large decline in housing wealth, minorities have less housing equity available to help pay for college expenses. Home equity allows parents to fund college expenses, but since a loss of home equity disproportionately affects minorities, this group will also be less likely to achieve higher education.

SUMMARY

It is fair to say that workers and families have been impacted by significant work-related changes, including mass layoffs and involuntary job displacement through shutdowns. Better planning and working alliances are needed to assist displaced workers from diverse backgrounds to adapt to job loss and thereby reduce the disproportionate stress in those families. While these policies have helped displaced workers adjust to involuntary joblessness, there is still a need for social support that helps minimize the damage to them. Workers and families can be more dramatically impacted when single-parent families have become jobless and are dependent on government assistance. It is also in the best interest of the whole society that businesses, organizations, and the government form collaborations and alliances that address the long-term needs and well-being of displaced workers.

This chapter focused on the long-term effects of involuntary unemployment on children. Not only does unemployment affect children during their childhood, but children who face parental unemployment have been shown to experience decreased earnings as adults. According to many findings, African Americans and other minorities have disproportionally lost more wealth and educational opportunities, due to the large decline in housing equity. For many of those families, home equity was the only money available to help pay for college expenses.

Economic downturns are not unlikely occurrences, and it will be necessary to prepare for the future by providing tools to protect people from adverse effects of booms and busts in the economy. Mallinckrodt and Bennett (1992) found that, during an economic downturn, displaced workers are often likely to develop problems that could influence their long-term physical or mental health. For example, those affected workers normally report loss of self-esteem and locus of control, and this increases the likelihood that those workers will become depressed. The depression itself could signal the beginning of deterioration in health and well-being over time. During an economic downturn, supportive relationships are important resources for displaced workers and for their families' well-being. There are data suggesting that people suffer in many ways beyond financial difficulty when they are separated from the workplace and lack support and affirming relationships.

REFERENCES

Arulampalam, W. (2001). Is unemployment really scarring? Effects of unemployment experiences on wages. *The Economic Journal, 111*, 585–606.

Carter, D., Simkins, B. J., & Simpson, W. G. (2003). Corporate governance board diversity and firm value. *Financial Review, 38*, 33–53.

Clark, A., Georgellis, Y., & Sanfey, P. (2001). Scarring: The psychological impact of past unemployment. *Economica, 68*, 221–241.

Clark, R. (2003). Self-reported racism and social support predict blood pressure reactivity in blacks. *Annals of Behavioral Medicine, 25*, 127–136.

Cox, T. H., & Blake, S. (1991). Managing cultural diversity: Implications for organizational competitiveness. *The Executive, 5*, 45–56.

Cutrona, C., Russell, D., & Rose, J. (1986). Social support and adaptation to stress by the elderly. *Psychology and Aging, 1*, 47–54.

data.ed.gov (2012). *Faith Opportunity Zone's early child initiatives.* Retrieved from <http://data.ed.gov/grants/investing-in-innovation/applicant/15711>.

DeNavas-Walt, C., Proctor, B. D., & Smith, J. C. (2011). *U.S. Census Bureau, current population reports, P60-239, income, poverty, and health insurance coverage in the United States: 2010.* Washington, DC: US Government Printing Office.

Diener, E., & Seligman, M. E. P. (2004). Beyond money: Toward an economy of well-being. *Psychological Science in the Public Interest, 5*, 1–31.

Equality and Human Rights Commission (2009). *Inquiry into race discrimination in the construction industry action plan.* Retrieved from <http://www.equalityhumanrights.com/uploaded_files/action_plan_v3.pdf>.

Espey, J., Harper, C., & Jones, N. (2010). Crisis, care and childhood: the impact of economic crisis on care work in poor households in the developing world. *Gender & Development, 18*, 291–307.

FIBCO Family Services Inc. (2012). *Meeting the needs of our community.* Retrieved from www.fibco.org.

Fine, M. G. (1996). Cultural diversity in the workplace: "The state of the field.". *Journal of Business Communication, 33*, 485–502.

Fleury, M. J., & Mercier, C. (2002). Integrated local networks as a model for organizing mental health services administration and policy. *Mental Health and Mental Health Services Research, 30*, 55–73.

Foster-Fishman, P. G., Berkowitz, S. L., Lounsbury, D. W., Jacobson, S., & Allen, N. A. (2001). Building collaborative capacity in community coalitions: A review and integrative framework. *American Journal of Community Psychology, 29*, 241–261.

Frisch, M. B. (2006). *Quality of life therapy: Applying a life satisfaction approach to positive psychology and cognitive therapy.* Hoboken, NJ: John Wiley & Sons, Inc.

Greenberg, J. (2012). *Diversity in the workplace: Benefits, challenges, and solutions.* Retrieved from <http://easysmallbusinesshr.com/2010/08/diversity-in-the-workplace-benefits-challenges-and-solutions/>.

Harvey, C. P., & Allard, M. J. (2012). *Understanding and managing diversity: Readings, cases, and exercises* (5th ed.). Boston: Pearson.

Holzer, H. (2010). The "Great Recession" and the well-being of American children. *Testimony of Harry J. Holzer before the U.S. Senate Subcommittee on Children and Families*, (Retrieved from http://www.help.senate.gov/imo/media/doc/Holzer.pdf).

Hossfeld, B. (2008). Developing friendships and peer relationships: Building social support with the Girls Circle program. In C. W. LeCroy, & J. E. Mann (Eds.), *Handbook of prevention and intervention programs for adolescent girls* (pp. 42–80). Hoboken, NJ: John Wiley.

Hudson, B., Hardy, B., Henwood, M., & Wistow, G. (1999). In pursuit of inter-agency collaboration in the public sector. *Public Management*, *1*, 235–260.

Irons, J. (2009). Economic scarring: *The long-term impacts of the recession*. Economic Policy Institute Briefing Paper #243. Retrieved from www.epi.org/publication/bp243/.

Isaacs J. B. (2011). *The recession's ongoing impact on America's children: Indicators of children's economic well-being through 2011*. Brookings Institution. Retrieved from <http://www.brookings.edu/research/papers/2011/12/20-children-wellbeing-isaacs>.

Janz, M. R., Soi, N., & Russell, R. (2009). *Collaboration and partnership in humanitarian action. World Vision International, Inter-Agency Working Group (IWG)*. Humanitarian Exchange Magazine. Retrieved from <http://www.odihpn.org/humanitarian-exchange-magazine/issue-45/collaboration-and-partnership-in-humanitarian-action>.

Johnson, P., Wistow, G., Schulz, R., & Hardy, B. (2003). Interagency and interprofessional collaboration in community care: the interdependence of structures and values. *Journal of Interprofessional Care*, *17*, 69–83.

Katz, L. F. (2010). *Long term unemployment in the great recession*. Testimony for the Joint Economic Committee U.S. Congress Hearing on "Long-Term Unemployment: Causes, Consequences and Solutions," Cannon House Office Building, Room 210, April 29, 2010. Retrieved from <http://scholar.harvard.edu/sites/scholar.iq.harvard.edu/files/lkatz/files/long_term_unemployment_in_the_great_recession.pdf>.

Lim, V. K. G., & Sng, Q. S. (2006). Does parental job insecurity matter? Money anxiety, money motives, and work motivation. *Journal of Applied Psychology*, *91*, 1078–1087.

Livingston, G., & Cohn, D. (2010). *Social and demographic trends: U.S. birth rate decline linked to recession*. Pew Research Center. Retrieved from <http://pewresearch.org/pubs/1552/birth-rates-united-states-decline-recession>.

Lyubomirsky, S., King, L., & Diener, E. (2005). The benefits of frequent positive affect: does happiness lead to success? *Psychological Bulletin*, *131*, 803–855.

Mallinckrodt, B., & Bennett, J. (1992). Social support and the impact of job loss in dislocated blue-collar workers. *Journal of Counseling Psychology*, *39*, 482–489.

Mask, D. (2007). *The medici effect: How workplace diversity improves creativity and performance*. Alliance Training and Consulting, Inc. Retrieved from <http://www.alliancetac.com/?PAGE_ID = 2311>.

Mirhaydari, A. (2012). *Are American workers getting lazy? MSN Money*. Retrieved from <http://money.msn.com/investing/are-american-workers-getting-lazy-mirhaydari>

Page, S. E. (2007). *The difference: How the power of diversity creates better groups, firms, schools, and societies*. Princeton, NJ: Princeton University Press.

Palma-Rivas, N. (1998). Current status and future trends of diversity initiatives in the workplace: Diversity experts' perspective. *Human Resource Development Quarterly*, *9*, 235–253.

Palme, M., & Sandgren, S. (2008). Parental income, lifetime income, and mortality. *Journal of the European Economic Association*, *6*, 890–911.

Robinson, G., & Dechant, K. (1997). Building a business case for diversity. *The Academy of Management Executive*, *11*, 21–31.

Root, K. A. (2006). Job loss, the family, and public policy. *Marriage & Family Review*, *39*, 11–26.

Social Planning Network of Ontario (2010). *Ontario social landscape: Socio-demographic trends and conditions in communities across the province.* Retrieved from <http://www.spno.ca/images/stories/pdf/reports/ontario-social-landscape-2010.pdf>.

Society for Human Resource Management (2010). *Workplace diversity practices: How has diversity and inclusion changed over time?* SHRM poll. Retrieved from <http://www.shrm.org/Research/SurveyFindings/Articles/Pages/WorkplaceDiversity Practices.aspx>.

Stevens, A. J., & Schaller, J. (2012). Short-run effects of parental job loss on children's academic achievement. *Economics of Education Review, 30*, 289–299.

Stice, E., Ragan, J., & Randall, P. (2004). Prospective relations between social support and depression: Differential direction of effects for parent and peer support? *Journal of Abnormal Psychology, 113*, 155–159.

Sullivan, D., & von Wachter, T. (2009). Job displacement and mortality: An analysis using administrative data. *Quarterly Journal of Economics, 124*, 1265–1306.

Taylor, P., Kochhar, R., Fry, R., Velasco, G., & Motel, S. (2011). *Wealth gaps rise to record highs between Whites, Blacks and Hispanics.* (Retrieved from http://pewsocialtrends.org/files/2011/07/SDT-Wealth-Report_7-26-11_FINAL.pdf). Pew Research Center Social & Dempographic Trends.

von Wachter, T., Song, J., & Manchester, J. (2009). *Long-term earnings losses due to mass layoffs during the 1982 recession: An analysis using US administrative data from 1974 to 2004.* Retrieved from citeseerx.ist.psu.edu/viewdoc/download?doi = 10.1.1.183.

Wolff, T. (2001). A practitioner's guide to successful coalitions. *American Journal of Community Psychology, 29*, 173–191.

Woodland, R. H., & Hutton, M. S. (2012). Evaluating organizational collaborations: Suggested entry points and strategies. *American Journal of Evaluation, 33*, 366–383.

Yap, M., Holmes, M. R., Hannan, C. A., & Cukier, W. (2010). The relationship between diversity training, organizational commitment, and career satisfaction. *Journal of European Industrial Training, 34*, 519–538.

Zhao, X., Lim, V. K. G., & Teo, T. S. H. (2012). The long arm of job insecurity: Its impact on career-specific parenting behaviors and youths' career self-efficacy. *Journal of Vocational Behavior, 80*, 619–628.

FURTHER READING

Aylsworth, J. (2009). Downsizing, stress and forgiveness: A US perspective. In S. J. Morgan (Ed.), *The human side of outsourcing: Psychological theory and management practice.* Oxford: Wiley-Blackwell (http://onlinelibrary.wiley.com/doi/10.1002/9780470749456.ch12/pdf).

Browning, M., Moller Dano, A., & Heinesen, E. (2006). Job displacement and stress-related health outcomes. *Health Economics, 15*, 1061–1075.

Hudson, B., Hardy, B., Henwood, M., & Wistow, G. (1997). Strategic alliances: Working across professional boundaries: Primary health care and social care. *Public Money & Management, 17*, 25–30.

McKee-Ryan, F. M., Virick, M., Prussia, G. E., Harvey, J., & Lilly, J. D. (2009). Life after the layoff: getting a job worth keeping. *Journal of Organizational Behavior, 30*, 561–580.

McKee-Ryan, F. M., & Kinicki, A. J. (2002). Coping with job loss: A life-facet perspective. In: C. L. Cooper, & I. T. Robertson (Eds.), *International review of industrial and organizational psychology 2002* (*Vol. 17*). Chichester, UK: Wiley <http://onlinelibrary.wiley.com/doi/10.1002/9780470696392.ch1/summary>.

APPENDIX A

The CES-D Depression Scale—Useful in Determining Worker Burnout

One of the most common screening tests for depression and burnout is the Center for Epidemiologic Studies Depression Scale (CES-D), originally developed by Lenore Radloff (1977) while she was a researcher at the National Institute of Mental Health. This quick self-test measures depressive feelings and behaviors during the past week. The test is in the public domain and does not require permission to use. Scoring instructions and the meaning of scores are given at the end of the test.

Almost 85% of those found to have depression after an in-depth structured interview with a psychiatrist will have a high score on the CES-D. However, about 20% of those who score high on the CES-D will have rapid resolution of their symptoms and will not meet full criteria for major or clinical depression. This is particularly important if you equate depression with burnout. Changes in job assignment, working conditions, and co-workers can quickly lead to improvements in burnout.

High scores should be viewed with concern and appropriate mental health professionals should be contacted to assess the level of depression; it's serious and there is potential for improvement through medication and/or counseling.

Taking the CES-D

Please note: This test will only be scored correctly if you answer each one of the questions honestly. It's usually best to give the first answer that comes to mind and not dwell on it. Circle the correct answer and then go to the scoring guide at the end of the test to calculate your score.

Questions

1. I was bothered by things that don't usually bother me.
   - **a.** Rarely or none of the time (<1 day)
   - **b.** Some or a little of the time (1–2 days)
   - **c.** Occasionally or a moderate amount of the time (3–4 days)
   - **d.** Most or all of the time (5–7 days)

2. I did not feel like eating; my appetite was poor.
  a. Rarely or none of the time (<1 day)
  b. Some or a little of the time (1–2 days)
  c. Occasionally or a moderate amount of the time (3–4 days)
  d. Most or all of the time (5–7 days)

3. I felt that I could not shake off the blues even with the help of my family or friends.
  a. Rarely or none of the time (<1 day)
  b. Some or a little of the time (1–2 days)
  c. Occasionally or a moderate amount of the time (3–4 days)
  d. Most or all of the time (5–7 days)

4. I felt that I was just as good as other people.
  a. Rarely or none of the time (<1 day)
  b. Some or a little of the time (1–2 days)
  c. Occasionally or a moderate amount of the time (3–4 days)
  d. Most or all of the time (5–7 days)

5. I had trouble keeping my mind on what I was doing.
  a. Rarely or none of the time (<1 day)
  b. Some or a little of the time (1–2 days)
  c. Occasionally or a moderate amount of the time (3–4 days)
  d. Most or all of the time (5–7 days)

6. I felt depressed.
  a. Rarely or none of the time (<1 day)
  b. Some or a little of the time (1–2 days)
  c. Occasionally or a moderate amount of the time (3–4 days)
  d. Most or all of the time (5–7 days)

7. I felt everything I did was an effort.
  a. Rarely or none of the time (<1 day)
  b. Some or a little of the time (1–2 days)
  c. Occasionally or a moderate amount of the time (3–4 days)
  d. Most or all of the time (5–7 days)

8. I felt hopeful about the future.
  a. Rarely or none of the time (<1 day)
  b. Some or a little of the time (1–2 days)
  c. Occasionally or a moderate amount of the time (3–4 days)
  d. Most or all of the time (5–7 days)

9. I thought my life had been a failure.
  a. Rarely or none of the time (<1 day)
  b. Some or a little of the time (1–2 days)

c. Occasionally or a moderate amount of the time (3–4 days)
d. Most or all of the time (5–7 days)

10. I felt fearful.
a. Rarely or none of the time (<1 day)
b. Some or a little of the time (1–2 days)
c. Occasionally or a moderate amount of the time (3–4 days)
d. Most or all of the time (5–7 days)

11. My sleep was restless.
a. Rarely or none of the time (<1 day)
b. Some or a little of the time (1–2 days)
c. Occasionally or a moderate amount of the time (3–4 days)
d. Most or all of the time (5–7 days)

12. I was happy.
a. Rarely or none of the time (<1 day)
b. Some or a little of the time (1–2 days)
c. Occasionally or a moderate amount of the time (3–4 days)
d. Most or all of the time (5–7 days)

13. I talked less than usual.
a. Rarely or none of the time (<1 day)
b. Some or a little of the time (1–2 days)
c. Occasionally or a moderate amount of the time (3–4 days)
d. Most or all of the time (5–7 days)

14. I felt lonely.
a. Rarely or none of the time (<1 day)
b. Some or a little of the time (1–2 days)
c. Occasionally or a moderate amount of the time (3–4 days)
d. Most or all of the time (5–7 days)

15. People were unfriendly.
a. Rarely or none of the time (<1 day)
b. Some or a little of the time (1–2 days)
c. Occasionally or a moderate amount of the time (3–4 days)
d. Most or all of the time (5–7 days)

16. I enjoyed life.
a. Rarely or none of the time (<1 day)
b. Some or a little of the time (1–2 days)
c. Occasionally or a moderate amount of the time (3–4 days)
d. Most or all of the time (5–7 days)

17. I had crying spells.
a. Rarely or none of the time (<1 day)

- **b.** Some or a little of the time (1–2 days)
- **c.** Occasionally or a moderate amount of the time (3–4 days)
- **d.** Most or all of the time (5–7 days)

18. I felt sad.
- **a.** Rarely or none of the time (<1 day)
- **b.** Some or a little of the time (1–2 days)
- **c.** Occasionally or a moderate amount of the time (3–4 days)
- **d.** Most or all of the time (5–7 days)

19. I felt that people disliked me.
- **a.** Rarely or none of the time (<1 day)
- **b.** Some or a little of the time (1–2 days)
- **c.** Occasionally or a moderate amount of the time (3–4 days)
- **d.** Most or all of the time (5–7 days)

20. I could not get "going".
- **a.** Rarely or none of the time (<1 day)
- **b.** Some or a little of the time (1–2 days)
- **c.** Occasionally or a moderate amount of the time (3–4 days)
- **d.** Most or all of the time (5–7 days)

Scoring

Scoring for all except questions 4, 8, 12, and 16:
- 0 points: Rarely or none of the time (<1 day)
- 1 point: Some or a little of the time (1–2 days)
- 2 points: Occasionally or a moderate amount of the time (3–4 days)
- 3 points: Most or all of the time (5–7 days).

For questions 4, 8, 12, and 16, the scoring is exactly the same except that it is reversed: "Most or all of the time" is scored 0 points, "Rarely or none of the time" is scored 3 points, etc. Roughly speaking, the higher the score, the greater the depressive symptoms.

What a score means

- Less than 15: Fairly normal range of emotion.
- 15–21: Mild to moderate depression. Further exploration of the reasons for the depression are explored and the potential for an increase in depressed feelings are evaluated. With this should come an evaluation of medical, social and psychological reasons for the depression and the potential for an evidence-based practice modality offering relief.

- Over 21: Possibility of major depression. Requires treatment and, as the score increases, an evaluation of potential risk in the form of self medicating with drugs and alcohol, risk of impulsive acts to relieve the depression, and suicide potential.

REFERENCE

Radloff, L. S. (1977). The CES-D scale: A self-report depression scale for research in the general population. *Applied Psychological Measurement*, *1*, 385–401.

APPENDIX B

Forced Early Retirement Stress Because of Burnout and Job Loss[1]

Early retirement is a complex issue for many older adults who may feel diminished and mistreated at work and see retirement as a way of coping with low morale and stress. Often it isn't a solution, since many early retirees have not thought through retirement as a lifestyle change and may still desire to work in new organizations but may believe that their age makes new employment unlikely. Financial incentive plans for early retirement that seem lucrative may in fact offer a person less financial security in the long run and reduced social security and pension benefits. Work is important to most people because it offers status and a daily schedule. When those two factors are taken away, many early retirees feel unimportant and confused about how to spend their day. As a nurse told a colleague when he began chatting about his plan to retire early, "You have 30 good years ahead of you." she said. "What are you going to do with yourself?" She was absolutely right and our colleague decided to handle his unhappiness with a current job by finding another job elsewhere, and it gave him 2 more years of work while he began careful planning for retirement and increased his savings.

Mor-Barak and Tynan (1993) suggest that retirement as early as 62 is an "artifact of the Social Security laws that has acquired certain conveniences, leading to its perception and adoption as 'normative' " (p. 49). They also says that it "enables employers to dispense with the services of older workers gracefully, avoiding the administrative difficulties of selectively firing often 'faithful' workers" (p. 49) while allowing older workers to "salvage" self-respect because retiring at a specific age means you are a member of a class of workers who were let go by mandate from the workforce rather than being individually removed.

[1] Parts of this appendix were taken, with permission, from Glicken, M. D. (2010). *Retirement for Workaholics: Life after work in a downsized economy.* Santa Barbara, CA: Praeger.

Maestas and Li (2007) studied what happened to workers who retire early because of burnout. They write that because burnout rises with continued exposure to stress at work, it should peak just prior to retirement, then decline after the individual leaves the workplace. An individual for whom burnout is high enough to induce retirement may later un-retire if he or she experiences boredom and believes that returning to work will outweigh any negative consequences of working. This notion of un-retiring should help many older workers experiencing burnout to realize that the desire to work often returns in time, and that retirement decisions based entirely on burnout may suggest that, leaves of absence, requests for work assignment changes, and cycling over to other types of work may be alternatives to retirement. Keep in mind that it may be more difficult to return to work, at least stimulating work, after you retire because breaks in a work record are often felt by employers to be a bad sign.

Forced retirement or retirement in which workers are given strong messages that they are unwanted have both been associated with greater difficulties in adjusting (Atchley, 1982; Walker, Kimmel, & Price, 1981), lower satisfaction with retirement (Isaksson, 1997), adverse psychological reactions (Sharpley & Layton, 1998), and increased stress (Isaksson, 1997; Sharpley & Layton, 1998).

Individuals who are forced to retire because of ill health, predictably report lower levels of morale (Braithwaite, Gibson, & Bosly-Craft, 1986), higher stress scores (Bossé, Aldwin, Levenson, & Workman-Daniels, 1991), and are at greater risk for emotional difficulties (Sharpley & Layton, 1998). Martin Mathews & Brown (1988) found that the lower the socioeconomic status of men, the more negative the impact of retirement overall, often because of a lack of planning, lower post-retirement income, early health problems, and few alternatives to work. Also, individuals who experience a substantial loss of income during retirement tend to experience poor morale (Richardson & Kilty, 1991) and poor adjustment (Palmore, Fillenbaum, & George, 1985). Many people who find their retirement plans changed because companies no longer honor pension plans or have grossly changed pension plans also report lower satisfaction with retirement and greater levels of stress.

Fletcher and Hansson (1991) found that retirees who expected to have very little personal control over their lives during retirement not only had more negative views of retirement but also feared the event. Glamser (1976) found that those expecting retirement to be a positive experience held a positive attitude about retirement, while those expecting retirement to be a negative adjustment held negative attitudes.

A Case Study of an Older Worker Considering Retirement Because of Burnout

Jason Stewart is a 63-year-old professor of counseling at a lower-level public university in the Midwest. He has been feeling burned out and unhappy about his job, believing that the students he trains are inferior and that most students have lost their idealism and only want to be private practitioners and make a great deal of money. He chose counseling as a career to help others and to make the world a better place—ideas that seem old fashioned in the current climate of cynicism and narcissism which he finds among the students he teaches. His feelings of burnout and unhappiness have been gaining in strength since Jason was passed over for the chairmanship of his department 5 years ago. He is now wondering if he should quit work completely or seek another job, and has come for retirement counseling to help him decide on a course of action. Jason has no hobbies other than reading mysteries, watching films, and writing articles and books. He wants the counselor to use a brief problem-solving approach that focuses on the present, doesn't assume that a problem has its origins in the past, and uses logical solutions.

The initial sessions went very well. Jason was highly motivated, did a great deal of reading about early retirement and older adult burnout, and found that it wasn't unusual for people in his field to feel burned out and unhappy with their jobs after many years of tough, loyal, and successful work without very much financial or emotional payoff. As Jason read, talked to the counselor, and made behavioral charts, he began to complain about feeling depressed. "I still don't know what to do," he said, and wondered if the counselor had any suggestions. He did. Why not enter the job market and see if he could find a job where his skills could be put to better use and where the students were stronger?

Jason did just that and much to his surprise he was a finalist for several very high-level positions in highly ranked universities. He spoke to the counselor about the experience. "I wanted something better, but now I'm scared. I don't think I want to work that hard, and I'm worried that having been in a mediocre university makes me unprepared to deal with high-level faculty and students. The thought of moving makes me feel old and tired."

The counselor listened to Jason for several sessions as he discussed his confusion and concerns about his job possibilities. She told him that it seemed as if the pull to stay was stronger than the pull to leave. Was there a way he could stay at his university and perhaps change what he was doing and begin to work less? Jason explored these options and came back with an idea:

"I found out that we have an early retirement plan where you can get your pension and social security and still work for 5 years up to 50% of the time and get paid using your current salary and benefit levels as a base. At the end of the 5-year period, you can work part-time but at a lower salary rate. I think I could do that, and maybe it would help me deal with retirement. The problem is that I don't want to keep teaching, so I went to my chair and discussed the plan. He wants me to spend the 50% time creating new curricula and trying to deal with the problem of too many poor students in the department. He doesn't think we have enough diversity and he wants to see more idealistic students and faculty. Everyone was feeling the same way I did, he told me, which was a great surprise to me. He said that the reason I was passed over for the chair's position had nothing to do with me or the faculty. The faculty wanted me but the administration wanted someone younger. It pissed me off to find out about ageism, but I had originally thought it was because they didn't like me. Having 5 years to ease myself into retirement would give me time to write books and to do some traveling. I live alone, and maybe it's time to find someone who can offer companionship and intimacy. I've put off those needs since I divorced 20 years ago, and I feel very lonely at times."

The counselor thought his idea was a good one and wondered how he might find someone to be in his life. "I was reading a mystery novel by the Swedish writer Henning Mankell called Firewall (1998)," he said. "His main character, a cop called Kurt Wallander, is like me: lonely and set in his ways but in need of someone in his life. The detective uses a dating service and finds someone. I started thinking about women who have given me some indication that they are interested in me. Maybe I'll just follow up and see if I can find someone that way. I don't think I could ever use a dating service at my age, so we'll see. And I need to start going to our national conferences. I met my wife that way and we did pretty well for almost 20 years; not bad in this day and age."

What to Do if You Experience Burnout or are Forced to Retire

Older workers often have little choice in whether they continue working full-time. As Mor-Barak and Tynan (1993) point out, "Despite this interest in continued employment by employers and older adults, older workers are more likely to lose their jobs than younger workers in instances such as plant closings and corporate mergers (Beckett, 1988)" (p. 45). The authors go on to say that many businesses can't or won't deal with life events faced by older workers such as "widowhood and caring for ailing spouses, and as a result many older workers are forced to retire earlier than planned" (p. 45).

Writing about the loss of work and its impact on older men, Levant (1997) says that as men lose their good-provider roles, the experience results in "severe gender role strain" (p. 221) which affects relationships and can be disruptive to the point of ending otherwise strong marriages. Because older adults are more likely to lose high-level jobs as a result of downsizing and age discrimination, social contacts decrease, and many otherwise healthy and motivated workers must deal with increased levels of isolation and loneliness. Schneider (1998) points out that many of us are workaholics and that, when work is taken away or jobs are diminished in complexity and creativity, many older adults experience a decrease in physical and mental health. And while early retirement is touted as a way to achieve the good life at an early age, the experience is a complex and even wrenching one in which older adults who are financially able to retire often have little ability to handle extra time, have failed to make sound retirement plans, and find out quickly that not working takes away social contacts, status, and a way to organize time.

For many healthy, work-oriented and motivated older adults, volunteer and civic roles are not at all what they are looking for. They want to continue to work, to contribute, and to receive the financial and social status and benefits related to work. However when full-time work isn't possible, Zedlewski and Butrica (2007) found that numerous studies supported the finding that work and formal volunteering improve health, reduce the risk of serious illness and emotional difficulties such as depression, and improve strength and cognitive functioning, while full retirement without work and early loss of jobs increased the probability of illness and emotional difficulties. Clearly, having something of value to do after retirement is a protective factor in keeping older adults healthy and emotionally engaged with the world around them.

REFERENCES

Atchley, R. C. (1982). Retirement: Learning the world of work. *Annals of the American Academy of Political and Social Sciences*, *464*, 120–131.

Beckett, J. O. (1988). Plant closing: How older workers are affected. *Social Work*, *33*, 29–33.

Bossé, R., Aldwin, C. M., Levenson, M. R., & Workman-Daniels, K. (1991). How stressful is retirement? Findings from the Normative Aging Study. *Journal of Gerontology*, *46*, 9–14.

Braithwaite, V. A., Gibson, D. M., & Bosly-Craft, R. (1986). An exploratory study of poor adjustment styles among retirees. *Social Science and Medicine, 23*, 493–499.

Fletcher, W. L., & Hansson, R. O. (1991). Assessing the social components of retirement anxiety. *Psychology and Aging, 6*, 76–85.

Glamser, F. D. (1976). Determinants of a positive attitude toward retirement. *Journal of Gerontology, 31*, 104–107.

Isaksson, K. (1997). *Patterns of adjustment to early retirement, Reports from the Department of Psychology* (828, 1–13). Stockholm, Sweden: Stockholm University.

Levant, R. F. (1997). The masculinity issue. *The Journal of Men's Studies, 5*(3), 221–229.

Maestas, N. & Li, X. (October 2007). *Burnout and retirement decision*. Michigan Retirement Research Center, University of Michigan.

Martin Matthews, A., & Brown, K. H. (1988). Retirement as a critical life event. *Research on Aging, 9*, 548–571.

Mor-Barak, M. E., & Tynan, M. (1993). Older workers and the workplace: A new challenge for occupational social work. *Social Work, 38*(1), 45–55, January.

Richardson, V. E., & Kilty, K. M. (1991). Adjustment to retirement: Continuity vs. discontinuity. *International Journal of Aging and Human Development, 33*, 151–169.

Schneider, K. J. (1998). Toward a science of the heart: Romanticism and the revival of psychology. *American Psychologist, 53*, 277–289.

Sharpley, C. F., & Layton, R. (1998). Effects of age of retirement, reason for retirement and pre-retirement training on psychological and physical health during retirement. *Australian Psychologist, 33*, 119–124.

Walker, J., Kimmel, D., & Price, K. (1981). Retirement style and retirement satisfaction: Retirees aren't all alike. *International Journal of Aging and Human Development, 12*, 267–281.

Zedlewski, S. R., & Butrica, B. A. (2007). Are we taking full advantage of older adults' potential? The Retirement Project: Perspectives of Productive Aging. *The Urban Institute, 9*, 1–8.

APPENDIX C

Managing Workers Using the New Interactive Technologies

INTRODUCTION

An essential aspect of effective supervision is the ability of workers and supervisors to communicate effectively with one another, but for what purpose, under what conditions, and in which context? With interactive technologies and the Internet, supervisors no longer need to supervise workers in face-to-face meetings but now have the freedom to use email, interactive television, websites, online courses for staff development, and any number of new and creative ways of communicating that are unrestricted by time and place. Are these methods effective and do they pose problems? This appendix will look at the new technologies and provide the current research on their effectiveness. Before we do that, however, let's consider the issue of communicating between supervisors and workers and what we hope to accomplish.

COMMUNICATING SUPERVISORY INTERVENTIONS

Loganbill, Hardy, and Delworth (1982) describe critical aspects of supervisor techniques or strategies that should be a part of any supervision experience. These aspects are not limited to a specific format but should be considered in evaluating the effectiveness of supervision through any medium and include the following.

1. Facilitative interventions are worker-centered and help workers learn and apply the necessary skills in the treatment process either in face-to-face meetings or in a more indirect way (memos, telephone conversations, and emails).
2. Interventions that use confrontation are used to examine and compare work because workers are experiencing conflict in their work-related relationships or because supervisors have concern about a worker's performance. This should always be done face-to-face.

Conceptual interventions are used when supervisors ask workers to think analytically or theoretically. In this type of interaction, group discussion, staff development, papers sent on the Internet to workers, staff meetings, and case presentations can all have a positive impact on workers if resistance isn't great. If it is, a confrontation might be needed to help a worker understand his or her resistance and to soften it so that new material can be integrated into the worker's application of treatment approaches.

1. Prescriptive interventions are a form of coaching workers to perform or eliminate certain behaviors. Loganbill et al. (1982) caution that prescriptive interventions lower morale when a supervisor always negates a worker's point of view in favor of that of the supervisor.
2. Catalytic interventions exist when a supervisor helps a worker understand something so very significant about a client that it could lead to a substantial breakthrough in the performance of the worker and result in important change in the client.

The Journal of Supervision (2004) reports that the average supervisor spends 80% of their time communicating: 10% writing, 15% reading, 25% listening, and 30% speaking. The Journal says that accurate and effective communication requires the following:

1. **Credibility:** Supervisors must be believable. If they make too many factual errors, workers will tend not to believe anything they say.
2. **Context:** Supervisors need to understand how workers view the organization and communicate in ways that workers find grounded in reality.
3. **Content:** Supervisors cannot assume that all workers know the significance of messages the supervisors send them. It is best to give a bit of history and then indicate why the information provided has relevance for the worker.
4. **Continuity and consistency:** You should not assume that one message may be enough to alter a worker's behavior. Reliance on a single communication effort may have a low success rate. Communication requires repetition to impact workers who are busy with their priorities.
5. **Channels:** Supervisors have many ways of communicating (email, memo, meetings, video conferences, etc.). It's important to know which of these channels is most likely to reach and motivate the highest number of workers.
6. **Capability of the audience:** Clarity of language is very important. Researchers know that when they give directions on how to fill out questionnaires that it's important to write them in a way an 8th grader

would understand and respond to accurately. Your language should be free of jargon and seldom use complex words that some workers may not know.

7. **Clarity:** I always have others read messages and provide feedback, particularly if the message has some emotional content that may be misunderstood. While I think I'm a good writer, my own emotions may affect what I say and how I say it. I also take some time to think about what I've said. Before sending the message, I mull it over and rewrite it a few times. First drafts are notorious for being insensitive and overwritten.

USING THE INTERNET AND INTERACTIVE TECHNOLOGIES FOR SUPERVISION

Can the Internet be used for many supervisory functions? Stofle and Hamilton (1998) believe that chat rooms can be used for certain supervisory functions, including those that center on cases: when confidentiality can be maintained by use of code words; for discussion of team functioning; and to discuss new approaches to treatment. The authors also believe that online supervision can replace face-to-face supervision when distances are great, as in rural areas or when students are placed in agencies removed from a central agency or educational site. But, they caution, online supervision requires a solid, trusting relationship and motivation. The authors agree, however, that a problem with using the Internet for supervision is the inability to see the non-verbal behavior of workers or supervisors, but they have devised a simple code to indicate emotions. Some examples are:

:) Smile
<g> Grin
:(Frown
;) Wink
:P Disappointed
:O Shocked
? What?/Explain/Why?

They believe the advantages and disadvantages of using the Internet for group supervisory sessions are as follows.

- **Disadvantages:** Lack of non-verbal cues; technical problems with the online process such as the server being busy or people getting bumped off; poor typing skills that take time away from the process or confuse meaning; space limitations that prevent the sender from sending the entire message and the receiver from responding; silence or inactivity between typed sentences can be interpreted as others not paying attention or being uninterested; distractions from other people nearby including family members or other workers.

- **Advantages:** Simplicity; convenience, since group supervision can be done anywhere at any time including when workers are at home; some things are easier to write than to say, particularly if you sense that others in the group will disapprove non-verbally in face-to-face group conference; the meeting is permanent since it can be saved and referred to in the future.

Miller, Miller, Burton, Sprang, and Adams (2003) evaluated the use of interactive TV in the training and supervision of health and mental health professionals in rural areas. They found the use of telecommunications technology providing information and care across distance to be an appropriate, cost-effective means of supporting patients and providers in the changing health care system. The authors studied a new clinical internship program in a rural setting, attempting to provide supervision for allied health interns in related specialties including speech pathology, physical therapy, occupational therapy, and psychology. The use of interactive technologies was augmented by face-to-face supervision, but when that wasn't possible because of distances and problems in traveling, supervision was done by secure email messages and interactive telephone calls (cameras hooked up to computers that allowed supervisors and students to talk to and see one another).

Eighty students were supervised by four professionals for 30 weeks. The supervision consisted of monthly group teleconferences (audio or, when necessary, video), weekly individual telephone supervision, and daily or as needed email supervision. Supervisors and clinicians had duplicate copies of tapes of the previous week's clinical encounters to facilitate supervision. Considering just the interactive portion of the experience, there were over 20,000 emails, 450 secured fax information forms, and 500 hours of psychotherapy videotape. Communications were catalogued in a searchable, analyzable database.

While there were many advantages to the use of interactive technologies, not least of which was to provide supervision to workers in rural or remote areas who might not otherwise be trained, the cost was not less than if supervisors were present onsite. However, the quality of the experience was highly rated by workers, and client care seemed consistent with onsite supervision. There were, however, some drawbacks.

The interactive format may not have allowed some interns to obtain the contact they might receive in a live face-to-face supervisory interaction regarding highly personal information (problems with countertransference, for example). Supervisees did not get all the supervisory time they needed, since interactive technology required good competencies and self-directed learning styles. Some interns, according to the authors, were not ready for this style of supervision. Technology was often plagued by problems and, because of this, immediate feedback was not always available. Interactive technologies are not as secure as onsite supervision, and client confidentiality may be a problem because of hackers and intrusive technologies that allow others to view, hear, or see supervisory conferences and emails.

In a further study of the use of interactive approaches to supervision, Gainor and Constantine (2002) compared two randomly selected cohorts of counseling psychology doctoral students to determine whether sensitivity to diversity increased if group composition included ethnic and racial diversity. One randomly selected group received their supervision in person while a second group received their supervision using the Internet. Both groups improved on tests to measure sensitivity to multiculturalism, but the face-to-face group improved more. The authors believe that the reasons why the in-person group had better improvement included the following.

- The lack of non-verbal cues to correctly perceive behavior in the web-based group made it difficult for supervisors to determine group members who were having difficulty with diversity.
- Critical information may be omitted in web-based groups because the group process is limited and the supervisor can't see behavior that may need to be followed up on.
- Ladany, Hill, Corbett, and Nutt (1996) found that a third of the students being supervised in their study using face-to-face supervision failed to disclose racial or ethnic bias against clients, and that this number could increase in web-based supervision.
- Robson and Robson (1998) suggest that, although computer technology can be used for intimate communication, impersonation and impersonalization may increase personal barriers to intimacy.
- Even though face-to-face supervision was more effective in improving multiculturalism, the authors are realistic about the benefits and suggest that supervision might be enhanced by using both direct contact and web-based supervision, particularly for those supervisory functions

that may be less emotional and complex (discussion of new procedures, for example).

- Gainor and Constantine (2003) note that, while their findings would suggest the superiority of face-to-face supervision, other researchers have had more positive experiences with web-based supervision. For example, Myrick and Sabella (1995) report that school counselor trainees and practicing counselors reported more advantages than disadvantages to web-based supervision, including more accessible assistance and encouragement, interpersonal closeness and openness, the ability to read and review at one's convenience, and spirited conversations.

There are important concerns about the use of web-based supervision that are quite apart from whether it is effective. Van Horn & Myrick (2001) raise concerns about inappropriate people accessing confidential information, particularly when others have access to computers used by supervisees (as in university or public library computer labs). The authors suggest that some trainees have very limited knowledge of computers and that confidential information may inadvertently be sent to others. How many of us have done this in our personal lives? I certainly have when I'm in a rush. And while we can expect most students to be very computer literate, older students often aren't, and some students have built up quite a negative reaction to technology in general and computers specifically that make their use very problematic.

On the other hand, I (Glicken) used a web-based approach to teaching a graduate research course by putting my notes on the web for every class meeting. The scores on research tests were almost 15% higher than before I used the web. Reading material rather than taking notes in class improves learning for many people. For that reason, among many others discussed here, you should consider web-based supervision as a way of enhancing learning but not as a substitute for face-to-face contact with workers who may need a more personal and confidential approach. Feedback that is highly personal or may include a negative confrontation is hurtful if received as an email message.

A Case Example: You be the Supervisor

You have been asked to provide input on a $300,000 state-funded grant to enable use of the Internet and various interactive technologies to provide services to frail elderly adults living some distance from your agency.

The purpose of the grant is to develop skill in workers and clients to use interactive video and audio (small cameras attached to computers that transmit video and audio over the telephone lines and can be recorded on video machines for workers to view if the worker isn't in the office). Interactive technologies would allow workers to evaluate clients on a day-by-day basis. If clients show deterioration, a worker could immediately be dispatched or emergency services could be contacted.

The current system allows workers to provide home visits at 2-month intervals. Everyone agrees that this is too little time to spend with frail, at-risk clients, but the idea of using technology to evaluate clients is a turnoff to your workers. They believe that it would change their jobs from something highly personal to something highly abstract and, while efficient, that it would be too distant from direct client contact to enjoy. Some of the workers have threatened to quit if the grant is funded. You've indicated to upper management that the grant isn't well thought of by your workers, but management argues that the grant will provide much more efficient practice, and if your workers don't like it, they can leave. This new system will allow for immediate contact with clients and direct response if clients are in crisis. It makes sense to use this approach given funding difficulties and the growing number of frail elderly clients living well into their 90s who live alone or with an equally frail spouse. Upper management also points out that it would be far cheaper to hire people without treatment experience, train them, and have them do client–worker contacts online. If clients need personal help, the agency can outsource the service to workers in private practice.

The grant is written with your help but minus worker feedback. When the grant is funded, you have responsibility for getting the reluctant workers on board.

Questions

1. Where do your allegiances lie? With the agency or with the workers?
2. Should you have done anything while the grant was being written to get your workers on board? If so, what, and why?
3. New technologies are likely to change the nature of work in the human services. How would you train workers to use interactive technologies?
4. Would it have helped to share the advantages of the grant with your workers and to focus on the fact that early intervention would improve effectiveness rates and save your client group a good deal of pain and suffering? Why or why not?
5. Do you think there is a real risk that workers will quit when you ask that they become involved in the application phase of the grant? What might you do to prevent this from happening?

REFERENCES

Gainor, K., & Constantine, G., Ph.D. (2003). Multicultural group supervision: A comparison of in-person versus web-based formats. *Professional School Counseling, 6*(2), 15–23.

Journal of Supervision (2004). Successful communication. *Supervision, 65*(11), 7–14.

Ladany, N., Hill, C. E., Corbett, M. M., & Nutt, E. A. (1996). Nature, extent, and importance of what psychotherapy trainees do not disclose to their supervisors. *Journal of Counseling Psychology, 43*, 10–24.

Loganbill, C., Hardy, E., & Delworth, U. (1982). Supervision: A conceptual model. *Counseling Psychologist, 10*, 3–42.

Miller, T., Miller, J., Burton, D., Sprang, R., & Adams, J. (2003). Telehealth: A model for clinical supervision in allied health. *Internet Journal of Allied Health Sciences and Practice, 1*(2), 1–11.

Myrick, R. D., & Sabella, R. A. (1995). Cyberspace: New place for counselor supervision. *Elementary School Guidance and Counseling, 30*, 35–44.

Robson, D., & Robson, M. (1998). Intimacy and computer communication. *British Journal of Guidance and Counselling, 26*, 33–41.

Stofle, G., & Hamilton, S. (1998). White hat communications. *The New Social Worker, 5*, 1–8.

Van Horn & Myrick (2001). *21st Century skills for school counselors.* Retrieved August 23, 2012 from <http://21stcenturyschoolcounselor.weebly.com/counselor-technology.html>.

INDEX

Note: Page numbers followed by "*b*" and "*t*" refer to boxes and tables respectively.

D

E

F

Q

R

S

T

U

V

W

Printed and bound by CPI Group (UK) Ltd, Croydon, CR0 4YY
08/05/2025
01865019-0001